INTERVENTIONAL CARDIOLOGY SECRETS

Eduardo de Marchena, M.D., FACC, FACP
Professor of Medicine and Surgery
Department of Medicine
University of Miami School of Medicine
Director of Interventional Cardiology
Jackson Memorial Hospital
Miami, Florida

Alexandre C. Ferreira, M.D.
Assistant Professor of Medicine
Division of Cardiology
Department of Medicine
University of Miami School of Medicine
Jackson Memorial Hospital
Miami, Florida

HANLEY & BELFUS
An imprint of Elsevier

HANLEY & BELFUS
An Imprint of Elsevier

The Curtis Center
Independence Square West
Philadelphia, Pennsylvania 19106

Note to the reader: Although the techniques, ideas, and information in this book have been carefully reviewed for correctness, neither the author nor the publisher can accept any legal responsibility for any errors or omissions that may be made. Neither the author nor the publisher makes any guarantee, expressed or implied, with respect to the material contained herein.

Library of Congress Control Number: 2003103378

INTERVENTIONAL CARDIOLOGY SECRETS　　　　　　**ISBN 1-56053-585-7**

Printed in the United States of America

Last digit is the print number: 9 8 7 6 5 4 3 2 1

CONTENTS

CONTRIBUTORS

Alexandre Abizaid, M.D., Ph.D.
Staff, Interventional Cardiology, Dante Pazzanese Institute of Cardiology, São Paulo, Brazil

Yeon S. Ahn, M.D.
Professor, Department of Medicine, University of Miami School of Medicine, Wallace H. Coulter Platelet Laboratory, Miami, Florida

David E. Allie, M.D.
Cardiovascular Surgeon and Director, Cardiothoracic and Vascular Surgery, Cardiovascular Institute of the South, Lafayette, Louisiana

Eric Auerbach, M.D.
Division of Cardiology, Department of Medicine, University of Miami School of Medicine; Jackson Memorial Hospital, Miami, Florida

Steven R. Bailey, M.D.
Professor of Medicine and Radiology, Department of Medicine, University of Texas Health Science Center, San Antonio, Texas

Glenn J. Barquet, M.D.
Division of Cardiology, Department of Medicine, University of Miami School of Medicine; Jackson Memorial Hospital, Miami, Florida

Gary J. Becker, M.D., FSIR, FACC, FACR
Assistant Medical Director and Medical Director of Research and Outcomes, Miami Cardiac and Vascular Institute, Baptist Hospital of Miami, Miami, Florida

James F. Benenati, M.D.
Associate Professor (voluntary), Department of Radiology, University of Miami School of Medicine; Interventional Radiologist, Miami Cardiac and Vascular Institute, Baptist Hospital of Miami, Miami, Florida

Deepak L. Bhatt, M.D.
Director, Interventional Cardiology Fellowship, Department of Cardiovascular Medicine, Cleveland Clinic Foundation, Cleveland, Ohio

H. Michael Bolooki, B.S.
Division of Thoracic and Cardiovascular Surgery, Department of Surgery, University of Miami School of Medicine; Jackson Memorial Hospital, Miami, Florida

Hooshang Bolooki, M.D., FACC, FRCS(C)
Professor of Surgery and Director, Adult Cardiac Surgery, Division of Thoracic and Cardiovascular Surgery, Department of Surgery, University of Miami School of Medicine; Attending Cardiac Surgeon, Jackson Memorial Hospital, Miami, Florida

Fernando A. Cura, M.D.
Staff, Department of Cardiology and Interventional Cardiology, Instituto Cardiovascular de Buenos Aires, Buenos Aires, Argentina

Eduardo de Marchena, M.D., FACC, FACP
Professor of Medicine and Surgery, Department of Medicine, University of Miami School of Medicine; Director of Interventional Cardiology, Jackson Memorial Hospital, Miami, Florida

Darwin Eton, M.D.
Associate Professor and Chief, Division of Vascular Surgery, Department of Surgery, University of Miami School of Medicine; Jackson Memorial Hospital; Cedars Hospital; Miami Veterans Affairs Medical Center, Miami, Florida

Jeffrey Scott Fenster, M.D.
Division of Cardiology, Department of Medicine, Jackson Memorial Hospital, Miami, Florida

Fausto Feres, M.D., Ph.D.
Staff, Interventional Cardiology, Dante Pazzanese Institute of Cardiology, São Paulo, Brazil

Alexandre C. Ferreira, M.D.
Assistant Professor, Division of Cardiology, Department of Medicine, University of Miami School of Medicine; Jackson Memorial Hospital, Miami, Florida

Christian Fierro-Renoy, M.D.
Assistant Professor, Department of Medicine, Hospital Metropolitano, Quito, Ecuador

Alejandro M. Forteza, M.D.
Associate Professor, Department of Neurology, University of Miami School of Medicine; Attending Physician, Jackson Memorial Hospital, Miami, Florida

Alvaro Galindo, M.D.
Associate Professor of Pediatric Cardiology, University of Miami School of Medicine; Jackson Memorial Hospital, Miami, Florida

Ronald B. Goldberg, M.D.
Professor, Department of Medicine, University of Miami School of Medicine; Jackson Memorial Hospital, Miami, Florida

Nilesh J. Goswami, M.D.
Interventional Cardiovascular Fellow, Division of Cardiology, Department of Medicine, University of Texas Health Science Center, San Antonio, Texas

Vivek J. Goswami, M.D.
Clinical Outcomes Research Fellow, Division of Cardiology, Department of Medicine, University of Texas Health Science Center, San Antonio, Texas

Lawrence L. Horstman, B.S.
Research Associate, Department of Medicine, University of Miami School of Medicine, Wallace H. Coulter Platelet Laboratory, Miami, Florida

Farouc A. Jaffer, M.D., Ph.D.
Division of Cardiology, Harvard Medical School; Massachusetts General Hospital, Boston, Massachusetts

Cesar Jara, M.D., FACC
Cardiovascular Service Center, St. Catherine Hospital, Community Health Care System, East Chicago, Indiana

Javier Jimenez, M.D.
Assistant Professor, Division of Cardiology, Department of Medicine, University of Miami School of Medicine; Jackson Memorial Hospital, Miami, Florida

Joaquin J. Jimenez, M.D.
Assistant Professor, Department of Medicine, University of Miami School of Medicine, Wallace H. Coulter Platelet Laboratory, Miami, Florida

Wenche Jy, Ph.D.
Research Assistant Professor, Department of Medicine, University of Miami School of Medicine, Wallace H. Coulter Platelet Laboratory, Miami, Florida

Samir R. Kapadia, M.D.
Acting Assistant Professor, Division of Cardiology, Department of Medicine, University of Washington School of Medicine, Seattle, Washington

Kushagra Katariya, M.D.
Assistant Professor, Division of Cardiothoracic Surgery, Department of Surgery, University of Miami School of Medicine; Jackson Memorial Hospital, Miami, Florida

Barry T. Katzen, M.D.
Associate Professor, Department of Radiology, University of Miami School of Medicine; Founder and Medical Director, Miami Cardiac and Vascular Institute, Baptist Hospital of Miami, Miami, Florida

Morton J. Kern, M.D.
Director, J. Gerard Mudd Cardiac Catheterization Laboratory, St. Louis University Health Sciences Center, St. Louis, Missouri

Suleiman M. Kharabsheh, M.D.
Interventional Cardiology Fellow, Division of Cardiology, Department of Medicine, Albert Einstein College of Medicine of Yeshiva University; Montefiore Medical Center, Bronx, New York

Margaret Kovacs, Ed.D., M.S.N.
Clinical Faculty, Biomedical Engineering Institute, Florida International University; Manager, Division of Clinical Research, Miami Cardiac and Vascular Institute, Baptist Hospital of Miami, Miami, Florida

Juan Carlos Londoño, M.D.
Interventional Cardiologist, Cardiac Catheterization Laboratory, Mount Sinai Medical Center, Miami Heart Institute, Miami, Florida

Maria Isabel López, M.D., FACC
Assistant Professor, Division of Cardiology, Department of Medicine, University of Miami School of Medicine; Jackson Memorial Hospital, Miami, Florida

Stephen Mallon, M.D.
Professor, Division of Cardiology, Department of Medicine, University of Miami School of Medicine; Director, Cardiac Catheterization, Jackson Memorial Hospital, Miami, Florida

Saqib Masroor, M.D., M.H.S.
Division of Cardiothoracic Surgery, Department of Surgery, University of Miami School of Medicine; Jackson Memorial Hospital, Miami, Florida

Sameer Mehta, M.D., FACC
Associate Professor, Division of Cardiology, Department of Medicine, University of Miami School of Medicine; Chief, Interventional Cardiology, Cedars Medical Center, Miami, Florida

Linda Mourant, R.N.
Outcome Coordinator, Department of Research and Outcomes, Miami Cardiac and Vascular Institute, Baptist Hospital of Miami, Miami, Florida

Debabrata Mukherjee, M.D.
Assistant Professor, Division of Cardiology, Department of Internal Medicine, University of Michigan Medical School, Ann Arbor, Michigan

Oscar C. Muñoz, M.D.
Division of Cardiology, Department of Medicine, University of Miami School of Medicine; Jackson Memorial Hospital, Miami, Florida

Robert A. O'Rourke, M.D., FACC, MACP
Charles Conrad Brown Distinguished Professor of Cardiovascular Disease, Division of Cardiology, Department of Medicine, University of Texas Health Science Center, San Antonio, Texas

Igor F. Palacios, M.D.
Associate Professor, Department of Medicine, Harvard Medical School; Director, Cardiac Catheterization Laboratories and Interventional Cardiology, Massachusetts General Hospital, Boston, Massachusetts

Juan A. Pastor-Cervantes, M.D.
Interventional Cardiologist, Our Lady of Lourdes Hospital; Southwest Medical Center; Lafayette General Hospital, Lafayette, Louisiana; Dauterive Hospital; Iberia Medical Center, New Iberia, Louisiana

Alex Powell, M.D.
Assistant Professor (voluntary), Department of Radiology, University of Miami School of Medicine; Miami Cardiac and Vascular Institute, Baptist Hospital of Miami, Miami, Florida

Joshua Purow, M.D.
Division of Cardiology, Department of Medicine, University of Miami School of Medicine; Jackson Memorial Hospital, Miami, Florida

Ramon Quesada, M.D., FACP, FACC, FCCP, FSCAI
Voluntary Assistant Professor, Division of Cardiology, Department of Medicine, University of Miami School of Medicine; Medical Director, Interventional Cardiology, Miami Cardiac and Vascular Institute, Baptist Hospital of Miami, Miami, Florida

Pranay T. Ramdev, M.D.
Assistant Professor, Division of Vascular Surgery, Department of Surgery, University of Miami School of Medicine; Jackson Memorial Hospital; Cedars Hospital, Miami, Florida

Luis E. Rechani, M.D.
Division of Cardiology, Department of Medicine, University of Miami School of Medicine; Jackson Memorial Hospital, Miami, Florida

Martha Reyes, M.D.
Research Coordinator, Department of Cardiology, Cedars Medical Center, Miami, Florida

Mustafa Ridha, M.D.
Consultant Cardiologist and Clinical Tutor, University of Kuwait Faculty of Medicine; Consultant Cardiologist, Department of Internal Medicine, Adan Hospital; Consultant Interventional Cardiologist, Chest Disease Hospital, Kuwait, Kuwait

Marco Roffi, M.D.
Department of Cardiology, University Hospital, Zurich, Switzerland

Jose G. Romano, M.D.
Assistant Professor, Department of Neurology, University of Miami School of Medicine; Attending Physician, Jackson Memorial Hospital, Miami, Florida

Ravish Sachar, M.D.
Interventional Cardiology Fellow, Department of Cardiovascular Medicine, Cleveland Clinic Foundation, Cleveland, Ohio

Tomas Salerno, M.D.
Professor of Surgery and Chief, Division of Cardiothoracic Surgery, Department of Surgery, University of Miami School of Medicine; Jackson Memorial Hospital, Miami, Florida

Johnny S. Sandhu, M.D.
Department of Radiology, University of Miami School of Medicine; Jackson Memorial Hospital, Miami, Florida

Neil Sawhney, M.D.
Division of Cardiology, Department of Medicine, Brown University School of Medicine; Rhode Island Hospital, Providence, Rhode Island

Alan Schob, M.D.
Assistant Professor, Department of Medicine, University of Miami School of Medicine; Chief, Cardiovascular Laboratory, Miami Veterans Affairs Medical Center, Miami, Florida

Rafael F. Sequeira, M.D.
Professor, Division of Cardiology, Department of Medicine, University of Miami School of Medicine; Jackson Memorial Hospital, Miami, Florida

Niranjan Seshadri, M.D.
Department of Cardiovascular Medicine, Cleveland Clinic Foundation, Cleveland, Ohio

Neerav Shah, M.D.
Division of Cardiology, Department of Medicine, University of Miami School of Medicine, Miami, Florida

Barry L. Sharaf, M.D., FACC
Associate Professor, Division of Cardiology, Department of Medicine, Brown University School of Medicine; Director, Angiographic Core Laboratory, Rhode Island Hospital, Providence, Rhode Island

Maria P. Solano, M.D.
Assistant Professor of Clinical Medicine, University of Miami School of Medicine; Jackson Memorial Hospital, Miami, Florida

Juan C. Sotomonte, M.D.
Division of Cardiology, Department of Medicine, University of Miami School of Medicine, Miami, Florida

Amanda Sousa, M.D., Ph.D., FACC
Director of Interventional Cardiology, Dante Pazzanese Institute of Cardiology, São Paulo, Brazil

J. Eduardo Sousa, M.D., Ph.D., FACC
Director, Dante Pazzanese Institute of Cardiology, São Paulo, Brazil

V.S. Srinivas, M.B., B.S.
Assistant Professor of Medicine, Division of Cardiology, Department of Medicine, Albert Einstein College of Medicine of Yeshiva University; Montefiore Medical Center, Bronx, New York

Cristiane Takita, M.D.
Assistant Professor, Department of Radiation Oncology, University of Miami School of Medicine; Sylvester Comprehensive Cancer Center, Jackson Memorial Hospital, Miami, Florida

Hassan Tehrani, M.B., Ch.B.
Division of Cardiothoracic Surgery, Department of Surgery, University of Miami School of Medicine; Jackson Memorial Hospital, Miami, Florida

Craig A. Thompson, M.D.
Division of Interventional Cardiology, Harvard Medical School; Massachusetts General Hospital, Boston, Massachusetts

On Topaz, M.D., FACC, FACP
Professor of Medicine, Division of Cardiology, Department of Internal Medicine, Medical College of Virginia, Virginia Commonwealth University; Director, Interventional Cardiology, McGuire Veterans Affairs Medical Center, Richmond, Virginia

Mauricio Velez, M.D.
Division of Cardiology, Department of Medicine, Jackson Memorial Hospital, Miami, Florida

Ajay K. Wakhloo, M.D., Ph.D.
Professor of Radiology and Neurological Surgery, Section of Neuroendovascular Surgery and Interventional Neuroradiology, Department of Radiology, University of Miami School of Medicine; Chief, Neuroendovascular Surgery and Interventional Neuroradiology, Jackson Memorial Hospital, Miami, Florida

Craig M. Walker, M.D.
Interventional Cardiologist and Medical Director, Cardiovascular Institute of the South, Lafayette, Louisiana

Christopher J. White, M.D.
Chairman, Department of Cardiology, Ochsner Clinic Foundation, New Orleans, Louisiana

Samir Yebara, M.D.
Research Coordinator, Department of Cardiology, Cedars Medical Center, Miami, Florida

Miguel Zabalgoitia, M.D.
Professor of Medicine (Cardiology) and Director of Echocardiography and Noninvasive Services, University of Texas Health Science Center, San Antonio, Texas

Juan Pablo Zambrano, M.D.
Division of Cardiology, Department of Medicine, University of Miami School of Medicine; Jackson Memorial Hospital; Veterans Affairs Medical Center, Miami, Florida

Gerald Zemel, M.D.
Medical Director, Interventional Radiology, Miami Cardiac and Vascular Institute, Baptist Hospital of Miami, Miami, Florida

PREFACE

The field of interventional cardiology is awash in a growing number of ingenious devices. This has led many to be lulled into the false belief that proficiency in interventional cardiology can be achieved solely by developing new catheter skills. As evidenced by the extensive material presented here, that is not the case. *Interventional Cardiology Secrets,* which uses the Socratic model of questions and answers, translates the vast vascular knowledge into usable wisdom, making it very attractive to practicing interventional cardiologists and interventional cardiologists in training. Our goal was to make this book comprehensive but cohesive. We are proud to present to the reader our view of the field of interventional cardiology, impervious to personal interest or commercial bias.

Eduardo de Marchena, M.D.
Alexandre C. Ferreira, M.D.

ACKNOWLEDGMENT

We would like to thank Gladys Molinares for her excellent secretarial assistance in the preparation of this book.

DEDICATION

To my parents for their guidance, support, and encouragement; to my teachers for their knowledge; to my patients for their confidence; and to my wife and children for keeping life fun.

ED

To my parents, Jose Carlos and Cleomar, for their thoughtful guidance; to my wife, Jacqueline, for her love and constant encouragement; and to our children, Gabriela, Isabela, and Felipe, for the joy and inspiration they brought to our lives.

ACF

I. Cardiac Catheterization

1. THE CARDIAC CATHETERIZATION LABORATORY: EQUIPMENT AND PERSONNEL

Glenn Barquet, M.D., and Stephen Mallon, M.D.

EQUIPMENT

1. How are x-rays generated for cineangiography?

1. A generator provides the power needed to produce x-rays. It is composed of a step-up transformer that converts line current into high voltage (70–120 kilovolts [kV]) and high current (300–800 milliamperes [mA]) needed to power the x-ray tube. The generator may be pulsed at up to 30 pulses per second to avoid motion artifact of objects moving at high speeds while maintaining a high degree of contrast.

2. X-ray tube composed of a glass or metal housed tube with a tungsten filament and disc accelerates electrons across an electrical field provided by the generator to produce x-rays. This is very inefficient, with only 1% of the electrical energy delivered to the tube being converted to x-rays and the remainder retained as heat.

2. How is the production of x-rays regulated to account for differing patient size and penetrance?

The automatic exposure control (AEC) is essentially the generator's brain. The AEC governs the generator and x-ray tube to produce the optimal combination of x-ray tube voltage, current, and exposure time for visualization of rapidly moving coronary arteries. If a decrease in light is sensed at the output end of the image intensifier, the AEC increases one of the three adjustable variables:

- **kV:** The energy of the x-ray photons thereby increasing penetration; this is the most commonly increased variable to avoid blackening
- **mA:** The electrical current flowing through the x-ray tube, thereby increasing the number of x-ray photons generated
- **msec:** The duration of the x-ray pulse is adjustable with more "on time" allowing a greater number of photons to pass through the patient

3. What component receives the x-rays for conversion into visible images?

The first component of the imaging chain is the image intensifier (II). The II is located opposite the x-ray tube above the patient. The II functions to receive the x-rays traveling through the patient (at the input phosphor) and converting the x-rays to visible light (at the output phosphor). The visible light may then be used to expose 35-mm cine film, produce digital images, or be converted into real-time fluoroscopic images by video cameras.

4. How is magnification achieved?

First, the field of view (FOV) is narrowed by automatic collimation of the exiting x-ray beam to the desired diameter. The central portion of the II input phosphor receives a smaller diameter beam that has exited the patient and uses electrostatic lenses to magnify the image reaching the output phosphor. For example, without magnification, 9-inch mode covers the entire input phosphor and produces an image measuring 1 inch in diameter for viewing at the output phosphor. At 6-inch mode, the x-ray beams cross-sectional area is decreased by 50% and only the central portion of the input phosphor is activated. The use of electrostatic lenses within the II magnifies the rays of light to the same 1-inch image at the output phosphor. Consequently, images are magnified because a smaller FOV is filling up the same output area of the II tube. Note that magnification should be used judiciously because it results in greater radiation exposure to the patient and staff.

5. Is there an alternative to the II for conversion of x-rays to viewable images?

Recent technology in the form of digital x-ray detectors allows "flat-panel" detector systems to convert incident x-rays into an array of discrete electrical signals. These signals can then be read individually, processed, displayed, and stored for review. The x-ray detector still converts x-rays to light. However, a matrix of light-sensitive cells receives the light and converts it to an array of digital values (ones and zeros). The resolution is dependent upon the number of light-sensitive cells within the matrix (ranging from 1000×1000 to 2000×2000).

6. How is light exiting the II viewed live on TV monitors and recorded either digitally or on 35-mm cine film?

Light exiting the II is received by one of two pickup tube video cameras (one for cine and one for fluoroscopy). Standard resolution for both fluoro and cine cameras is 525 lines per video frame or high resolution ($\sim$ 1000 lines per video frame). During fluoroscopy, essentially all light from the II is sent to the television camera. During cineangiography, a partially silvered mirror is flipped into the light path to divert 90% of the light to the cine camera for image acquisition (either digitally or on 35-mm film). The remaining 10% of the light in the II is directed toward the television camera for real-time fluoroscopy. For digital systems, the video camera functions as the analog signal source for processing by online computers into digital images. Alternatively, a solid-state image sensor (e.g., CCD camera) may be used to receive incident light from the II to produce digital images.

7. Name the equipment labeled in the catheterization laboratory below.

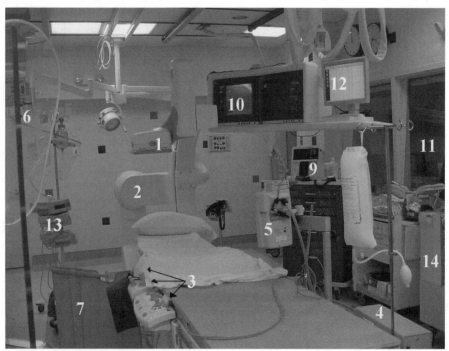

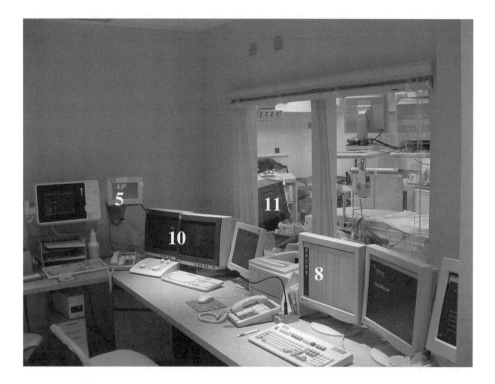

1. Flat panel x-ray detector
2. Gantry to allow for complex angulations
3. Patient support table with panning controls
4. Junction box for connection of pressure transducers to physiologic recorders
5. Angiographic injector and controls
6. Ceiling supported transparent leaded x-ray shield
7. Subtable leaded curtain shield
8. Physiologic pressure recorder behind leaded wall
9. Defibrillator and crash cart
10. High-resolution fluoroscopy and playback video monitor
11. Leaded glass control room window
12. Tableside physiologic monitor
13. Infusion pumps (non–free flowing)

8. What advantages does a digital system using CCD cameras have over traditional 35-mm cine angiography?

The advantages of the CCD camera are simpler design, smaller size, improved dynamic range, better spatial resolution, no temporal lag, longer life, and lower cost. The radiation exposure is lower with digital systems and avoids the need for handling and disposing of hazardous chemicals needed for 35-mm film processing (e.g., silver).

9. What is a collimator, and how does collimation differ from edge filtration?

A collimator consists of motor-driven symmetrical lead shields that "crop" the beam exiting the x-ray tube, thereby defining the beams cross-sectional area. Wedge-shaped edge filters function as partially absorbent shields that attenuate the passage of raw radiation through lucent lung fields that would otherwise produce bright spots ("burn-out"), limiting detailed imaging of adjacent coronary arteries. In addition to improved imaging, proper collimation reduces radiation exposure to the patient and staff because scatter is proportional to the x-ray beam area.

10. Has a universal standard been developed for digital angiography?

Yes. The Digital Imaging and Communication in Medicine (DICOM) standard was developed as the universal method for archiving cardiac angiography. DICOM also allows for seamless exchange of digitally recorded procedures between laboratories and health care systems.

PERSONNEL

11. Who can perform interventional catheterizations as a primary operator?

1. An attending physician is generally in charge of the procedure (primary operator). Physicians should be credentialed and experienced in interventional techniques. The attending must be BC/BE, state licensed, and meet ACC/AHA guidelines.

2. A teaching attending physician instructs graduate physicians in the performance of the procedure and transmission of information to trainees. He or she must be present for all critical aspects of the procedure.

3. The primary role of the cardiovascular trainee (fellow) is to acquire mastery of interventional techniques. Trainees may perform all functions of the procedure as the primary operator but only under the supervision of a credentialed physician who assumes responsibility for the procedure's results.

12. Who can assist the primary operator in the performance of cardiac catheterizations?

1. A secondary operator is an additional attending or physician extender who assists the primary attending physician. He or she should not take credit for the case for the purpose of fulfilling minimum performance volume requirements.

2. A physician extender (physician's assistant and nurse practitioner) functions as secondary operator and should be proficient in both the technical and cognitive aspects of cardiac catheterization. Extenders should never be primary operators.

13. What is the role of the laboratory director?

The laboratory director is in charge of policy development, quality control, and fiscal administration. He or she should be board certified and thoroughly trained in cardiac radiographic imaging and radiation protection and should have at least 5 years of catheterization experience. The director is charged with granting privileges to applicant physicians, as well as supervision and implementation of new technologies.

14. What background training do cardiac catheterization laboratory nurses have?

Many different kinds of nurses work in cardiac catheterization laboratories, including nurse practitioners, registered nurses, licensed vocational or practical nurses, and nursing assistants. Previous training should include critical care experience, direct current cardioversion, knowledge of cardiovascular medications, ability to start intravenous infusions, familiarity with sterile technique, hemostasis methods, invasive monitoring of pressures, knowledge of devices (stents, IVUS, vascular catheters, size correlation of guidewires and adaptors, and manipulation of manifolds). During the procedure, the nurse should have no other responsibility than to monitor and observe the patient's status. Acute cardiac care, including advanced cardiac life support and related therapeutics, is essential in the event of patient decompensation.

15. Who is charged with guiding the use of radiological equipment?

The radiological technologist (RT) is an instrumental figure in the cardiac catheterization laboratory who guides the use of and care for radiological equipment. RTs should be experienced in radiographic and angiographic imaging principles and techniques. RTs should be experienced in the proper function of x-ray generators, cine pulse systems, image intensification, automatic image processing equipment, pressure injection systems, video systems, and cameras. If cine film is used, at least one technologist should be skilled as a darkroom technician. Radiation quality control and safety in the form of day-to-day calibration of equipment and the use of sensitometric or densitometric equipment and data is a must. Additionally, RTs should be skilled in online image processing, image enhancement, stenosis quantification, and volume analysis.

16. What additional staffing is instrumental in order to properly operate a cardiac catheterization laboratory?

1. A laboratory technologist should be skilled in managing blood samples (e.g., ACT, co-oximetry) and performing blood gas measurements and calculations. He or she should be qualified to monitor and record electrocardiographic and hemodynamic data. Skill and experience in interpreting rhythms, artifact, and pressure wave forms is critical in order to accurately and immediately report significant changes to the attending physician.

2. With the current move toward digital catheterization laboratories, a dedicated computer technician with computer skills is beneficial in facilitating computer archiving, troubleshooting, image storage, and maintenance of the digital patient database, as well as production of compact discs.

BIBLIOGRAPHY

1. Baim DS, Grossman W: Cardiac Catheterization, Angiography, and Intervention, 6th ed. Philadelphia, Lippincott Williams & Wilkins, 2000.
2. Bashore TM, Bates ER, Berger PB, et al: American College of Cardiology/Society for Cardiac Angiography and Interventions Clinical Expert Consensus Document on cardiac catheterization laboratory standards. A report of the American College of Cardiology Task Force on Clinical Expert Consensus Documents. J Am Coll Cardiol 37:2170–2214, 2001.
3. Limacher MC, Douglas PS, Germano G, et al: ACC expert consensus document. Radiation safety in the practice of cardiology. American College of Cardiology. J Am Coll Cardiol. 31:892–913, 1998.
4. Moore RJ: Imaging Principles of Cardiac Angiography. New York, Aspen Publishers, 1990.
5. Pepine CJ, Hill JA, Lambert CR: Diagnostic and Therapeutic Cardiac Catheterization, 3rd ed. Philadelphia, Lippincott Williams & Wilkins, 1998.

2. RADIATION PRINCIPLES AND SAFETY

Glenn Barquet, M.D., and Stephen Mallon, M.D.

1. What is radiation?

The process of emitting radiant energy in the form of waves or particles. It is divided into ionizing and non-ionizing radiation.

    a. Non-ionizing: Ultrasound, magnetic resonance imaging (MRI), laser beams, microwaves

    b. Ionizing: Any electromagnetic or particulate energy capable of producing ions by interaction with matter and capable of producing biological injury. (e.g., x-rays, gamma rays)

2. What are the units used for quantifying radiation exposure?

    1. Roentgen (R): Measure of exposure; the amount of ionization that the beam produces in air

    2. Radiation absorbed dose (rad): Measure of absorbed dose; how much heating the radiation beam produces in each gram of a specified material

    3. Gray (Gy): International system of units (SI) equivalent of rad; 1 Gy = 100 rads

    4. Radiation equivalent in man (rem): Dose equivalent; takes into account the different degrees of damage produced by different types of radiation (i.e., alpha particles vs. x-rays): SI unit = Sievert (Sv); 1 Sv = 100 rem; for purposes of x-ray exposure, 1 rem = 1 rad

    5. Effective dose equivalent (EDE): Measured also in rem or Sv; introduced by the National Council on Radiation Protection (NCRP) as a weighted average of the physical distribution of radiation and the relative radiosensitivity of different organs

3. What are typical ranges of exposure for staff working in a cardiac catheterization laboratory?

GROUP	MS/YR	MREM/YR
Physician	2–60	200–6000
Nurses	8–16	800–1600
Technologists	2	200
Assistant technicians	0–2	0–200

Note that background radiation exposure to the average person is 200 mrem/year.

4. What is the estimated probalility of developing a fatal cancer from radiation exposure?

LIFETIME DOSE EQUIVALENT (REM)	FATAL CANCER, %
0.1	0.004
1.0	0.04
10.0	0.4
100.0	4.0

As measured outside the shield, without use of thyroid shielding. Note that true dose equivalent may be overestimated by a factor of 6 because of monitoring outside lead aprons. The background lifetime risk of spontaneously occurring fatal cancer is one in five or 20%.

5. What are the recommended upper limits of radiation exposure?

	LIMIT
Average operator exposure per interventional cardiac catheterization	0.004–0.016 rem
Maximum annual recommended exposure for medical workers	5 rem/year
Maximum lifetime accumulated exposure for medical workers	1 rem × age (in years) or 50 rem
Maximum fetal exposure	0.05 rem/month or 0.5 rem total

6. In what ways can radiation cause biological injury?
1. Stochastic effects: All-or-none phenomenon with the target of injury being DNA. The probability of stochastic effects' occurring increases as the cumulative radiation exposure increases without an established threshold level of exposure. Examples include cancer and genetic effects.
2. Nonstochastic effects (deterministic effects): Dose dependent and result in cell death. These effects are seen upon crossing a particular threshold level of radiation exposure. The greater the radiation exposure, the greater the amount of injury. Examples include skin erythema, desquamation, cataracts, marrow suppression, organ atrophy, gonadal injury, sterility, and fibrosis.

7. What genetic risks exist with radiation exposure before conception and during pregnancy?
The natural risk of spontaneous genetic mutation in humans is 6%. Assuming appropriate shielding with lead aprons, the annual gonadal dose equivalent of an invasive cardiologist is in the range of 70–160 mrem per year. The risk of serious birth defects in future offspring of irradiated parents is estimated to be 2×10^{-5} to 3×10^{-5} per rem.

The estimated risk of a congenital malformation or of developing a malignancy after in utero exposure of 1 rem is about 1 in 500 (0.2%). The risk of mental retardation extrapolated from Hiroshima data is about 0.4 % per rem of exposure. Japanese survivor information also suggests a loss of approximately 20–30 IQ points per rem. Therefore, recommendations call for no more than 0.5 rem for the entire pregnancy or < 0.05 rem/month (measured by waist dosimeter under a protective apron).

8. How can people limit their occupational exposure to radiation?
1. They can limit the time of fluoroscopy and cine. Although fluoroscopic radiation results in about 1/10 the exposure per second compared with cine, liberal use of fluoroscopy is often the source of greater radiation exposure.
2. Distance-x-ray beams travel in straight but divergent directions as they leave the x-ray tube and collimator. Therefore, greater distance from the x-ray source equates to less radiation as divergence allows for an exponential decrease in the number of x-ray photons per unit area (inverse square law).

$$X = 1/d^2$$
$$X = \text{exposure, d} = \text{distance}$$

3. Barriers: Proper collimation and copper filters, as discussed earlier, help limit exposure. Additional barrier methods to shield from radiation include side table drapes, ceiling-mounted acrylic shields, lead aprons, thyroid collars, and protective eyewear. Additional reduction in exposure can be achieved by keeping the image intensifier as close to the patient as possible and using higher kVp (less mA), lower framing rates, limiting the use of magnification, avoiding redundant views, and using pulsed fluoroscopy.

9. Describe how x-rays scatter upon interaction with a patient's body.
As illustrated in the figure at the top of the next page, radiation scatter is not uniform. Scatter propagates in waves or isoexposure curves with increasing distance form the patient, leading to exponential decrease in radiation exposure. Note also the contour of the waves, with the greatest radiation exposure occurring at table level because of unabsorbed scatter.

10. How much radiation is a patient exposed to in a typical cardiac catheterization, and what are the potential complications?
The radiation risk to a patient undergoing a cardiac catheterization with 10 minutes of fluoroscopy and 1 minute of cine run time is estimated to be 40–100 R at the skin (4000–10,000 R cm^2). This is equivalent to 150–400 chest x-rays. The risk of developing a solid carcinoma or leukemia from such exposure is 1.25×10^{-4}. Dermatologic complications may be immediate, with skin necrosis in extreme cases with lengthy cine or fluoro time or longer term, as in the case of radiation dermatitis. Filtration of lower energy photons using aluminum sheets provides for greater penetrance of the x-ray beam, thereby limiting the local skin dose equivalent.

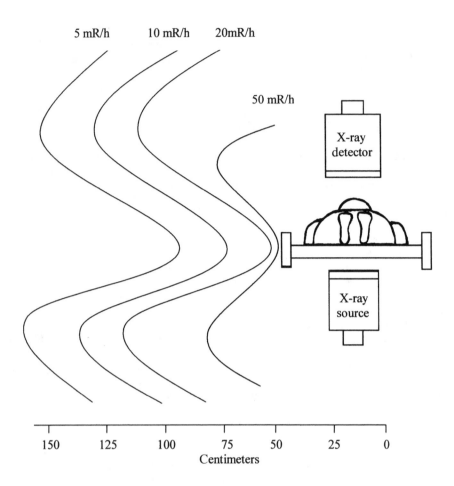

11. Which angiographic view exposes the operator to the greatest radiation, and why?

The cranial left anterior oblique (LAO) because most x-ray scatter occurs at the entry surface of the patient. The nearer the operator is to the x-ray tube (not the II), the greater the exposure. In cranial LAO, the x-ray tube is closest to the operator and accounts for 2.6 to 6.1 times greater exposure to the operator versus right anterior oblique (RAO) caudal.

12. How is radiation exposure to staff monitored?

Either film badges (less expensive) or transluminescent dosimeter badge are worn. It is recommended that two badges be worn during cardiac catheterizations, one at the thyroid shield and the second at the waist below the lead apron. The front of the TLD or film badge should face the direct line of scattered x-rays.

13. How does patient size affect operator exposure to radiation?

Cases involving larger patients expose the operator and staff to greater levels of radiation. Two factors accounting for this are greater scatter of radiation with larger patients and obligatory AEC increases in voltage or current in order to produce satisfactory images.

14. What amount of radiation exposure is associated with the development of cataracts?

The minimum one-time dose of radiation associated with the development of a progressive cataract is 200 rads. Higher total doses may be tolerated without development of cataracts if spread over a longer period of time. The recommended maximum dose equivalent to the lens is 15 rem/year. Use of leaded glasses is recommended to reduce the risk of cataract development.

BIBLIOGRAPHY

1. Baim DS, Grossman W: Cardiac Catheterization, Angiography, and Intervention, 6th ed. Philadelphia, Lippincott Williams & Wilkins, 2000.
2. Balter S, Sones FM, Brancato R: Radiation exposure to the operator performing cardiac angiography with U-arm systems. Circulation 58:925–932, 1978.
3. Bashore TM, Bates ER, Berger PB, et al: American College of Cardiology/Society for Cardiac Angiography and Interventions Clinical Expert Consensus Document on cardiac catheterization laboratory standards. A report of the American College of Cardiology Task Force on Clinical Expert Consensus Documents. J Am Coll Cardiol 37:2170–2214, 2001.
4. Limacher MC, Douglas PS, Germano G, et al: ACC expert consensus document. Radiation safety in the practice of cardiology. American College of Cardiology. J Am Coll Cardiol. 31:892–913, 1998.
5. Moore RJ: Imaging Principles of Cardiac Angiography. New York, Aspen Publishers, 1990.
6. Pepine CJ, Hill JA, Lambert CR: Diagnostic and Therapeutic Cardiac Catheterization, 3rd ed. Philadelphia, Lippincott Williams & Wilkins, 1998.

3. DIAGNOSTIC ANGIOGRAPHY

Niranjan Seshadri, M.D., and Deepak L. Bhatt, M.D.

1. What are the indications for coronary angiography?

Coronary angiography is currently the gold standard for defining the coronary anatomy. The American College of Cardiology has established guidelines for the performance of coronary angiography. The accepted indications for angiography after an acute myocardial infarction (MI) are primary percutaneous intervention for ST segment elevation MI, cardiogenic shock complicating an acute MI, recurrent ischemia after ST segment elevation MI, persistent chest pain or an abnormal functional study after fibrinolysis, and before surgery for mechanical complications of MI. Coronary angiography is indicated in unstable angina in patients with high-risk or intermediate risk features or refractory to medical therapy. Other indications are suspected Printzmetal's angina, abnormal stress test result with high-risk features, sudden cardiac death or ventricular arrhythmias without an obvious precipitating factor, congestive heart failure with accompanying ischemia or angina, patients requiring valve surgery or adult patients with angina requiring repair of a congenital anomaly, suspected stent thrombosis, recurrent angina within 9 months of a percutaneous intervention, and planned high risk non-cardiac surgery (i.e., vascular surgery) in patients with angina or a positive stress test result.

There are other situations in which coronary angiography is frequently performed; however, there is a lack of agreement of definite benefit. These indications include rescue percutaneous intervention for failure of reperfusion with thrombolytics, improvement of class III or IV angina to a higher class with medical therapy, abnormal stress test result with low-risk features, class I or II angina intolerant to medical therapy, perioperative MI, and yearly angiography after heart transplantation.

2. When is non-ionic contrast dye indicated?

Several types of intravascular radiocontrast dyes are available. These dyes differ mainly in their osmolality, with the newer non-ionic agents having an osmolality approaching that of blood. Whenever possible, ionic contrast is preferred because of the significantly increased cost of non-ionic agents. The side effects of ionic agents are mainly related to their hypertonicity, which may cause hypotension, bradycardia, myocardial depression, nausea and vomiting, and increased intravascular volume. Therefore, non-ionic contrast dye is indicated in patients with suspected significant left main coronary artery stenosis, severe left ventricular dysfunction and New York Heart Association class IV heart failure, and severe aortic stenosis. Other potential side effects of ionic contrast agents such as anaphylactoid reactions and renal dysfunction have not been shown to be eliminated by the use of non-ionic contrast agents. However, in patients who have had previous anaphylactoid reactions to ionic contrast agents and preexisting renal insufficiency (serum creatinine > 2 mg/dL), non-ionic contrast dye is indicated to reduce the potential for these complications.

3. What are the common congenital coronary anomalies?

Common coronary anomalies could easily be missed if the operator does not have a reasonable level of suspicion in cases in which coronary arteries are missing or an area of the myocardium appears underperfused. The most common anomaly is absent left main trunk (0.47%); the left anterior descending and left circumflex coronary arteries originate separately from the left sinus of Valsalva. Other common coronary anomalies include origin of the left circumflex coronary artery from the right sinus of Valsalva (0.45%), origin of the right coronary artery from the ascending aorta above the sinus (0.18%), and origin of the right coronary artery from the left sinus of Valsalva (0.13%). An infrequent anomaly is the origin of the left main trunk from the right sinus (0.02%). In these cases, the course of the left main artery is usually through the septum; in rare cases, the left main passes between the aorta and the pulmonary artery.

4. How is aortic regurgitation graded on aortography?

Aortography is useful for assessing the aortic valve, defining aortic aneurysms or dissection, nonselectively identifying suspected anomalous takeoffs of coronary arteries, or nonselectively identifying graft vessels that are difficult to engage.

The grading of aortic insufficiency is done on a scale of 1+ to 4+, with 1+ being mild and 4+ being severe aortic insufficiency. If there is trace amount of contrast dye in the left ventricle that clears in one beat, it is graded as 1+ aortic insufficiency. In 2+, or moderate aortic insufficiency, there is mild left ventricular opacification that does not clear in one beat. In moderate to severe or 3+ aortic insufficiency, ventricular opacification equals that of the aortic root. In 4+ aortic insufficiency, ventricular opacification is greater than that of the aortic root.

5. How is mitral insufficiency graded on ventriculography?

With left ventriculography, the mitral valve apparatus can be seen in both the left and right anterior oblique views. In the 30-degree right anterior oblique view, there is overlap of the mitral valve with the aorta and the left atrium. The 50-degree left anterior oblique view with 15- to 20-degree cranial angulation may be used to avoid the overlap that occurs in the right anterior oblique view. Angiographically, mitral insufficiency is quantitated on a scale of 1+ to 4+, with 1+ representing mild, 2+ moderate, 3+ moderate to severe, and 4+ severe mitral insufficiency. In 1+ mitral insufficiency, there is mild opacification of the left atrium that often clears in one beat. In 2+ mitral insufficiency, there is moderate left atrial opacification that is of lesser intensity than the left ventricle. In 3+ mitral insufficiency, there is opacification of the left atrium equal to that of the left ventricle. In 4+ mitral insufficiency, there is complete opacification of the left atrium greater in intensity than that of the left ventricle.

6. How is coronary dominance determined?

The artery that gives off the posterior descending artery, which supplies the posterior interventricular groove, determines coronary dominance. In most people (85%), the posterior descending artery comes off the right coronary artery, making the anatomy right dominant. In 7% of individuals, the circulation is codominant. In these cases, the posterior descending artery comes off from the right coronary artery and the left circumflex coronary. In 8% of cases, the left circumflex coronary artery is the dominant vessel.

7. What do damping and ventricularization of the pressure waveform indicate?

A dampened pressure waveform (i.e., a decrease in the catheter tip systolic pressure) or a ventricularized pressure waveform (i.e., a decrease in the catheter tip diastolic pressure) usually indicates that the catheter tip is either deep seated, restricting coronary inflow, or the tip is against the wall. It also indicates the possibility of significant left main stenosis. The catheter is gently withdrawn with a slight clockwise or a counterclockwise rotation. With this manipulation, the pressure waveform should return to normal if the catheter tip is against the wall or is deep seated in the vessel. If significant left main stenosis is suspected, the catheter tip is pulled back and a short cine run is performed; alternatively, the catheter is withdrawn into the left sinus and a nonselective injection of the left main trunk may be performed (a left anterior oblique caudal view may be particularly useful).

8. What are the complications of coronary arteriography?

With currently available technology, coronary arteriography is a very safe procedure. The complications, although infrequent, can potentially be serious. They include death (0.1%), stroke (0.05%), and MI (0.05%). Coronary dissection rarely occurs and is usually the result of injecting contrast dye into a catheter that is not coaxial to the coronary artery. Coronary artery spasm, usually of the right coronary artery, is a less serious complication that is treated by withdrawing the catheter out of the coronary artery and injecting intracoronary nitroglycerin. Patients with preexisting renal failure may have worsening of kidney function; in certain high-risk patients (e.g., diabetics, dehydrated patients), contrast dye may precipitate renal failure. The risk of emergency coronary artery bypass grafting caused by a procedural complication is extremely low (~ 0.1% of all percutaneous interventions and even lower in diagnostic angiography). The risk of ventricular fibrillation during left heart catheterization is 0.5%. Use of ionic contrast dye in patients with severe heart failure or renal failure may result in fluid overload and pulmonary edema. The peripheral vascular complications associated with left heart catheterization include femoral pseudo-aneurysms, arteriovenous fistulas, arterial thrombosis, and distal showering of emboli. There is an increased risk of vascular complications such as arterial thrombosis with the brachial or radial approach compared with the femoral approach. Other potential complications include risk of infections, femoral neuropathy, and allergy to contrast dye.

9. What is myocardial bridging?

Myocardial bridging occurs when an epicardial coronary artery dips below part of the myocardial tissue. This occurs most commonly in the distribution of the mid left anterior descending artery. This is recognized angiographically when the artery appears to have an area of stenosis only during systole (Fig. 1). In hypertrophic cardiomyopathy patients, the septal perforators may exhibit a similar phenomenon. Myocardial bridging rarely causes true ischemia. However, some patients have been treated with coronary artery bypass surgery or stenting.

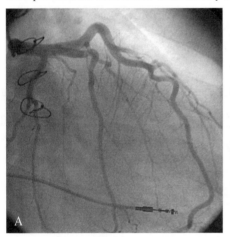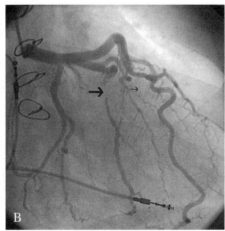

FIGURE 1. Myocardial bridging. Right anterior oblique view of the left coronary artery in diastole (A) and in systole (B). In systole, there is focal stenosis of an epicardial coronary artery (B, *large arrow*) and septal perforators (B, *small arrow*). Courtesy of Sasan Ghaffari, M.D., Cleveland Clinic Foundation.

10. What are the commonly used views for the left coronary artery?

The first view of the left coronary system should be one that shows the course of the left main coronary artery. Most operators prefer either a straight posteroanterior (PA) or a 20-degree right anterior oblique and 20-degree caudal view to show the left main trunk. Caudal views are generally good for visualizing the circumflex coronary artery, and cranial views are good for visualizing the left anterior descending artery and its branches. The 20-degree right anterior oblique, 20-degree caudal projection, which shows the left main trunk well, is also a good view for the proximal circumflex. In this view, portions of the left anterior descending artery (LAD) may also be visualized. A straight 30-degree caudal view is also useful for looking at the left circumflex coronary artery. For the LAD, a straight PA view with a 40-degree cranial angulation shows the mid and distal portions well. To separate out the diagonals from the LAD, a 30-degree right anterior oblique angulation with a 25-degree cranial tilt is very useful. In this view, the diagonals are placed above the LAD. A 40-degree left anterior oblique view with a 25- to 30-degree cranial angulation is another good view for separating the diagonals from the LAD. The 45-degree left anterior oblique with 30-degree caudal angulation, the so-called "spider shot," lays out the left main trunk and the proximal LAD and circumflex artery. With this view, the origins of the diagonal branches are also well seen. A view with 40-degree left anterior oblique angulation shows the mid portions of the LAD and circumflex coronary artery. These are the standard views for visualizing the left coronary system.

11. What are the commonly used views for the right coronary artery?

The right coronary artery is viewed in straight right and left anterior oblique (35- to 40-degree) projections. The right anterior oblique view shows the proximal and mid portions well. In this view, the posterior descending artery and the posteroventricular branches of the right coronary artery are also well seen. A 40-degree left anterior oblique view shows the mid portion of the right coronary artery well. The bifurcation of the right coronary artery, posterior descending artery, and posteroventricular branches are best seen in the PA view with a 40-degree cranial angulation.

12. How are coronary stenoses quantified?

To accurately assess severity of coronary stenoses, it is important to obtain at least two orthogonal views of each coronary segment of interest. With only one projection, eccentric lesions may be missed. Lesion severity is based on a reference diameter, which is usually the most normally appearing segment. However, this method of estimation does not take into account factors such as presence of diffuse disease, arterial remodeling, and the physiologic significance of stenoses. Another useful method of quantitating stenoses is to compare the reference vessel and lesion diameter with the catheter diameter (a 6-French catheter has an external diameter of 2 mm). Based on the diameter of the reference vessel, lesions are graded in percent of "normal," the "normal" being the diameter of the reference vessel. Core laboratories doing quantitative coronary angiography use calipers, a more accurate method of measurement.

13. How is coronary vasospasm provoked in catheterization laboratories?

In patients with suspected coronary vasospasm, medications such as methylergonovine may be used in a catheterization laboratory to provoke coronary spasm. After ruling out stenoses angiographically, intravenous methylergonovine (0.2 mg) is administered. If the patient develops chest pain or has ST elevation on the electrocardiogram, the coronaries are visualized again. In case of true coronary spasm, this maneuver causes a focal area of stenosis angiographically (Fig. 2); and this is usually relieved with intracoronary nitroglycerin. Calcium channel blockers are good long-term medications for patients with coronary vasospasm.

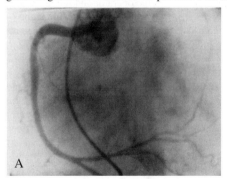 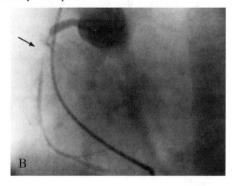

FIGURE 2. Coronary spasm provoked by ergonovine. Left anterior oblique view of the right coronary artery before (A) and after (B) the administration of ergonovine. After administration of ergonovine, there is diffuse spasm of the right coronary artery with a greater focal involvement of the proximal portion of the artery (B, *arrow*). (Courtesy of Frederick A. Heupler Jr, M.D., and Sasan Ghaffari, M.D., Cleveland Clinic Foundation.)

14. In what situations should left ventriculography be avoided?

Performing left ventriculography is potentially hazardous in patients with critical aortic stenosis (aortic valve area < 0.75 cm^2), significant left main disease, severe left ventricular dysfunction with a left ventricular end-diastolic pressure > 25 mm of Hg, and in those with a mechanical aortic valve.

15. How is coronary air embolism recognized and treated?

One of the potentially serious complications of coronary angiography is the inadvertent injection of air during selective coronary arteriography or during ventriculography. When advancing a catheter in the aorta and connecting it to the manifold and flushing with saline, great care should be exercised to prevent accidental introduction of air bubbles. As an additional precautionary measure, the syringe should be at a 45-degree angle to the patient while injecting contrast dye into the coronary circulation. Air bubbles appear as radiolucent shadows.

Patients with air embolism in the coronary circulation may have sudden onset of chest pain and transient ST segment elevation. These patients should be given either sublingual or intracoronary nitroglycerin and saline should be flushed down the coronary artery to help dislodge the air embolus downstream. The most serious sequelae of air embolism during ventriculography is embolism to the brain. Patients may exhibit sudden onset of agitation, confusion, or a focal neurologic deficit. A hyperbaric oxygen chamber may be used to treat selected patients.

16. What are the contraindications for coronary angiography?

The only absolute contraindication for coronary angiography is patient refusal to undergo the procedure. Other relative contraindications are shown in the following table.

Relative Contraindications for Coronary Arteriography

Coagulopathy (international normalized ratio > 1.8; platelet count $< 50,000$)
Increasing serum creatinine level
Severe contrast dye allergy
Active systemic infection
Local infection at the access site
Severe electrolyte imbalance
Digitalis toxicity
Severe peripheral vascular disease
Uncontrolled severe hypertension

17. What can be done to minimize radiation exposure?

It is extremely important to minimize radiation exposure of the operator and the laboratory personnel because exposure to radiation is cumulative. The primary source of radiation is the x-ray generator under the catheterization laboratory table. The greater the distance of the image intensifier from the patient and the more oblique the projection, the higher the radiation scatter. Cineangiography generates five times the radiation as fluoroscopy. Radiation exposure may be limited by using leaded aprons with at least a 0.5-mm lead lining, thyroid lead shields, lead eye glasses (0.5 mm thick lead equivalent glasses), using collimators, limiting fluoroscopy and cineangiography time, reducing the distance between the patient and the image intensifier, setting up shots that require minimal panning, and using lead table shields to minimize radiation from under the table. Thyroid shields and lead aprons should be checked under fluoroscopy at least once a year to ensure that there are no cracks in the lead lining.

18. What are the precautions to be taken in patients with iodine dye allergy, and how is it treated?

If a patient reports prior significant adverse reaction to contrast agents, steps to prevent adverse reactions on subsequent exposure to contrast agents include premedicating the patient and the use of non-ionic contrast agents during coronary angiography. Patients are premedicated with prednisone (usually 40 mg orally every 6 hours for four doses) or hydrocortisone (100 mg intravenously at least 6 hours before the procedure) and cimetidine (20 mg orally) and with diphenhydramine (Benadryl) 50 mg intravenously. In patients reporting prior severe allergy to contrast agents, giving a 0.5 cc test dose and observing the patient for a few minutes may be prudent.

Allergic reactions to contrast agents may manifest as hives and itching, which usually respond to Benadryl. Severe reactions such as oropharyngeal edema, bronchospasm, and hypotension require prompt treatment with 0.5 cc of 1:1000 epinephrine administered subcutaneously. In some cases, endotracheal intubation and aggressive fluid resuscitation may be required.

19. What are the angiographic views for visualizing coronary artery bypass grafts?

For visualization of the body of arterial and venous bypass conduits, left and right anterior oblique projections are generally used. Using the same projections for visualizing the native coronary circulation and the graft conduits simplifies the interpretation of coronary angiograms. For example, if the native circumflex is best seen in an right anterior oblique caudal projection, a graft to one of the circumflex branches may be best seen in this view. Other views may be used to open up specific segments. For example, the anastomotic site of the left internal mammary artery graft to the LAD is best seen in a straight lateral view. Good views for grafts to the diagonal branches are cranial right and left anterior oblique views. For a graft to the distal right coronary artery, the cranial left anterior oblique and lateral views are generally useful.

BIBLIOGRAPHY

1. Baim DS, Grossman W: Grossman's Cardiac Catheterization, Angiography and Intervention, 6th ed. Philadelphia, Lippincott Williams & Wilkins, 2000, pp 211–322.
2. Bhatt DL: Left heart catheterization. In Marso SP, Griffin BP, Topol EJ (eds): Manual of Cardiovascular Medicine. Philadelphia, Lippincott Williams & Wilkins, 2000, pp 700–721.
3. Bhatt DL, Heupler FA, Jr: Coronary angiography. In Topol EJ (ed): Textbook of Cardiovascular Medicine, 2nd ed. Philadelphia: Lippincott Williams & Wilkins, 2002, pp 1635–1650.
4. Kern MJ: The Cardiac Catheterization Handbook, 3rd ed. St. Louis, Mosby, 1999.

4. HEMODYNAMIC SUPPORT INTRA-AORTIC BALLOON PUMP AND CARDIOPULMONARY BYPASS

Hooshang Bolooki, M.D., and H. Michael Bolooki, B.S.

1. What are the indications for emergency use of intra-aortic balloon pump (IABP) in the cardiac catheterization laboratory?

There are two major categories of indications for the use of IABP. The first is in patients who are unstable (by hemodynamic criteria) as a result of myocardial ischemia or infarction and require counterpulsation on an **elective** basis prior to cardiac catheterization or early after the study has initiated.

The second is the **emergency** use of IABP in patients who become hemodynamically unstable as a result of a catastrophic occurrence while diagnostic studies or percutaneous revascularization measures are in progress or completed. In general, when there is time to perform hemodynamic measurements, the indications for the use of the IABP are based on established criteria by Myocardial Infarction Research Units (MIRU) in the early 1970s. These hemodynamic criteria, which have remained unchanged over the years, include a decrease in systolic blood pressure to less than 90 mmHg, left ventricular end diastolic pressure (or pulmonary wedge pressure) greater than 18 mmHg, cardiac index of less than $1.8L/min/m^2$, and tachycardia (pulse rate >110). Time constraints and urgency may not allow completion of these measurements in the cardiac catheterization laboratory unless the data are available on-line. Frequently, only the arterial blood pressure and heart rate readings are noted. The two parameters, along with clinical presentation of acute coronary syndrome, where there is no response to initial administration of pressor agents and coronary vasodilators are an indication for the use of intra-aortic balloon pump in most emergent situations. Additional indications include a mean arterial blood pressure of less than 60 mmHg associated with significant cardiac arrhythmia especially when ventricular tachyarrhythmia develops. This device would alleviate the left ventricular arrhythmia if it were due to an imbalance in myocardial oxygen supply and demand. Counterpulsation with IABP can maintain a constant intra-arterial pressure, which would allow sufficient time to implement for other measures such as optimized drug treatment, management decisions, use of percutaneous PCP bypass, or surgical intervention. IABP and PCP bypass can serve as temporary support measures to surgical intervention.

Certain cardiac rhythms such as atrial fibrillation with a fast response and ventricular tachyarrhythmia (especially multi-focal and with a fast rate) may interfere with the function of the intra-aortic balloon pump. However, these do not constitute a contraindication to its use. In fact, counterpulsation therapy may serve as an effective measure to remedy this atrial or ventricular arrhythmia of ischemic etiology. Because of simplicity of application of IABP, a detailed hemodynamic study prior to its use has not been strictly applied and in fact in unstable patients, is probably unnecessary. Use of IABP frequently prevents development of severe cardiac decompensation and cardiac arrest. In our experience, IABP can be used during CPR because chest compression results in a signal that can trigger the balloon device. The combination of chest compression and balloon inflation results in a sequential rise in intra-aortic blood pressure mimicking counterpulsation as is seen during normal cardiac systole. With development of ventricular fibrillation, cardioversion should be promptly employed and IABP assist continued.

2. Describe the hemodynamic consequences of diastolic augmentation.

The IABP is the only counterpulsation device that is clinically available and has been utilized in millions of cardiac patients worldwide. The immediate visible effects of diastolic augmentation is that the arterial blood pressure curve pattern is changed from a single sinusoid pattern into a double humped curve with the first impulse indicating the opening of the aortic valve (cardiac systole) followed by a sharp V (dicrotic notch) and a second hump due to inflation of the intra-aortic balloon. This is followed by a marked decline in the intra-aortic pressure as a result of balloon deflation. Balloon deflation should coincide with the end of isometric contraction of the left ventricle (peak dp/dt) and the instant of opening of the aortic valve. Deflation of the balloon creates a negative pressure within the aorta and assists in ventricular emptying (after load reduction) and a decrease in subsequent arterial systolic pressure (systolic unloading). This change in the arterial pressure curve is associated with a decrease in end-diastolic intra-aortic pressure and to an extent the mean arterial blood pressure. Similarly, there is a marked decrease in afterload, in peripheral resistance, and in peak systolic intra-ventricular pressure while simultaneously there is an improvement in systolic output of the left ventricle. There is also a decrease in the left ventricular end diastolic pressure and volume as well as dp/dt. The pulmonary wedge pressure, the pulmonary artery systolic pressure, and the heart rate also decrease. Cardiac output increases, and urinary flow as well as cerebral perfusion may improve markedly. Most frequently myocardial oxygen supply and demand equation improves, leading to a marked decrease in myocardial ischemic changes. In a patient with coronary artery disease, IABP has a significant salutary effect (like water on fire).

3. Should all patients who receive IABP support in the catheterization laboratory go directly to the O.R. for definitive surgical treatment and emergent coronary bypass?

The need for intra-aortic balloon pump does imply urgent operative intervention. After placement of balloon assist, in an unstable patient, it is possible to successfully complete the diagnostic studies and/or the endovascular myocardial revascularization once clinical and hemodynamic stability has been achieved. If clinical stability continues and the involved coronary artery has a TIMI III blood flow, the patient may be observed in the coronary care unit. The intra-aortic balloon pump can be discontinued once it is obvious that urgent or emergent surgical intervention is not planned. In patients after PTCA, a second cardiac catheterization may be necessary to ascertain the patency of the instrumented vessel.

All patients who have additional coronary lesions requiring bypass grafting should have the operative procedure performed (depending upon their degree of instability) immediately after PTCA urgently or emergently. In these patients, in the operating room, after the coronary bypass procedure is completed, the intra-aortic balloon pump is not discontinued. The IABP is removed after 24–36 hours of postoperative observation if the patient's general condition remains stable.

The emergent coronary bypass procedure should be done with extreme care utilizing arterial grafts to the extent possible allowing only short periods of myocardial ischemia. Frequently, patients with failed PTCA have received long-acting (oral) antiplatelet agents (clopidogrel). This drug is associated with extensive postoperative bleeding and may delay the surgical intervention for 5–7 days. Use of short acting agents such as GP IIIb/IIa inhibitor is not a contraindication to urgent (within 4–6 hours) surgical intervention, although it results in larger blood loss postoperatively than is normally observed.

4. What are the early complications of intra-aortic balloon counterpulsation?

The early complications of intra-aortic balloon counterpulsation are similar to those of percutaneous placement of PCP bypass catheters. In general, decrease in distal arterial blood flow results in leg ischemia (approximately 11% in patients who receive intra-aortic balloon counterpulsation) and very rarely results in limb loss (less than 1%). Fasciotomy of the affected leg and assessment of distal pulses with a Doppler probe are helpful in preventing major complications. Delayed complications include localized hematoma of the groin area and lymphorrhagia. These can be successfully treated with minimal surgical intervention.

The use of intra-aortic balloon pump may cause peripheral neuropathy involving the leg and rarely the spinal column. Peroneal nerve palsy or paresis with foot drop is seen, and at times femoral nerve palsy may result in numbness of the frontal area of the affected thigh as well as a reduction in patellar reflex. Intimal debris from the aorta during IABP may cause shower emboli and localized infarction of various organs. This complication is frequently seen in patients who remain in a state of severe cardiac failure unresponsive to medical management.

5. What are the indications and the results of emergency percutaneous establishment of cardiopulmonary bypass?

Emergency percutaneous cardiopulmonary bypass (PCPB) is generally used for patients who are not responsive to cardiopulmonary resuscitation (CPR). This indication can be broadened to include some patients who have had cardiac arrest for periods longer than 10 minutes. However, in our experience, the possibility of neurologic survival once the period of CPR is beyond 10 minutes is less than 5%. This is especially true for patients who have had cardiac standstill (asystole) as opposed to patients who are in ventricular fibrillation that responds to electrical cardioversion. Patients with cardiac standstill need to have a cardiac pacemaker (inserted percutaneously by subxiphoid approach) to produce a heart rhythm. Patients who respond rapidly to these measures may also respond favorably to the use of PCPB. Use of cardiopulmonary bypass is usually associated with various degrees of cerebral edema. Cerebral edema is also seen after prolonged CPR. Their combination results in neurological dysfunction with protracted recovery time. This deficit is frequently discovered after the acute phase and may be associated with a prolonged vegetative state requiring respiratory and renal support if cardiac function has recovered.

Early complications associated with emergency percutaneous CP bypass include inability to pass the arterial and venous cannulae through the femoral artery and vein. With failure of percutaneous attempts at cannulation, a surgical cut down at the groin area is needed. The femoral artery may be diseased and not suitable to accommodate the large (14 F) cannula safely. Perforations of the femoral artery and the femoral vein have been seen in emergent situations. Correct positioning of the cannula within the selected vessel is mandatory to establishing the cardiopulmonary bypass. Otherwise, the opposite femoral artery and vein should be cannulated. With femoral vessel perforation, the patient should be taken to the operating room and the iliac vessels and at times the retroperitoneal structures should be explored. An attempt is made to repair the femoral and the iliac artery and vein promptly. These dissections of themselves are time consuming and extensive and require a great deal of meticulous hemostasis.

Late complications of percutaneous CP bypass include lymphorrhagia, wound infection, and femoral arterial false aneurysm formation. Arteriovenous (AV) fistula may develop a few weeks after the cannulae have been removed. Percutaneous removal of these cannulae is not recommended because of a definite possibility of hemorrhage, false aneurysm formation, as well as development of AV fistula. The fistula, at times, is large and has a palpable thrill. To prevent rupture, urgent surgical management is mandatory.

Damage to the femoral nerve (directly or due to pressure from a groin hematoma) is associated with sensory losses in the frontal surface of mid thigh area. Chronic venous stasis due to occlusion of the femoral or iliac vein is also seen.

Iliofemoral venous thrombosis may occur, which may lead to pulmonary embolism or distal phlegmasia. It is important that in these patients, when they are in the operating room, the area below the knee (the calf) is examined, and since there are periods of prolonged ischemia of the leg, we suggest lower leg fasciotomy, to prevent leg and foot ischemia. After removal of the cannulae, the distal pulses and the venous circulation in the posterior tibial and dorsalis pedis areas should be monitored. Venous flow should be maintained with measures such as sequential leg compression devices and intravenous heparin or injections of low molecular weight heparin as well as antiplatelet agents (when there are no contraindications). Venous flow is also monitored with Doppler studies.

6. What are the clinical presentations of intra-aortic balloon perforation during counterpulsation? How should it be managed?

Passage of the intra-aortic balloon catheter through a guiding sheath prevents injury to the balloon section of the catheter due to intra-arterial hard plaques. However, balloon catheter passage by sheathless technique should be done extremely carefully to prevent balloon injury and perforation. Balloon perforation in the course of intra-aortic balloon counterpulsation is identified with the appearance of blood within the balloon catheter lumen and with gradual decline in diastolic augmentation pressure. Upon the observation of blood in the lumen of the catheter, one should suspect balloon perforation and immediately proceed with removal of the balloon catheter. If the patient is unstable and needs the circulatory assist with the intra-aortic balloon counterpulsation, another balloon catheter should be placed through the opposite femoral artery and the perforated balloon removed after the guide wire for the new balloon catheter is in place. This should be done very quickly, and after injection of heparin into the catheter lumen to prevent blood clotting within the balloon. Otherwise, the balloon may not be deployed from the femoral artery without causing significant laceration and injury to the iliac and femoral arteries. If the balloon catheter withdrawal is not easy, removal should be done in the operating room after exposing the iliac and the femoral arteries. Major injuries to the iliac arteries have occurred as a result of forceful removal of clotted balloon catheter. A balloon catheter that is clotted may be treated with the use of tPA injection into the balloon catheter. Once lysis of the clot has occurred, attempt is made to gradually remove the catheter. The surgical team should be prepared to explore the iliac artery and the lower abdominal aorta if the balloon catheter does not deploy. If removal of the balloon catheter has resulted in dissection or tear of the iliac artery, the distal vessel should be bypass grafted to improve the distal blood flow. A Fogarty catheter may be used to open the proximal lumen and to extract any clots. At times, preparations should be made to bypass graft the distal femoral artery with a cross leg graft.

7. Define the leg compartment syndrome and describe its management.

A patient who is receiving counterpulsation with an IABP is in constant danger of leg ischemia. This may develop in spite of detection of a satisfactory distal Doppler pulse. Viability of the ischemic leg is dependent upon the degree of collateral circulation in the groin area (circumflex iliac and pudendal vessels) as well as the small blood flow through the femoral artery around the balloon catheter. The first indication of pending compartment syndrome is leg pain in the calf area. Associated hypothermia of the leg and poor capillary filling are the next stage of progression to limb loss. Eventually the foot looses its neurologic (motor and sensory) function, at which time there has been a significant delay in diagnosis of severe leg ischemia. An initial finding in compartment syndrome is increase in interstitial pressure in each of the calf compartments where long flexor muscles are located within a tight osteo-fascial compartment. The inter-compartment pressure normally is about 3–8 mmHg. With compartment syndrome, which results in muscle edema, compartment pressure increases initially to 15–25 mmHg and then to >30 mmHg. At that stage, there is little arterial inflow into the leg or venous effluent. By prompt 3-quadrant fasciotomy in the operating room or urgently at the bedside, the pressure build up is released and the muscles are allowed to bulge, allowing some arterial in-flow and venous out-flow.

The incision over the skin and the fascia is left open and is dressed in a sterile fashion. The muscles are usually discolored. The release of pressure may cause the return of Doppler pulse and possibly the neurologic function if the period of ischemia has been less than 6–8 hours. This procedure frequently has resulted in saving the patient's leg.

BIBLIOGRAPHY

1. Arafa OE, Pedersen TH, Svennevig JL, et al: Vascular complications of the intra-aortic balloon pump in patients undergoing open-heart operations. 15 years experience. Ann Thorac Surg 67:645–561, 1999.
2. Bolooki H: Circulatory assist device for the management of intractable ventricular tachyarrhythmia. Cardiac Electrophysiol Rev 5:361–362, 2001.
3. Bolooki H: Clinical application of intra-aortic balloon pump. In Physiology of Balloon Pumping, 3rd ed. Armonk, NY, Futura Publishing, 1998, pp 109–162.
4. Christenson JT, Cohen M, Ferguson JJ III, et al: Trends in intra-aortic balloon counterpulsation complications and outcomes in cardiac surgery. Ann Thorac Surg 74:1086–1091, 2002.
5. Eisenberg MS, Mengert TJ: Primary care: Cardiac resuscitation. N Engl J Med 344:1304–1313, 2001.

6. Fasseas P, Cohen M, Kopistansky C, et al: Pre-operative intra-aortic balloon pump counterpulsation in stable patients with left main coronary disease. J Invas Cardiol 13:679–683, 2001.
7. Ferguson JJ, Cohen M, Freedman RJ, et al: The current practice of intra-aortic balloon counterpulsation. Results from the Benchmark Registry. J Am Coll Cardiol 38:1456–1462, 2001.
8. Jorgensen EO: Neurological and circulatory outcomes of cardiopulmonary resuscitation in progress: Influence of pre-arrest and arrest factors. Resuscitation 36:45–49, 1998.
9. Robertson RM: Sudden death from cardiac arrest: Improving the odds. N Engl J Med 343:1259–1260, 2000.

II. Coronary Artery Disease

5. CORONARY BLOOD FLOW PHYSIOLOGY

Morton J. Kern, M.D.

1. Why are measurements of coronary physiology needed?

Coronary angiography remains the standard for the diagnosis of epicardial coronary disease. However, precise quantification of stenosis severity is limited by the inability to provide accurate two- or three-dimensional resolution on coronary "luminograms." The limitations of coronary angiography have been well documented by comparisons with intravascular ultrasound and ischemic stress testing. It is well known that angiography fails to provide critical details regarding the arterial wall and lumen morphology and that it fails to accurately describe the forces acting on blood flow to predict flow limitations in all but the most extreme ends of the spectrum of stenoses. Together with direct measurement of coronary blood flow velocity and distal perfusion pressures, coronary angiography allows interventional cardiologists to have complete assessments of both coronary anatomy and physiology.

Angiography repeatedly fails clinicians; a typical remark is, "I can't really tell if this lesion is severe; let's take another view" (Fig. 1). After three or four more views with different angulations, the lesion is no better visualized. At this point, there should be little doubt that the physician cannot accurately gauge the true nature of the lesion in question. Intracoronary physiologic techniques overcome the failings of lumenography. Measuring coronary blood flow and pressure provides unique information that complements the angiographic evaluation and in most cases facilitates decision making regarding appropriateness of medical or interventional therapy.

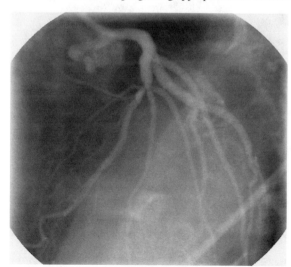

FIGURE 1. Angiogram of difficult lesion at trifurcation. Does angiographic finding reveal physiology significance of lesion?

2. What factors regulate coronary blood flow?

Coronary blood flow is closely matched to myocardial oxygen demand. Myocardial demand is determined by three factors: heart rate, contractility, and left ventricular (LV) wall stress (blood pressure [BP] and LV volume). The physiologic mechanisms for the coupling of coronary blood flow to myocardial metabolism can be reviewed in detail elsewhere. Coronary blood flow is controlled principally by coronary arterioles, which are richly innervated with receptors from both divisions of the autonomic nervous system and are sensitive to many endogenous physiologic vasodilators, including adenosine. Coronary blood flow is the sum of three resistances; R_1, the epicardial arteries; R_2, the arterioles; and R_3, the intramyocardial capillary system. For the most part, the normal large epicardial conduit arteries offer minimal resistance to coronary blood flow. Arteriolar vasodilation can increase blood flow more than threefold. However, in the presence of hemodynamically significant epicardial stenosis, the R_1 resistance increases and the arterioles maximally vasodilate. Coronary blood flow becomes limited and under conditions of increased oxygen demand, a mismatch between oxygen delivery and demand occurs, resulting in angina.

3. Why is there a pressure gradient across a stenosis?

Pressure is normally transmitted equally from the aorta throughout all coronary arteries. An epicardial coronary artery stenosis produces resistance and energy loss, which results in post-stenotic pressure loss. A decrease in perfusion pressure varies exponentially with flow across a stenosis (Fig. 2). The stenosis causes flow turbulence, frictional losses, and separation forces, which result in energy loss as heat is dissipated and causes a loss of pressure distal to an epicardial stenosis. The distal pressure loss creates a pressure gradient between the aorta and the distal region of the involved coronary artery. Angina is produced when the lower limit of perfusion pressure distal to a critical epicardial stenoses results in inadequate arteriolar vasodilation to provide the necessary level of coronary flow.

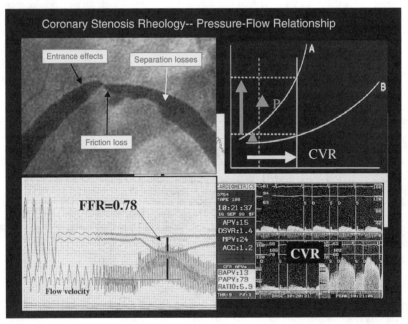

FIGURE 2. Factors from angiographic anatomy contributing to resistance to blood flow. Stenosis causes resistance by friction from entrance effects, separation, and turbulence (*top left*). Two similar diameter lesions can produce two different pressure-flow resistance curves (*top right*). Flow and pressure measurements show how FFR is obtained (*bottom left*). Doppler coronary flow velocity signals used to measure coronary flow reserve (CVR) (*bottom right*).

4. What is coronary vasodilatory reserve (CVR), and what are factors that influence it?

CVR is the ratio of maximal hyperemic to basal coronary blood flow. CVR is subject to variations in conditions, which may alter resting flow and limit maximal hyperemic flow. In animals and young adults, CVR may be > 4. In patients with normal coronary arteriography and chest pain syndromes, CVR is 2.7 ± 0.6. In patients with non-obstructive coronary disease, CVR averages 2.5 ± 0.95. In patients with orthotopic heart transplantation and normal arteries, CVR is 3.1 ± 0.9. CVR values < 2.0 are associated with microvascular disease and occur in approximately 12% of chest pain patients with normal arteries. CVR may be reduced in patients with essential hypertension and normal coronary arteries and in patients with aortic stenosis and normal coronary arteries.

Basal flow is influenced by myocardial oxygen demand (i.e., heart rate [HR], BP, contractility). Tachycardia increases basal flow; coronary flow reserve is reduced by 10% for each 15 beats of heart rate. Increasing mean arterial pressure reduces maximal vasodilatation, reducing hyperemia with less alteration in basal flow. Hyperemic flow is related to maximal vasodilatory capacity of the microcirculatory bed and is affected by left ventricular hypertrophy, diabetes mellitus, infarction, and ischemia.

Patient age affects CVR. Weineke et al. examined CVR in patients in 242 unobstructed coronary arteries in 141 patients and found that individual CVR values obtained at different basal average peak velocities could be transformed and corrected for patient age relating them to a mean basal average peak velocity (BAPV) of 15 cm/sec and age of 55 years ($CVR_{corr} = 2.85 * CVR_{measured} * 10^x$, where $X = 0.48 \log (BAPV) + 0.0025 * age - 1.16$). Use of the corrected CVR standardizes for variations in basal average peak velocity and patient age and may discriminate between intrinsic and extra cardiac factors impairing CVR.

5. How does diabetes affect CVR?

CVR is diminished in patients with diabetes, especially in those with diabetic retinopathy. Akasaka et al. compared 29 patients with diabetes mellitus (18 with diabetic retinopathy) with 15 control patients with chest pain and normal coronary arteries. The diabetic retinopathy was nonproliferative in all 18 patients studied. CVR was measured in the angiographically normal segment of the left anterior descending coronary artery in patients at rest and during maximal hyperemia induced with 0.014 mg/kg of intravenous (IV) adenosine. Volumetric coronary blood flow was significantly reduced during hyperemia (107 ± 23 and 116 ± 18 vs. 136 ± 17 mL/min, respectively) and was higher at baseline (58 ± 16 and 45 ± 12 vs. 37 ± 10 mL/min, respectively) in diabetic patients with and without retinopathy compared with control groups ($P < 0.05$ for both diabetic groups). CVR was also significantly lower in diabetic patients with and without retinopathy compared with the control patients (1.9 ± 0.4 and 2.8 ± 0.3 vs. 3.3 ± 0.4; $P < 0.01$, respectively). Advanced diabetic retinopathy is a significant marker of impaired CVR.

6. How does hyperlipidemia affect CVR?

Hyperlipidemia and increased blood flow viscosity decrease CVR. Rim et al., found a strong negative correlation between CFR and blood viscosity in nine dogs whose serum triglyceride levels were experimentally increased. Whereas myocardial vascular resistance increased with increasing triglyceride levels, hyperemic myocardial blood flow decreased ($R = -0.64$). The decrease in hyperemic myocardial blood flow was associated with a decrease in blood velocity ($R = 0.56$), observations confirmed by direct intravital microscopic observation in mice. The authors concluded that whereas increasing lipid levels in a fully dilated normal coronary bed caused no change in large or small vessel dimensions, an increase in blood viscosity caused capillary resistance to increase, attenuating hyperemic coronary blood flow.

7. How do beta-blockers affect CVR?

Beta-blocking agents, a key in the management of myocardial ischemia, modulate CVR through incompletely understood pathophysiologic mechanisms. Beta-blockers potentiated CVR. CVR was examined in 23 symptomatic patients undergoing PCI 1 minute after vessel occlusion,

after administration of intracoronary adenosine, and again before and after 5 mg of IV metoprolol. CVR was 2.1 at rest and increased to 2.7 after metoprolol administration ($P = 0.002$). The
postischemic CVR (after angioplasty balloon deflation) increased from 2.6 to 3.3 ($P < 0.001$) and
was significantly higher than CVR regardless of metoprolol. Coronary vascular resistance decreased after beta-blocker administration, from 3.4 ± 2.0 to 2.3 ± 0.7 mm Hg *sec/cm (Fig. 3).
Metoprolol increased in postischemic and pharmacologic CVR.

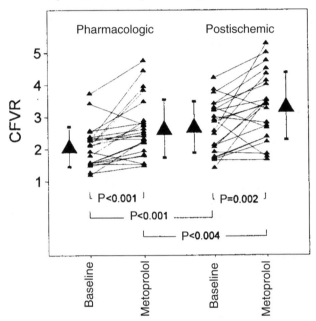

FIGURE 3. Pharmacologic and post-ischemic coronary flow velocity reserve (CFVR) increased significantly
from 2.1 ± 0.6 to 2.6 ± 0.9, respectively, from 2.7 ± 0.8 to 3.3 ± 1.0 after intravenous administration of
5 mg metoprolol. In two patients, there was no change in pharmacologic CFVR, but in another two patients,
there was even a decrease in CFVR after beta-blockade. Postischemic CFVR was generally higher than pharmacologic CFVR. (Reproduced with permission from Billinger M, et al: Do beta-adrenergic blocking agents
increase coronary flow reserve? J Am Coll Cardiol 38:1866–1871, 2001.)

8. What is the effect of gender on CVR?

As part of the Women's Ischemic Syndrome Evaluation (WISE) study, Reis et al. examined
48 women with chest pain, normal coronary arteries, or minimal luminal irregularities with CVR.
Sixty percent of women with CVR < 2 had a hyperemic velocity of 89% of baseline but no change
in cross-sectional vessel area. Forty percent of women with CVR, averaging 3.24, had increases
in coronary flow velocity and a cross-sectional area by 179% and 17%, respectively. In these
women, a CVR of 2.2 provided a high sensitivity and specificity (90% and 89%, respectively) for
the diagnosis of microvascular dysfunction. Failure of epicardial coronary artery to dilate at least
9% was also a sensitive (79%) and specific (79%) surrogate marker of microvascular dysfunction. The attenuated epicardial coronary dilatory response likely represented significant microvascular dysfunction in women with chest pain and no obstructive coronary artery disease.

9. What is relative coronary flow velocity reserve, and when is it used?

Because CVR is a two-component system (i.e., epicardial and microvascular), there is un-
certainty accepting an abnormal CVR as the sole indicator of lesion significance. To measure lesion severity independent of the microvascular influence, a relative CVR (rCVR), defined as the
ratio of maximal flow in the coronary with stenosis (Q^S) to flow in a normal coronary without

stenosis (Q^N) has been used. rCVR is independent of the aortic pressure, heart rate, and microvascular abnormalities and is well suited to assess the physiologic significance of target coronary stenoses when an adjacent nondiseased reference coronary artery is available. rCVR is the ratio of CVR_{target} to CVR in an angiographically normal reference vessel, with (rCVR = $(Q^s/Q_{base}) / (Q^N/Q_{base}) = (CVR_{target}/CVR_{reference})$. Basal flow in the two vessels is assumed to be similar; therefore, rCVR mathematically resembles Gould's derivation. rCVR cannot be used in patients with three vessel coronary disease who have no suitable reference vessel. rCVR relies on the assumption that the microvascular circulatory response is uniformly distributed among the myocardial beds, thus rCVR is of no value in patients with myocardial infarction or LV regional dysfunction or those with heterogeneous microcirculatory responses. The assumption that microvascular responses throughout the LV or between the right ventricle (RV) and LV are uniform has been questioned because of the flow heterogeneity and regional difference in coronary blood flow and myocardial oxygen consumption, explaining why the non-ischemic threshold range for rCVR in patients is so large at 0.65 to 1.0.

10. What is pressure-derived fractional flow reserve (FFR), and how is it used?

Myocardial perfusion is closely linked to myocardial ischemia and is directly dependent on the coronary "driving" pressure associated with three major coronary vascular resistances (i.e., epicardial, arteriolar, and intramyocardial capillary resistance). The myocardial perfusion pressure is reduced when an epicardial stenosis causes pressure loss distal to the stenosis in proportion to the flow rate. If the myocardial bed resistances are stimulated to maximal hyperemia and remain constant, then the poststenotic hyperemic coronary artery pressure represents the maximal achievable perfusion available in that vessel and can be used to estimate normal coronary blood flow.

Using coronary pressure measured at constant and minimal myocardial resistances (i.e., maximal hyperemia), Pijls et al. derived an estimate of the percentage of normal (i.e., in the theoretical absence of the stenosis) coronary blood flow expected to go through a stenotic artery, called the fractional flow reserve (FFR). The FFR, calculated as the ratio of the poststenotic or distal coronary pressure to aorta pressure (as the pressure in an unobstructed artery, i.e., the theoretical normal artery pressure) obtained at sustained minimal resistance (i.e., maximal hyperemia), reflects both antegrade and collateral myocardial perfusion rather than merely transstenotic pressure loss (i.e., a stenosis pressure gradient). Because it is calculated only at peak hyperemia, FFR is further differentiated from CVR by being largely independent of basal flow, driving pressure, heart rate, systemic blood pressure, or status of the microcirculation. The FFR—but not the resting pressure or hyperemic pressure gradient—is strongly related to provocable myocardial ischemia (FFR < 0.75) established by rigorous comparisons with different clinical stress testing modalities in patients with stable angina (Fig. 4).

Defining CVR, rCVR, FFR

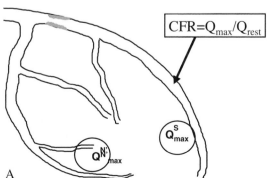

$$CFR = Q_{max}/Q_{rest}$$

Q^s_{max}

Q^N_{max}

A

FIGURE 4. *A*, Definitions of coronary flow reserve (CFR) = maximal flow (Q max) / resting flow (Q max) in target artery. (*continued*)

Defining CVR, rCVR,
FFR

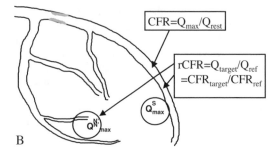

B

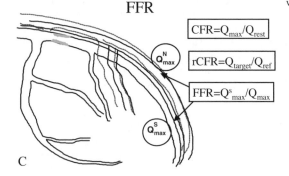

FIGURE 4. (*continued*) B, Relative CFR (rCFR) = maximal flow in target vessel (Q target) / maximal flow in normal reference vessel (Q ref). C, Fractional flow reserve (FFR) = maximal flow in stenotic vessel (Q^s max) / maximal flow in same vessel without stenosis (Q^n max).

Defining CVR, rCVR,
FFR

C

11. Are FFR and rCVR independent of the microcirculation?

Both FFR and rCVR are theoretically independent of hemodynamic and microcirculatory changes, and unlike CVR, should be strongly correlated. Baumgart et al. demonstrated that absolute CVR did not correlate with FFR. FFR and rCVR did show a correlation both to percent area stenosis ($r = 0.89$ and $r = 0.79$; $P < 0.0001$) and to each other. There was a strong linear relationship between FFR and rCVR (0.91; $P < 0.0001$) but not absolute CVR, as expected, because of the influence of variable microvascular flow. Correlation between both FFR and rCVR was good, indicating the limited influence of the microcirculation on these variables for lesion assessment.

12. How does FFR relate to CVR?

A normal FFR indicates the conduit resistance is not a major contributing factor to perfusion impairment and that focal conduit enlargement (e.g., stenting) would not restore normal perfusion regardless of microcirculatory abnormalities. Patients with microvascular disease have a discordance between FFR and CVR. Meuwissen, et al. compared FFR and CVR in 126 patients with intermediate stenosis. In 27% of patients, there was disagreement between FFR and CFR. Patients with normal FFR (> 0.75) but abnormal CVR (< 2.0) had a larger variability in minimum microvascular resistance (2.42 1+ 0.77 vs. 1.91 ± 0.70 mm Hg cm^{-1}. sec^{-1}; $P = 0.034$) compared with those with normal CVR regardless of the FFR (Fig. 5). This variance suggests that microvascular resistance modulates the relationship between FFR and CFR; therefore, both techniques should be considered for complete lesion assessment.

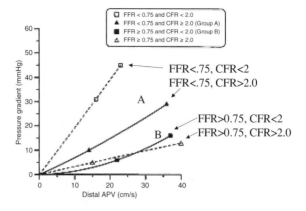

FIGURE 5. Pressure gradient-flow velocity relation showing average data at baseline and hyperemia for all groups. Lines are quadratic fits of form $y = ax + bx^2$. (Reproduced with permission from Meuwissen J, Chamuleau AJ, Siebes M, et al: Role of variability in microvascular resistance on fractional flow reserve and coronary blood flow velocity reserve in intermediate coronary lesion. Circulation 103:184–187, 2001.)

13. Can I use FFR in patients with microvascular disease?

The reliability of fractional flow reserve measurements in patients with microvascular disease was examined by Claeys et al. Intracoronary pressure and flow during maximal and submaximal hyperemia was recorded simultaneously across 21 infarct- and 19 noninfarct-related stenoses, before and after intervention. The decline in coronary flow from 48 mL/min during maximal hyperemia to 36 mL/min during submaximal hyperemia was associated with a small decrease in translesional pressure gradient (22 ± 12 mm Hg to 19 ± 12 mm Hg; $P = 0.02$) and a small increase in the mean distal arterial pressure ratio (FFR) from 77% to 81% ($P = 0.003$). In 21 noninfarct-related lesions versus 22 matched infarct-related lesions with similar percent diameter stenoses, the presence of microvascular dysfunction indicated no difference between the FFR in those with and without myocardial infraction (MI) at 0.79 ± 1.12 versus 0.83 ± 1.12 ($P =$ NS). These data suggest that the application of standard FFR calculations in a more general population of ischemic heart disease can include patients with microvascular disease. However, continued caution should be used for the current physiologic criteria in patients with profound microvascular disease, acute or remote myocardial infarction (MI), and unstable angina.

14. How can physiologic techniques be used to differentiate focal from diffuse atherosclerosis?

Diffuse atherosclerosis, rather than a focal narrowing, is characterized by a continuous and gradual pressure recovery (distal to proximal) without a localized, abrupt increase in pressure related to isolated focal narrowing. Using continuous hyperemic pressure measurement during sensor wire pullback from a distal to proximal location, the impact of a specific area or the presence of diffuse disease can be documented. A diffusely diseased atherosclerotic coronary artery can be viewed as a series of branching units, diverting and gradually distributing flow along the longitudinally narrowing conduit length. The perfusion pressure gradually diminishes along the artery. In this artery, FFR is reduced but unassociated with a focal stenotic pressure loss. Thus, mechanical therapy directed at a presumed focal plaque to reverse such abnormal physiology would be ineffective to restore normal coronary perfusion.

De Bruyne et al. documented abnormal epicardial coronary resistance in patients with diffuse athersclerosis but normal coronary angiography (Fig. 6). Coronary pressure and fractional flow reserve as measures of coronary conductance were obtained in 37 arteries without atherosclerosis (group 1) and 106 nonstenotic arteries in 62 patients with a significant angiographic stenosis in another coronary artery (group 2). Hyperemic pullback gradients from distal to proximal were compared. An FFR near unity (ranging from 0.92 to 1.0) was found in group 1, indicating no resistance to flow in truly normal arteries. However, FFR was significantly lower in group 2 (ranging from 0.69 to 1.0). In 57% of arteries in group 2, FFR was lower than the lowest value in group 1. In 8% of arteries in group 2, FFR was < 0.75 without evident focal stenosis in any segment (Fig. 7). The investigators concluded that diffuse coronary atherosclerosis without focal narrowing by angiography caused a graded continuous pressure decrease along the course of the artery. The resistance to flow contributes to myocardial ischemia and has consequences with relation to selection of percutaneous intervention or medical therapy.

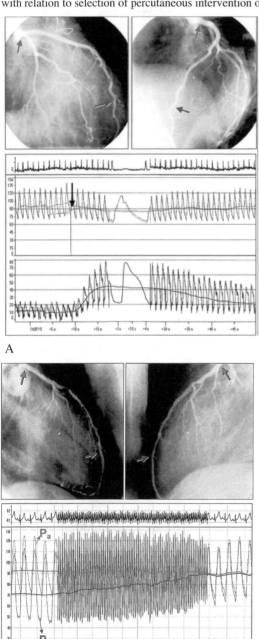

A

B

FIGURE 6. *A,* Normal coronary angiogram (*upper panels*), simultaneous aortic and distal coronary pressures (*top tracings*), and coronary flow velocity (*bottom*) recordings in a 55-year-old patient 3 weeks after orthotopic cardiac transplantation. No pressure gradient was measured during an adenosine-induced fourfold increase in coronary blood flow velocity between the proximal and distal left anterior descending artery. Normal coronary arteries do not cause appreciable resistance to blood flow. *Arrows* show the exact locations of aortic and distal coronary pressure measurements. Reproduced with permission from De Bruyne et al. Circulation 104:2401–2406, 2001. *B,* Example of a 44-year-old man with stable angina pectoris. A tight stenosis in the mid right coronary artery was treated by angioplasty. The coronary angiogram of the left anterior descending artery (LAD) (*upper panels*) did not show any focal stenosis, but luminal irregularities suggested diffuse atherosclerosis. Aortic and distal coronary pressures recordings (*lower panel*) during adenosine-induced maximal hyperemia show a pressure gradient of 23 mm Hg (corresponding to a fractional flow reserve of 0.76) when the pressure sensor is located in the distal LAD. When the sensor is slowly pulled back, a graded, continuous increase in distal coronary pressure is observed, which indicates diffuse atherosclerosis, not focal stenosis. *Arrows* show the exact locations of aortic and distal coronary pressure measurements. (Reproduced with permission from De Bruyne B, et al: Abnormal epicardial coronary resistance in patients with diffuse atherosclerosis but "normal" coronary angiography. Circulation 104:2401–2406, 2001.)

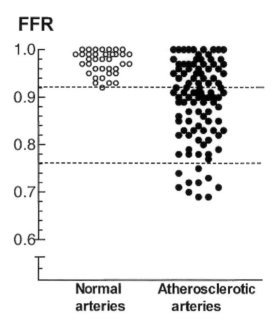

FFR

FIGURE 7. Individual values of fractional flow reserve (FFR) in normal arteries and in atherosclerotic coronary arteries without focal stenosis on arteriogram. The *upper dotted line* indicates the lowest value of FFR in normal coronary arteries. The *lower dotted line* indicates the 0.75 threshold level. (Reproduced with permission from De Bruyne B, et al: Abnormal epicardial coronary resistance in patients with diffuse atherosclerosis but "normal" coronary angiography. Circulation 104:2401–2406, 2001.)

15. What are the clinical data supporting use of coronary physiology for lesion assessment in the catheterization laboratory?

From numerous studies over the past decade, coronary physiologic measurements are now associated with significant data supporting four major clinical outcomes (Table 1). For lesion assessment before intervention, strong correlations exist between myocardial stress testing and FFR or CVR. An FFR of < 0.75 identifies physiologically significant stenoses associated with inducible myocardial ischemia, with high sensitivity, specificity, positive predicted value, and overall accuracy. An abnormal CVR (< 2.0) corresponded to reversible myocardial perfusion imaging defects with similarly high sensitivity, specificity, and predictive accuracy (Table 2).

Using coronary physiology thresholds, the outcome of deferring coronary interventions for intermediate stenoses with normal physiology are remarkably consistent, with clinical event rates of < 10% over a 2-year follow-up period. Despite the excellent safety of the deferred approach, some patients may still have recurrent angina, requiring continued medical therapy (Fig. 8). Similar to other clinical tests at a single point in time, in-laboratory measurements may not reflect the episodic ischemia of daily life. Physiologic thresholds have been validated by ischemic stress testing and clinical outcomes to support decisions to defer intervention while continuing medical therapy for endothelial dysfunction, hypertension, hyperlipidemia, and episodic coronary vasoconstriction.

Table 1. Catheter-based Anatomic and Physiologic Criteria Associated with Clinical Outcomes

APPLICATION	IVUS	CVR	RCVR	FFR
Ischemia detection	< 3–4 mm²	< 2.0	< 0.08–0.65	< 0.75
Deferred angioplasty	> 4 mm²	> 2.0	—	> 0.75
Endpoint of angioplasty	—	> 2.0–2.5 with < 35% DS	—	> 0.90
Endpoint of stenting	> 9 mm² > 80% ref area, full apposition	—	—	> 0.94–0.96

Modified from Kern MJ: Coronary physiology revisited: Practical insights from the cardiac catheterization laboratory. Circulation 101:1344, 2000.

Table 2. Comparison of Stress (Ischemia) Testing and Directly Measured Coronary Blood Flow Physiology

AUTHOR	YEAR	(N)	ISCHEMIC TEST	PHYSIOLOGIC THRESHOLD	SENSITIVITY	SPECIFICITY	PV+	PV−	ACCURACY
Poststenotic									
Miller	1994	33	Adeno/dipy MIBI	< 2.0	82	100	100	77	89
Joye	1994	30	Exercise thallium	< 2.0	94	95	94	95	94
Deychak	1995	17	Exercise thallium	< 1.8	94	94	100	91	96
Heller	1995	100	Exercise thallium	< 1.8	89	92	96	89	92
Danzi	1998	30	Dipy echo	< 2.0	91	84	—	—	87
Schulman	1997	35	Exercise ECG	< 2.0	95	71	—	—	86
Donahue	1996	50	Exercise/pharm thallium	< 2.0	98	76	88	88	—
Piek	1999	225	Exercise ECG	< 2.1	76	76	80	73	—
Abe	2000	46	Exercise thallium	< 2.0	83	95	—	—	88
Duffy	2001	43	Stress echo	< 2.0, rCVR < 0.75	80	93	—	—	81
Chamuleau	2001	127	Dipy MIBI	CVR < 2.0, rCVR < 0.75	100	76	—	—	69
El Shafei	2001	53	Exercise/pharm thallium	CVR < 0.20, rCVR < 0.75	71	83	81	74	75
					63	88	83	70	—
FFR									
Pijls et al.	1995	45	Four test standard*	< 0.75	88	100	100	88	93
de Bruyne et al.	1995	60	Exercise ECG	< 0.72	100	87	—	—	—
Bartunek	1999	37	Dobu/exercise Echo	< 0.68	95	90	—	—	—
Chamuleau	2001	127	Dipy MIBI	< 0.75	—	—	—	—	75
Caymaz	2000	30	Exercise thallium	< 0.75	—	—	91	100	—
Fearon	2000	10	Exercise thallium	< 0.75	90	100	—	—	95
De Bruyne et al.	2001	57	SPECT in AMI	< 0.75	82	87	—	—	—
Abe	2000	46	Exercise thallium	< 0.75	83	100	—	—	—

Adeno/dipy MIBI = adenosine or dipyridamole sestamibi scan; CFR = coronary vasodilatory reserve; dobu = dobutamine; sens = sensitivity; spec = specificity; PV+/PV− = predictive value positive/negative; pharm = pharmacologic. *Four tests were ECG, echo, pacing, nuclear stress tests.

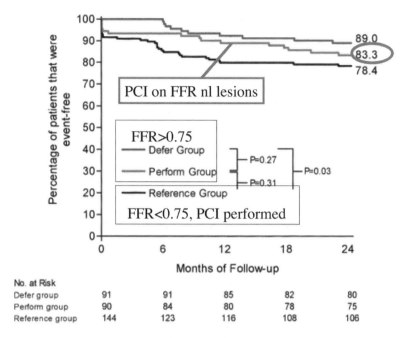

FIGURE 8. Kaplan-Meier survival curves for freedom from adverse cardiac events during 24 months of follow-up for three groups. (Modified with permission by Bech GJ, et al: Fractional flow reserve to determine the appropriateness of angioplasty in moderate coronary stenosis: A randomized trial. Circulation 103:2928–2934, 2001.)

16. How do pressure and flow wires measure the collateral circulation?

The collateral circulation can be described by intracoronary pressure and flow relationships. Ipsilateral collateral flow and contralateral arterial responses have been described in numerous studies using both pressure and flow to provide new information regarding mechanisms, function, and clinical significance of collateral flow in patients and provide new insights into coronary artery disease. For example, Seiler et al. examined coronary pressure and flow in 51 patients with coronary artery stenosis treated by percutaneous transluminal coronary angioplasty. Simultaneous measurements were used to calculate collateral flow indices (CF1) using velocity (V) or pressure (P). Both CFI_v and CFI_p (CFR_p is the FFR collateral as described by Pijls et al.) were compared with conventional methods for collateral assessment using ST segment elevation > 1 mm on IC or surface electrocardiogram (ECG) during coronary occlusion with balloon angioplasty. In 11 patients without ECG signs of ischemia during coronary occlusion, relative collateral flow amounted to 46% as determined by pressure flow indices. Patients with insufficient collaterals ($n = 40$) had CFI values of 18%. Using a CFI of 30%, sufficient and insufficient collaterals could be diagnosed with 100% sensitivity and 93% specificity by IC Doppler and 75% sensitivity and 92% specificity by IC pressure measurements. There was good agreement between Doppler and pressure CFI velocity ($P = 0.08+0.8$ CFI pressure; r = 0.80; $P = 0.0001$). The investigators concluded that intracoronary flow velocity or pressure measurements during routine coronary occlusion represent an accurate and a quantitative method for assessing the collateral coronary artery circulation in humans.

Furthermore, the pressure-derived collateral flow index (CFI_i) can be used as a parameter of microvascular dysfunction during acute MI. Yamamoto et al. measured pressure-derived collateral flow index and acute infarction in 48 patients undergoing stenting for reperfusion. Myocardial contrast echo was also performed to compare perfusion collateral flow index by pressure and left ventricular wall motion at day 1 with day 28. Investigators found that CFI_i was significantly higher in patients without myocardial reflow than those with myocardial reflow. There was a significant inverse correlation between the extent of functional improvement, implying that a higher collateral flow index by pressure was associated with a worse functional improvement. The authors concluded that during acute MI, CFI_p is unlikely to reflect collateral function but seems to increase with the severity of microvascular dysfunction. Because a high CFI_p was associated with poor functional recovery, it may useful to estimate prognosis in these individuals.

17. What is new in coronary physiology research?

Continued investigations in coronary physiology (simultaneous pressure and flow measurements) further advanced in our understanding of both epicardial and microcirculatory disturbances in patients with coronary artery disease. For example, one of the most recent innovations is the testing of coronary thermodilution to assess flow reserve using a temperature-sensitive pressure guidewire. In an *in vitro* model, absolute volume flow was compared with the inverse mean transit time of a thermodilution curve, obtained after a bolus injection of 3 mL of saline at room temperature. A strong correlation was found between absolute flow and the inverse mean transit time, when the temperature sensor > 6 cm from the injection site. In six of the instrumented dogs, FFR (ranging from 0.19 to 0.98), had a significant linear correlation between flow velocity and inverse transit time. A significant correlation between CFR by Doppler was calculated from the ratio of hyperemic to resting velocity, and CFR by thermodilution calculated as the ratio of hyperemic transit times was found (Fig. 9). These data validated the thermodilution principle to assess CFR. Because the pressure-temperature sensor is available on a commercially used angioplasty guidewire, the technique holds potential for simultaneous measurements of CFR and FFR.

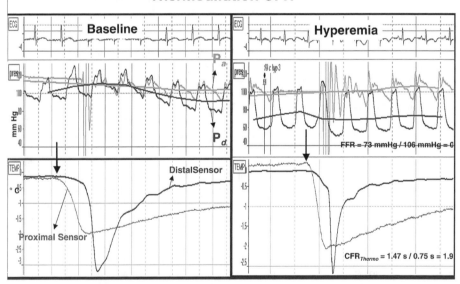

Simultaneous Pressure-Derived FFR and Thermodilution CFR

FIGURE 9. Correlation between $CFR_{Doppler}$ and CFR_{thermo} in dogs. (Reproduced with permission from De Bruyne B, Pijls N, Smith L, et al: Coronary thermodilution to access flow reserve experimental validation. Circulation 104:2003–2006, 2001.) (*continued*)

18. Is the lesion in Figure 1 significant?

The FFR in all three branches was > 0.90 (Fig. 10).

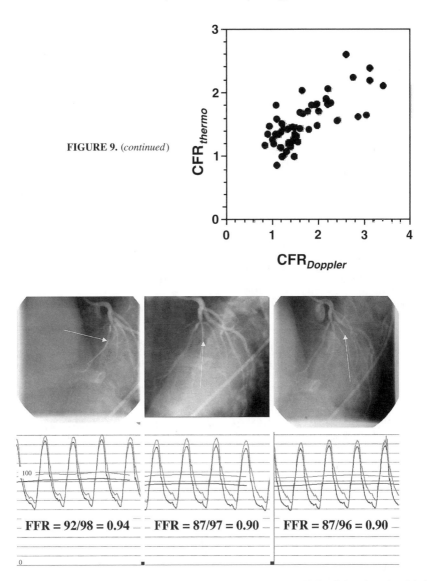

FIGURE 9. (continued)

FIGURE 10. For trifurcation lesion, fractional flow reserve is normal (> 0.90) in all three branches. Medical therapy is recommended. (Angiogram and FFR measurements courtesy of Dr. Bernard De Bruyne.)

BIBLIOGRAPHY

1. Akasaka T, Yoshida K, Hozumi T, et al: Retinopathy identifies marked restriction of coronary flow reserve in patients with diabetes mellitus. J Am Coll Cardiol 30:935–941, 1997.
2. Baumgart D, Haude M, Goerge G, et al: Improved assessment of coronary stenosis severity using the relative flow velocity reserve. Circulation 98:40–46, 1998.
3. Billinger M, Seiler C, Fleisch M, et al: Do beta-adrenergic blocking agents increase coronary flow reserve? J Am Coll Cardiol 38:1866–1871, 2001.
4. Claeys M, Bosmans J, Hendrix J, Vrints C: Reliability of fractional flow reserve measurements in pa-

tients with associated microvascular dysfunction: importance of flow on translesional pressure gradient. Cathet Cardiovasc Intervent 54:427–434, 2001.

5. De Bruyne B, Bartunek J, Sys SU, et al: Simultaneous coronary pressure and flow velocity measurements in humans: feasibility, reproducibility, and hemodynamic dependence of coronary flow velocity reserve, hyperemic flow versus pressure slope index, and fractional flow reserve. Circulation 94:1842–1849, 1996.

6. De Bruyne B, Hersbach F, Pijls N, et al: Abnormal epicardial coronary resistance in patients with diffuse atherosclerosis but "normal" coronary angiography. Circulation 104:2401–2406, 2001.

7. De Bruyne B, Pijls N, Smith L, et al: Coronary thermodilution to access flow reserve experimental validation. Circulation 104:2003–2006, 2001.

8. El-Shafei A, Chiravuri R, Stikovac MM, et al: Comparison of relative coronary Doppler flow velocity reserve to stress myocardial perfusion imaging in patients with coronary artery disease. Cathet Cardiovasc Intervent 53:193–201, 2001.

9. Feigl EO: Coronary physiology. Physiol Rev 63:1–205, 1983.

10. Gould KL, Kirkeeide RL, Buchi M: Coronary flow reserve as a physiologic measure of stenosis severity. J Am Coll Cardiol 15:459–474, 1990.

11. Gould KL, Lipscomb K, Hamilton GW: Physiologic basis for assessing critical coronary stenosis: instantaneous flow response and regional distribution during coronary hyperemia as measures of coronary flow reserve. Am J Cardiol 33:87–94, 1974.

12. Joye JD, Cates CU, Farah T, et al: Cost analysis of intracoronary Doppler determination of lesion significance: preliminary results of the PEACH study. J Invasc Cardiol 1:27, 1995.

13. Kern MJ: Coronary physiology revisited: practical insights from the cardiac catheterization laboratory. Circulation 101:1344–1351, 2000.

14. Kern MJ, Bach RG, Mechem C, et al: Variations in normal coronary vasodilatory reserve stratified by artery, gender, heart transplantation and coronary artery disease. J Am Coll Cardiol 28:1154–1160, 1996.

15. Kern MJ: Focus for the new millennium: diffuse coronary artery disease and physiologic measurements of severity. Am Coll Cardiol Curr J Rev March/April 13–19, 2000.

16. McGinn AL, White CW, Wilson RF: Interstudy variability of coronary flow reserve: influence of heart rate, arterial pressure, and ventricular preload. Circulation 81:1319–1330, 1990.

17. Meuwissen J, Chamuleau AJ, Siebes M, et al: Role of variability in microvascular resistance on fractional flow reserve and coronary blood flow velocity reserve in intermediate coronary lesion. Circulation 103:184–187, 2001.

18. Piek JJ, van Liebergen RAM, Koch KT, et al: Clinical, angiographic and hemodynamic predictors of recruitable collateral flow assessed during balloon angioplasty coronary occlusion. J Am Coll Cardiol 29:275–282, 1997.

19. Pijls NHJ, Bech GJW, el Gamal MIH, et al: Quantification to recruitable coronary collateral bloo flow in conscious jumans and its potential to predict future ischemic events. J Am Coll Cardiol 25:1522–1528, 1995.

20. Pijls NH, De Bruyne B, Peels K, et al: Measurement of fractional flow reserve to assess the functional severity of coronary-artery stenoses. N Engl J Med 334:1703–1708, 1996.

21. Pijls NH, Van Gelder B, Van der Voort P, et al: Fractional flow reserve: a useful index to evaluate the influence of an epicardial coronary stenosis on myocardial blood flow. Circulation 92:3183–3193, 1995.

22. Reis SE, Holubkov R, Lee JS, et al. for the WISE Investigators: Coronary flow velocity response to adenosine characterizes coronary microvascular function in women with chest pain and obstructive coronary disease. J Am Coll Cardiol 33:1469–1475, 1999.

23. Rim S, Leong-Poi H, Lindner J, Wei K, et al: Decrease in coronary blood flow reserve during hyperipidemia is secondary to an increase in blood viscosity. Circulation 104:2704–2709, 2001.

24. Seiler C, Fleisch M, Billinger M, Meier B: Simultaneous intracoronary velocity- and pressure-derived assessment of adenosine-induced collateral hemodynamics in patients with one- to two-vessel coronary artery disease. J Am Coll Cardiol 34:1985–1994, 1999.

25. Seiler C, Fleisch M, Garachemani A, Meier B: Coronary collateral quantitation in patients with coronary artery disease using intravascular flow velocity or pressure measurements. J Am Coll Cardiol 32:1272–1279, 1998.

26. Topol EJ, Nissen SE: Our preoccupation with coronary luminology. The dissociation between clinical and angiographic findings in ischemic heart disease. Circulation 92:2333–2342, 1995.

27. Van Liebergen RAM, Piek JJ, Koch KT, et al: Hypermic coronary flow after optimized intravascular ultrasound-guided balloon angioplasty and stent implantation. J Am Coll Cardiol 34:1899–1906, 1999.

28. Wieneke H, Haude M, Ge J, et al: Corrected coronary flow velocity reserve: a new concept for assessing coronary perfusion. J Am Coll Cardiol 35:1713–1720, 2000.

29. Yamamoto K, Ito H, Iwakura K, et al: Pressure-derived collateral flow index as a parameter of microvascular dysfunction in acute myocardial infarction. Am Coll Cardiol 38:1383–1389, 2001.

6. ENDOTHELIAL FUNCTION

Juan Pablo Zambrano, M.D., and Alexandre C. Ferreira, M.D.

1. What is the endothelium?

Since the pioneering work of Furchgott and Zawadzki in 1980, the endothelium has been recognized as a major regulator of vascular hemostasis. Endothelial cells, as the inner lining of blood vessels, are strategically located between circulating blood cells and the vascular smooth muscle. In a person with a body weight of 70 kg, the endothelium covers an area of approximately 700 m^2 and weights about 1.0 to 1.5 kg. The functional integrity of the endothelium is crucial for the maintenance of blood flow and antithrombotic capacity because the endothelium releases humoral factors that control relaxation and contraction, thrombogenesis and fibrinolysis, and platelet activation and inhibition. Thus, the endothelium contributes to blood pressure control, blood flow, and vessel patency.

2. Where does nitric oxide (NO) come from?

NO is produced from the amino acid L-arginine by the constitutively expressed enzyme, endothelial nitric oxide synthase (eNOS), and is released in response to stimuli to act on the endothelial cell surface. The enzyme is located within caveolae in the plasma membrane, bound to caveolin. It is inactive in this form, but an increase in endothelial intracellular calcium results in calmodulin formation, which displaces caveolin and activates the enzyme. Stimuli that increase calcium include receptor-mediated agonists (e.g., acetylcholine and substance P) as well as physical stimuli (e.g., shear stress).

3. How does NO exerts its action?

NO is a freely diffusible gas and has actions both within the lumen and on surrounding smooth muscle cells and tissues. It diffuses to adjacent smooth muscle where it increases guanylate cyclase activity, resulting in greater concentrations of cyclic $3'$, $5'$-guanosine monophosphate (cGMP). Cyclic GMP reduces intracellular calcium within the smooth muscle cell, causing smooth muscle relaxation.

4. What is NG-monomethyl-l-arginine (l-NMMA)?

It is possible to block competitively the production of NO with arginine analogues such as l-NMMA, and this has permitted the study of the functions of NO in humans. For example, l-NMMA infusion into the brachial artery of healthy volunteers causes a reduction in forearm blood flow, demonstrating the fundamental role of NO in the regulation of basal vascular tone.

5. What determines the bioactivity of NO, and how does it interact with free radicals?

NO bioactivity is determined by factors that influence its production as well as those that influence its breakdown. An essential cofactor that alters eNOS activity is tetrahydrobiopterin, which has been shown to restore NO bioactivity in patients with hypercholesterolemia and in smokers. One of the most interesting and potentially important regulators is the superoxide anion. This is produced under physiologic conditions as part of the normal metabolism and can react with other free radical species or is broken down by superoxide dismutase to produce hydrogen peroxide and oxygen. The hydrogen peroxide is then further broken down to oxygen and water by catalase. Superoxyde (O_2^-) and NO are unstable and react to produce peroxynitrite, which may produce other oxidant species. The activity of the endothelial-bound superoxide dismutase (ecSOD) enzyme is closely associated with conduit vessel NO-dependent endothelial function. In disease states associated with reduced NO bioactivity, there is evidence of increased oxidative stress; this is caused by the reactive species that inactivate NO.

6. What are the other possible biological effects of NO?

In addition to its vascular effects, NO is a potent inhibitor of leucocyte adhesion and platelet activation.

7. What is endothelin?

The endothelins are a group of similar 21 amino-acid peptides (endothelin 1, 2, and 3). Endothelin-1 is the most important of these and was first isolated form cultured porcine endothelial cells in 1988. Endothelin-1 is synthesized from preproendothelin-1 within vascular endothelial cells by the action of endothelin-converting enzyme (ECE). Endothelin is the most potent endogenous vasoconstrictor discovered to date (100-fold greater potency than noradrenaline).

8. How does endothelin exert its effect?

Two endothelin receptors have been identified, ET-A and ET-B. ET-A receptors are the predominant subtype and are present on vascular smooth muscle cells. Stimulation of ET-A receptors results in vasoconstriction. ET-B receptors are present both in endothelial cells, where they mediate vasodilation (through the release of NO and prostacyclin), and on smooth muscle cells, where they mediate vasoconstriction.

Endothelin is not stored but is rapidly synthesized within the endothelial cells in response to stimuli such as ischemia, hypoxia, and shear stress. Endothelin acts locally in a paracrine fashion. Endothelin is released predominantly abluminally (i.e., toward the smooth muscle cell), making plasma levels unreliable for predicting overall synthesis of endothelin. Despite this, plasma levels of endothelin correlate well to the severity of heart failure and ischemia. The plasma half-life of endothelin-1 is 4 to 7 minutes, with 80% being cleared by the lungs on first pass. Despite the short half-life, the actions of endothelin are prolonged after binding to receptors, with vasoconstrictor effects lasting 60 minutes or more.

9. What are the functional properties of the vascular endothelium?

PROPERTY	MEDIATORS
Modulation of thromboresistance	
Antiplatelet	Prostacyclin
	Nitric oxide
	Ecto-ADPase (CD39)
Anticoagulant	Heparin-like proteoglycans
	Thrombomodulin
	Protein C
	Tissue factor inhibitor
	VonWillebrand factor
Profibrinolytic	Tissue plasminogen activator
	Urokinase
Antifibrinolytic/prothrombotic	Plasminogen activator inhibitor 1/fibrinogen, tissue factor, thromboxane A_2, free oxidant radicals, endothelin 1
Modulation of vascular tone	Prostacyclin (−)
	Nitric oxide (−)
	Endothelial-derived hyperpolarizing factor (−)
	Bradykinin (−)
	C-natriuretic peptide (−)
	Angiotensin II (+)
	Adrenomedulin (+)
	Endothelin 1 (+)
	Prostaglandin H2 (+)
	Free oxidant radicals (+)
Modulation of smooth muscle cell growth	Heparin-like molecules (−)
	Nitric oxide (−)
	Transforming growth factor beta (−)
	Platelet-derived growth factor A/B (+)
	Basic fibroblast growth factor (+)
	Insulin-like growth factor (+)
Selective permeability barrier	Junctional proteins
	Endocytic receptors
	Cell surface glycocalix

(continued)

PROPERTY	MEDIATORS
Leukocyte recruitment	Inducible endothelial leukocyte adhesion molecules (P and E selectins, ICAM-1, VCAM-1)
	Chemoattractant/activators interleukin 8, monocyte chemoattractant protein; platelet activating factor, nuclear factor kappa-B)
Angiogenesis	Vascular endothelial growth factor

10. What are the methods available to assess endothelial function?

Invasive coronary vascular testing
    Conduit vessels: Ach, L-NMMA, FMD, cold pressor test, mental stress
    Resistance vessels: Ach, L-NMMA, cold pressor test, mental stress, CFR
Noninvasive coronary vascular testing
    PET: CFR, cold pressor test
    Echocardiography: CFR
    Phase-contrast MRI: CFR
Peripheral arterial assessment
    Conduit vessels: conduit artery FMD by noninvasive ultrasound
    Resistance vessels: forearm blood flow by plethysmography (Ach, L-NMMA)
    Cutaneous microcirculation: laser Doppler flowmetry
    Peripheral pulse waveform analysis: photoplethysmography
Circulating biomarkers
    Asymmetric dimethyl arginine, serum nitrate
    High-sensitivity C-reactive protein
    Endothelin-1
    Hematologic markers: vWF, PAI-1, tPA, thrombomodulin,
    Soluble cell adhesion molecules: ICAM-1, VCAM-1, E-selectin, P-selectin

Ach = acetylcholine; CFR = coronary flow reserve; FMD = flow-mediated dilation; ICAM = intercellular adhesion molecule; L-NMMA = NG monomethyl-L-arginine; MRI = magnetic resonance imaging; PAI = plasminogen activator inhibitor; PET = positron emission tomography; tPA = tissue plasminogen activator; VCAM = vascular cell adhesion molecule; vWF = von Willebrand factor.

11. What is the clinical relevance of the tests for endothelial function?

It is not entirely clear, but the currently available measures of endothelial function are predictive of long-term outcome in individual subjects. Although preliminary data from studies of the coronary circulation are encouraging, larger studies are required with noninvasive techniques. Several studies are underway to determine if brachial ultrasound might predict individuals at increased risk, but endothelial function testing can not yet be used in the clinical arena.

12. What is the role of endothelial dysfunction in pathophysiology of cardiovascular disease?

Although studies often report endothelial dysfunction as a loss of vasodilatory capacity, the term encompasses a generalized defect in all the homeostatic mechanisms. *Endothelial dysfunction* is a broad term that implies diminished production of or decreased availability of nitric oxide (NO) or imbalance in the relative contribution of endothelium derived relaxing and contracting factors (ET-1, angiotensin, and oxidants). Endothelial dysfunction has been implicated in the pathogenesis and clinical course of all known cardiovascular disease and is associated with future risk of cardiovascular events. It is now clear that impaired endothelial function in disorders such as atherosclerosis, hypertension, and heart failure leads to hypoperfusion, vascular occlusion, and end-organ damage.

13. What conditions are associated with endothelial dysfunction?

Atherosclerosis, hypercholesterolemia (high low-density lipoprotein (LDL) cholesterol, low high-density lipoprotein (HDL) cholesterol, high lipoprotein (a), small dense LDL-C, oxidized LDL cholesterol), high homocysteine levels, aging, smoking (active and passive), postmenopausal state or estrogen deficiency, family history of coronary artery disease, diabetes mellitus, hypertension, left ventricular hypertrophy, angina pectoris (stable and unstable), acute myocardial infarction, variant angina, obesity, physical inactivity, depression, metabolic syndrome, ischemia-reperfusion, transplant atherosclerosis, cardiopulmonary bypass, increased C-reactive protein, congestive heart failure, renal failure, postprandial state, vasculitis, preeclampsia, Kawasaki's disease, Chagas disease, infections.

14. Why is endothelial activation a crucial step in the pathophysiology of atherogenic risk factors?

Alterations of the endothelial integrity by cardiovascular risk factors initiates a variety of active processes such as inflammation, proliferation, or apoptosis, which are relevant to the endothelial surface as well as adjacent cells in the vessel wall. Thus, damage of the endothelium leads to an "endothelial activation," which determines the milieu within the vascular wall. The imbalance of the redox equilibrium (equilibrium between NO and reactive oxygen species) toward oxidative stress is initially limited to the endothelial cell layer, providing the basis for atherosclerotic plaque development. However, later, with the progression of the atherosclerotic plaque, the oxidative stress extends from the endothelium into the vascular wall and determines the plaque architecture as well as plaque vulnerability.

15. What are the inflammatory consequences of endothelial activation?

Reduced NO bioactivity, in line with enhanced oxidative stress, stimulates the production of cytokines such as interleukins, tumor necrosis factor alpha, and interferon, thereby attracting monocytes. Induction of adhesion molecules, such as vascular cell adhesion molecule (VCAM) or intercellular adhesion molecule (ICAM), supports migration of monocytes into the vessel wall, where they change into macrophages. Thus, endothelial activation has characteristic features of an inflammatory process. Furthermore, the redux equilibrium induces pro-inflammatory cytokines, leading to CRP production in the liver, an unspecific inflammatory marker. However, CRP is not only a systemic marker of endothelial activation but also plays an active role locally in the vasculature by inducing expression of the adhesion molecules on the endothelial surface, binding to macrophages and activating the complement system.

Therefore, permanent interaction exists between systemic factors and local endothelial and vessel wall processes.

16. What are the proliferative consequences of endothelial activation?

Reduced NO bioactivity or increased oxidative stress leads to tyrosine nitration of proteins in the vessel wall and interacts with redox-sensitive gene expression. A redox imbalance, toward oxidative stress, activates nuclear factor-κB system, a transcriptional protein, increasing proliferation of smooth muscle and other cells (a common denominator of endothelial activation, possibly causally linked to adhesion molecule expression). Whereas NO reduces proliferation of vascular smooth muscle cells and migration of monocytes, endothelin-1, and angiotensin II, associated with oxidative stress, exert proatherosclerotic effects on the vasculature. Unlimited cell proliferation is counteracted by cell apoptosis (i.e., programmed cell death) in order to maintain cellular homeostasis. Whereas, oxidized LDL cholesterol and angiotensin II promote apoptosis, endothelial NO inhibits apoptosis of endothelial cells.

BIBLIOGRAPHY

1. Anderson T: Endothelial function, introduction. Coron Artery Dis 12:431–433, 2001.
2. Caterina R: Endothelial dysfunctions: common demoninators in vascular disease. Curr Opin Clin Nutr Metab Care 3:453–467, 2000.
3. Farouque H: The assessment of endothelial function in humans. Coron Artery Dis 12:445–454, 2001.
4. Goodwin A: Role of endogenous endothelin in coronary flow in health and disease. Coron Artery Dis 12: 517–524, 2001.
5. Kharbanda R: Function of healthy endothelium.
6. Luscher T, Barton M: Biology of the endothelium. Clin Cardiol 20S:II-3–II-10, 1997.
7. Sherman D: Exercise and endothelial function. Coron Artery Dis 11:117–122, 2000.
8. Verma S: Fundamentals of endothelial function for the clinical cardiologist. Circulation 105:546–549, 2002.

7. STAGES OF CORONARY ATHEROSCLEROSIS

Juan Pablo Zambrano, M.D., and Eduardo de Marchena, M.D.

1. Why is important to understand the pathophysiology of coronary atherosclerosis?

It is important because coronary atherosclerosis (CA) is the most common cause of ischemic heart disease, and plaque disruption with superimposed thrombosis is the main cause the acute coronary syndromes (ACS), including unstable angina, myocardial infarction (MI), and sudden death.

2. When did the first description of atherosclerosis take place?

In mid to late 1800s, light microscopy features of atherosclerosis were discovered as Virchow and others used techniques that were novel at the time for paraffin embedding, sectioning, and staining of tissues.

3. What does the word *atherosclerosis* mean?

Atherosclerosis implies mature plaques. Mature plaques typically consist of two main components: *atheromatous* "gruel," which is lipid rich and soft, and *sclerotic* tissue, which is collagen rich and hard.

4. What is the key question in the phenomena of atherosclerosis that determines the occurrence of events?

The key question is not why atherosclerosis develops but rather why after decades of indolent growth, the mature plaque suddenly become complicated by life-threatening thrombosis. The composition, thrombogenicity, and vulnerability of the plaque—rather than its volume or the consequent severity of stenosis produced—have emerged as being the most important determinants for the development of the thrombus-mediated ACS.

5. What are the phases and lesion morphology progression of coronary atherosclerosis, according to gross pathological and clinical findings?

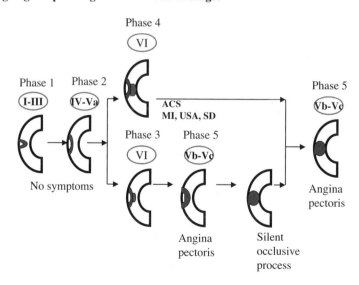

MI = myocardial infarction, SD = sudden death; USA = unstable angina. (Modified from Corti R, Fuster V, Badimon JJ, et al: New understanding of atherosclerosis (clinically and experimentally) with evolving MRI technology in vivo. Ann NY Acad Sci 947:181–198, 2001.)

6. Which pathologic processes are involved in atherosclerosis?
- Inflammation: Increase endothelial permeability, endothelial activation, and monocyte recruitment
- Growth: Smooth muscle cell proliferation, immigration, and matrix synthesis
- Degeneration: Lipid accumulation
- Necrosis: Possibly related to cytotoxic effects of oxidized lipids
- Calcification and ossification: Active rather than dystrophic process
- Thrombosis: Platelet recruitment and fibrin formation

7. What constitutes *plaque initiation* in atherosclerosis?
Plaque initiation occurs during the phase 1 of atherosclerosis, which consists of eccentric thickening of the intima at the level of the artery bifurcations followed by accumulation of lipids in the intima caused by an imbalance between lipid deposition and removal. This process is preceded by endothelial dysfunction caused by disturbances in patterns of blood flow at bending points and near bifurcations of the arterial tree, facilitating the entry of monocytes and plasma lipids and proteins in to the arterial wall. These phenomena can occur as early as during infancy.

8. What does *remodeling* mean in atherosclerosis?
Remodeling is the compensatory enlargement that occurs in the early stages of atherosclerosis. This process could be outward, in which the plaque progresses without compromising the lumen (positive remodeling), or inward (negative remodeling). The former is difficult to identify with angiography.

9. How does phase 2, or *lipid core formation,* occur, and what are the characteristics of the type of plaques found in this phase?
Scattered pools of extracellular lipids progress to a large, confluent accumulation of a free cholesterol with its esters forming the lipid core. Phase two is constituted by the type IV and Va plaques; their importance is that the phase two lesions are considered vulnerable and at high risk for disruption and thrombosis because of their thin caps and accumulations of macrophages and mast cells. The type IV lesions have a high extracellular lipid content intermixed with fibrous tissue beneath a fibrous cap; the type Va contains a larger lipid rich core within a thin fibrous cap. These lesions are clinically relevant because they may precede in up to two thirds of the cases to ACS.

10. What types of lesions are directly related to the occurrence of ACS?
In the stage of *plaque disruption and thrombus formation,* the phases 3 and 4 represent the sudden disruption or erosion of atherosclerotic plaques that in phase 4 leads to acute occlusive thrombosis, or so-called complicated type VI lesion, which is associated with the acute onset of cardiovascular events. On the other hand a small, nonocclusive, and often asymptomatic thrombus is seen in the uncomplicated type VI lesion of phase 3.

11. How does the thrombotic phenomena take place, and when is thrombus growth seen?
Disruption of the fibrous cap overlying an atheromatous core allows contact between blood and thrombogenic gruel; this activates the platelets and coagulation cascade. The adjacent clot is mainly composed of fibrin and platelets, but the rest of the thrombus is characterized by fibrin enmeshed with red blood cells. Thrombus growth occurs in cases of major plaque disruption, lipid extrusion, vasospasm and flow, low fibrinolytic activity, procoagulant states and high tissue factor activity, high levels of fibrinogen, and reactive platelets.

12. What is the importance of the tissue factor?
The lipid core of type IV and V lesions is rich in tissue factor that acts as a primary cell-associated activator of the coagulation cascade and thrombin generation. Apoptotic cells are the source of tissue factor, and macrophages coexpressing tissue factor and caspase-3 (a marker of apoptosis) are mostly localized in these lipid rich areas. The effect of tissue factor is counteracted

by the tissue factor pathway inhibitor (TFPI) expressed in the adventitial layer of the large arteries as well as macrophages in focal areas throughout the plaque, and it regulates procoagulant activity and thrombotic events within atherosclerotic plaques.

13. What does phase 5, or *plaque growth*, constitute?

This phase involves the progression to advanced atherosclerotic plaques through organization (histologic transformation) of thrombi. This gives the plaque certain histopathologic characteristics depending on the age of the thrombus.

14. What imaging techniques are used in the evaluation of the high-risk or vulnerable plaque?

- X-ray angiography
- Intravascular ultrasound
- Angioscopy
- Thermography
- Optical coherence computed tomography
- Raman spectroscopy
- Near-infrared spectroscopy
- Surface and transesophageal ultrasound
- Ultrafast computed tomography
- Nuclear scintigraphy
- Magnetic resonance imaging

BIBLIOGRAPHY

1. Corti R, Fuster V, Badimon J, et al: New understanding of atherosclerosis with evolving MRI technology in vivo. Ann NY Acad Science 947:181–198, 2001.
2. Falk E, Shah PK, Fuster V: Coronary plaque disruption. Circulation 92:657, 1995.
3. Fayad Z, Fuster V: Clinical Imaging of the high risk or vulnerable atherosclerotic plaque. Circ Res 89: 305–316, 2001.
4. Fuster V: Mechanisms leading to myocardial infarction: insights from studies of vascular biology. Circulation 90:2126–2146, 1994.
5. Fuster V, Badimon L, Badimon J, Chesebro JH: The pathogenesis of CAD and ACS. N Engl J Med 326: 242–250, 310–318, 1992.
6. Nezelof C, Seemayer TA: The history of pathology: an overview. In Damjanov I, Linder J (eds): Anderson's Pathology. St Louis, Mosby, 1996, pp 1–11.

8. PLATELETS, COAGULATION, AND THROMBOSIS

Wenche Jy, Ph.D., Joaquin J. Jimenez, M.D., Lawrence L. Horstman, B.S., and Yeon S. Ahn, M.D.

1. What are the main players in blood clotting (thrombosis)?

Formation of blood clots (i.e., thrombi) in coronary arteries is a major cause of acute coronary syndromes. The three main players in this process are the vascular endothelial cells (ECs), platelets, and the soluble coagulation proteins. These "three players" interact strongly and are modulated by other players such as inflammatory cytokines, leukocytes, and the complement system. For example, *endothelial injury* (which may include plaque rupture) can induce *platelet activation* caused by thrombin generated from tissue factor (TF), leading to platelet–platelet interaction (aggregation) and platelet–EC adhesion, eventuating in a *platelet plug* at the site of injury. A platelet plug consists of lacelike layers of activated platelet membranes bound to the injured endothelium. Activated platelets can, in turn, initiate *blood coagulation,* which acts like glue to seal off holes in the platelet plug, trapping red cells and transforming them to a firm jellylike clot. These events can occur in other sequences. In normal physiology, blood clotting prevents blood loss and protects tissue to allow repair of injury; however, in pathologic conditions, the clot may extend to occlude the entire lumen of the vessel (i.e., thrombosis), leading to ischemia of myocardium.

2. How does endothelial injury lead to blood clotting?

The normal intact vascular endothelium is an anticoagulant and antiadhesive surface, preventing its interaction with platelets, leukocytes, clotting factors, and as a barrier to substances such as collagen, fibronectin, and TF in the subendothelium. Healthy ECs also secrete nitric oxide (NO) to dilate blood vessels, prostacyclin to inhibit platelet activation, antithrombin III to attenuate coagulation, and tissue plasminogen activator (G-PA) to enhance fibrinolytic activity. EC-bound thrombomodulin and endothelial protein C receptor (EPCR) function in the protein C/S anticoagulation pathway, and tissue factor pathway inhibitor (TFPI) blocks activity of TF-VIIa and FXa.

When ECs are injured, they lose many of these properties, becoming procoagulant, proadhesive, proinflammatory, and prothrombotic. For example, denudation of the EC layer exposes collagen, allowing adhesion and aggregation of platelets with formation of a platelet plug, nidus of thrombus. Stimulated EC also secrete von Willebrand factor (vWF) to promote platelet adhesion; express TF to promote coagulation; and expose normally hidden phosphatidyl serine, a procoagulant phospholipid. At the same time, stimulated ECs shed (vesiculate) numerous tiny membrane vesicles, termed *endothelial microparticles* (EMPs), which express many EC membrane proteins (including TF) and which can activate monocytes to further augment the procoagulant and inflammatory reactions proximal to the activated or injured endothelial surface.

3. How do platelets become activated?

Platelets, or thrombocytes, are small ($\sim$2 μm), smooth, discoid cells circulating innocuously at the periphery of the blood stream (more concentrated near the vessel wall); the larger ($\sim$7 μm) and more numerous red cells (RBCs) preferentially flow in the center of the stream. Subtle changes in endothelial surface are first sensed by platelets passing near the vessel wall. Unless activated, platelets do not participate in biologic reactions or pathologic processes.

Despite their tiny size, activation of platelets is a complex process. The platelet plasma membrane expresses numerous receptors and adhesins for interaction with their respective ligands (Table 1). Upon receptor binding to an activating ligand (e.g., thrombin, collagen), intracellular signal transduction is initiated, resulting in the activated state. Platelet activation results in dramatic changes in shape and adhesive properties as well as secretion of granule contents. In addition, they shed submicroscopic membrane-derived microparticles, termed *platelet microparticles* (PMPs). Together with activated platelet membranes, PMPs provide the major anionic phospholipid sites for assembly of the vitamin K–dependent clotting factors, promoting coagulation (Fig. 1).

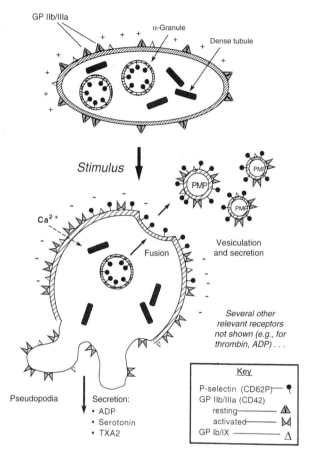

FIGURE 1. Principal events in platelet activation. When resting platelets are stimulated by agonists such as thrombin, collagen, or adenosine diphosphate (ADP), they undergo many morphologic and biochemical changes.

Activated platelet membranes and platelet microparticles (PMPs) are the major contributors of procoagulant (anionic) phospholipids required for blood clotting (see Fig 2).

Key events in platelet activation include (1) calcium influx and release of intracellular calcium stores from the dense tubules; (2) protrusion of pseudopodia; (3) secretion of granules (alpha and dense), including ADP, serotonin, and fibringogen; (4) activation of receptors, notably, modification of thrombin receptors and GP IIb/IIIa; (5) membrane "flip-flop," or exposure of normally in-facing anionic (procoagulant) phospholipids (e.g., phosphatidyl serine) to the plasma side; (6) appearance on the membrane surface of several other normally hidden receptors, such as P-selectin (CD62P) from the alpha granule; (7) synthesis and release of TxA$_2$; and (8) vesiculation of numerous tiny PMPs.

This is a simplified diagram. Not shown are many other receptors by which activated platelets are involved with blood clotting, such the thrombin receptor, ADP receptor, and so on.

4. How do platelets adhere to and aggregate at sites of endothelial injury?

In this context, the two major platelet surface glycoproteins are GP IIb/IIIa (integrin $\alpha_{IIb}\beta_3$) and GP Ib/IX. GP IIb/IIIa is the fibrinogen receptor: bound fibrinogen can bridge two or more

Table 1. Some Key Platelet Receptors

LIGAND	RECEPTOR	DISORDERS OR FUNCTIONS
Activation:		
Collagen	GP Ia/IIa, IIb/IIIa, IV, VI	Familial bleeding
Thrombin	PAR-1, 2, 3, 4	Familial bleeding
ADP	P2Y1, P2X1	Familial bleeding
Thromboxane A_2	TxA_2 receptor	Familial bleeding
Epinephrine	alpha-2-adrenergic receptor	Familial bleeding
Adhesion / aggregation:		
Fibrinogen	GP IIb/IIIa	Glanzmann's thrombasthenia (aggregation defect)
vWF	GP Ib/IX	Bernard-Soulier syndrome
Endothelial cells	PECAM-1 (CD31)	Endothelial adhesion
PSGL (leukocytes)	P selectin (CD62P)	Leukocyte adhesion
IC	Fc-gamma type II	Immune (e.g., HIT)

ADP = adenosine diphosphate: GP = glycoprotein; HIT = heparin-induced thrombocytopenia; IC = immune complex; PSGL = vWF = von Willebrand factor.

platelets together to form platelet aggregates. Aggregation is inhibited if GP IIb/IIIa is absent or dysfunctional, as in Glanzmann's thrombasthenia, a congenital bleeding disorder, or in treatment with ReoPro (abciximab), a monoclonal humanized (chimeric) monoclonal antibody (7E3 Fab) against GP IIb/IIIa, which has proved highly effective in the treatment of patients with acute coronary ischemia.

GP Ib/IX is the platelet adhesin mediating adhesion to the endothelium via von Willebrand (vWF). In the congenital bleeding disorder, Bernard-Soulier syndrome, this molecule is absent or dysfunctional, impairing platelet–EC adhesion. Studies in progress toward blocking this receptor promise new antithrombotic therapies for treatment of patients with acute coronary syndrome (ACS).

Activated platelets, including those adherent to injured endothelium, secrete thromboxane A_2, serotonin, and adenosine diphosphate (ADP), serving to recruit more platelets to the site of injury and enlarging the aggregate. In pathologic states (e.g., thrombotic, ischemic), the platelet plug may extend across the entire lumen, blocking blood flow.

5. What are the essential components of blood coagulation?

At risk of oversimplifying, the essential components are the major coagulation proteins, calcium, and suitable phospholipid (PL) membrane (i.e., anionic, notably phosphatidyl serine) (Fig. 2). It is important to recognize that the major coagulation reactions actually occur via anionic PL membrane-bound complexes of several protein clotting factors, as indicated in Figure 2. The main sources of procoagulant PL are activated platelets and their microparticles (PMPs), traditionally known as *platelet factor 3* (PF3), but other cells (e.g., leukocytes, ECs, RBCs) can also contribute significant procoagulant PL if suitably stimulated. Procoagulant PL cannot initiate coagulation. Not shown are the several complex reaction systems that oppose and inhibit coagulation that are activated at the same time, limiting and attenuating the spread of clotting.

6. What are the tenase and prothrombinase complexes?

The vitamin K–dependent clotting factors (i.e., II, VII, IX, X) are all posttranslationally modified to contain one or more gla domains (γ-carboxyglutamic acid), which function to bind them to anionic PL surfaces via Ca^{2+} (see Fig. 2). When thus bound, they are locally highly concentrated and positioned to interact with one another, assembling into protein complexes that perform the catalytic duties of coagulation. The factor-X activating complex is called the *ten-ase complex,* and the complex that activates prothrombin to thrombin is called the *prothrombinase* complex. Accordingly, blood clotting proceeds mainly in the vicinity of the platelet plug, near the site of endothelial injury, seldom extending to occlude the entire lumen of the vessel. However, in thrombotic conditions, thrombi can grow to occlude the entire vessel, resulting in ischemia and tissue damage (see Fig. 2).

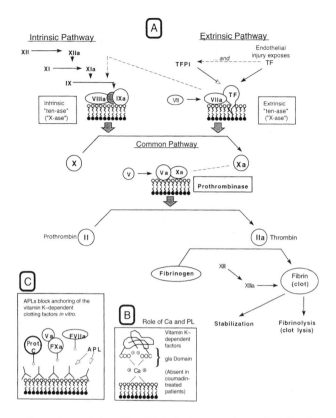

FIGURE 2. *A,* Outlines of coagulation. Simplified clotting cascade, emphasizing the critical role of membrane-associated complexes.

Only certain anionic membrane phospholipids (PLs$^{(-)}$) such as phosphatidyl serine (PS) have significant clotting activity, but these are hidden in resting cells, comprising the inner (cytoplasmic) leaflet of the bilayer. Activated platelet membranes are the major physiologic source of PLs$^{(-)}$, but activated leukocytes and injured endothelium can also contribute to this activity. Additionally, all of these cells release microparticles—platelet microparticles (PMPs), endothelial microparticles (EMPs), leukocyte microparticles (LMPs)—that further contribute.

The tenase and prothrombinase complexes are examples of membrane-associated clotting complexes.

B, Vitamin K–dependent factor binding to phospholipids. Vitamin K–dependent factors have a post-translationally modified amino acid, the *gla domain,* that anchors the protein to phospholipids (PLs$^{(-)}$ (anionic PL) in the presence of Ca^{2+}. Accordingly, the concentration of activated clotting factors on the PL$^{(-)}$ surface are locally highly concentrated, maximizing the rate of the clotting cascade. (Blood concentrations of activated clotting factors are extremely low, so clotting cannot proceed in flowing blood, being restricted to the PL$^{(-)}$ neighborhood; usually the platelet plug forms near the site of vessel injury.)

Coumadin impairs formation of gla domains of the vitamin K dependent factors, preventing them from binding to the PL$^{(-)}$ surface; therefore, clotting cannot proceed.

C, Presumed mechanism of lupus anticoagulant (LAC). In antiphospholipid syndrome (APS), the presence of antibodies against phospholipids (PL$^{(-)}$) (or any of several proteins that bind to PL$^{(-)}$) impede anchoring of activated clotting factors by competing for the same PL$^{(-)}$ sites. This leads to prolonged prothrombin time and partial thromboplastin time. Paradoxically, however, patients with APS seldom bleed; instead, they are prone to severe thrombosis. One popular explanation is that certain natural anticoagulants, especially proteins C/S, that also anchor to and require PL$^{(-)}$, are unable to exert their normal anticoagulant effect if those sites are blocked.

No attempt has been made to indicate recent revisions to the traditional "cascade" concept. Recent findings suggest that the intrinsic pathway does not initiate coagulation but instead serves a regulatory function and participates in fibrinolysis. Not shown are thrombin feedbacks, components of the fibrinolytic systems, inhibitory systems (e.g., AT-III, heparin cofactor II, protein C/S/TM system, protein C inhibitor, C1 inhibitor), and other details.

7. What tests should be given when PT and activated PTT (aPTT) are prolonged?

The intrinsic coagulation pathway involves more steps than the extrinsic (TF-initiated) pathway. Accordingly, aPTT, which screens the intrinsic pathway ($\sim$ < 35 sec) is normally longer than the PT ($\sim$ < 15 sec) which screens the extrinsic pathway. Prolonged PT suggests that certain factors (i.e., II, VII, X) may be deficient (< 30% of normal) or that inhibitors of these factors may be present. On the other hand, prolonged aPTT indicates that intrinsic factors may be deficient (< 30%) or inhibitors present. When both the PT and aPTT are prolonged, all of above must be considered or the presence of inhibitors of the common pathway (inhibitors to I, II, X) may be indicated.

8. How do you determine the cause of prolonged PT or aPTT?

To help decide the cause of prolonged PT or aPTT, a mixing test must be peformed. In a mixing test, patient plasma is mixed with equal volume of normal plasma. If the 50% normal plasma corrects the prolonged PT or aPTT, one or more clotting factors are deficient ($\sim$ < 30%) or dysfunctional. (Blood from patients taking coumadin usually normalizes in mixing tests.) If the mixing test does not correct the prolonged time, inhibitors are present. Further tests can be ordered to identify specific factor deficiency or inhibitor responsible. For instance, in the case of FVIII inhibitors, addition of FVIII will correct prolonged aPTT. Probably the most commonly encountered inhibitor is lupus anticoagulant (LA or LAC).

9. What is lupus anticoagulant and how is it tested?

LA or LAC was first described in patients with systemic lupus erythematous (SLE) but was subsequently found in many conditions without lupus; therefore, the term is a misnomer that persists for historical reasons. Much evidence identifies LAC as one or more antiphospholipid antibodies (APLAs), but debate continues about its precise identity, and the coagulation-based LAC test remains superior to immunologic (e.g., enzyme linked immunosorbant assay [ELISA]) tests for APLA in predicting thrombosis.

In this condition, the presence of antibodies reacting against anionic phospholipids (PLs) apparently blocks sites needed for anchoring the vitamin K–dependent clotting factors to the PL surface, thereby prolonging the PT or aPTT (see Fig. 2B). To establish the presence of LAC, the 50:50 mixing test should remain prolonged and it should be shown that excess PL can correct the prolongation (by sopping up the APLA). This latter test—antibody neutralization with excess PL—is now often done using a proprietary hexagonal phase PL, but classically, activated platelets were used.

Patients with LAC rarely bleed despite prolonged coagulation time. On the contrary, they tend to develop thrombotic complications. There are many theories to explain these paradoxical phenomena. Natural anticoagulants such as protein C and S also require anchoring to the PL surface, and this is hindered by APLA, impairing the function of this natural anticoagulant. APLAs may also bind to and activate platelets and endothelium to promote thrombosis. There is also a suggestion that APLAs impair fibrinolysis.

10. What is antiphospholipid syndromes (APS)?

This syndrome is defined by a thrombotic condition of unknown etiology associated with positive test result for one or more APLA. APLAs are detected by ELISA, and multiple target antigens are often seen. Cardiolipin (CL) is the most frequently tested antigen, followed by β2GP1. However, antibodies to many other PL-binding proteins have been detected in APS, including prothrombin (FII), FVII, and annexin V, as well as several pure PL such as phsophatidyl serine (PS) and phosphatidyl ethanolamine (PE). Exactly which antigens are most important, which exhibit LAC activity, and how many antigens should be tested are all controversial questions. FVII as an antigen in APS has most recently been identified, and its clinical significance is under investigation.

Patients with APS are often positive for LAC. It is generally believed that positive LAC with positive β2GP1 indicates high risk for thrombosis. Because APS is the most common acquired thrombophilia, these tests should be performed on those who present with thrombotic events without well-known risk factors, especially in non-elderly individuals.

11. What are the opposing forces in blood coagulation?

A number of natural anticoagulants exist that oppose procoagulant activity. They are chiefly antithrombin III (AT-III), heparin cofactor II, the protein C/S thrombomodulin system, and tissue factor pathway inhibitor (TFPI), produced mainly on endothelium. In addition, the fibrinolytic system works on fibrin, the endproduct of blood coagulation, to dissolve already formed (or incipiently forming) blood clots.

AT-III binds to the catalytic site of thrombin to inactivate it, and this is greatly potentiated by heparin. AT-III also inhibits IXa, Xa. AT-III deficiency is associated with high risk of thrombosis. Heparin cofactor II is also potentiated by heparin, but its physiologic role appears less important. Protein C and its cofactor, protein S, work to inactivate FVa after activation by thrombomodulin (TM) at or near the endothelium. Activated proteins C and S also inactivate FVIIIa. The net result is to slow or shut down coagulant activity (i.e., thrombin formation). Patients with protein C or S deficiency suffer from thrombotic complications. TFPI, which inactivates FXa as well as TF-VIIa, has come to light more recently and is still under investigation. TFPI is likely to have major physiologic importance *vis a vis* thrombosis and coronary artery disease. Other natural inhibitors include complement C1 inhibitor against FXIIa and alpha-1 antitrypsin against FIXa.

The fibrinolytic system: As fibrin forms, endothelial cells release t-PA, which converts the zymogen, plasminogen, to plasmin. After plasmin is bound to fibrin, it is protected from its inhibitor, alpha-2-antiplasmin, and degrades cross-linked fibrin, giving rise to soluble fibrin degradation products (FDP) such as D-dimer. Assay of D-dimer is increasingly used for detection of thrombi. Urokinase is a second endogenous plasminogen activator (u-PA).

Both t-PA and u-PA are inhibited by specific inhibitors, mainly PAI-1 and PAI-2. The former is produced in the endothelium but also other tissues, and the latter is found in leukocytes and is abundant in placenta.

12. How is platelet activation detected?

Platelet activation is viewed as a harbinger of thrombosis. Numerous tests are claimed to be useful in detecting platelet activation, including measurement of platelet secretory products in blood or urine, enhanced sensitivity to platelet aggregation, and secretion in response to agonists. However, these methods have not found wide clinical application because they are too cumbersome or their results have been inconsistent. Some clinically methods useful are:

Circulating platelet aggregates: Circulating platelet aggregates are presumed to reflect abnormal platelet "stickiness." We have described a simple flowcytometric assay of platelet aggregates in plasma and have validated it by showing elevations in patients in various thrombotic states such as thrombotic thrombocytopenic purpura (TTP).

PMPs: Activated platelets release membrane fragments (microparticles) (see Fig. 1). PMPs can be readily measured by flow cytometry, so they constitute a useful marker of platelet activation. Elevated PMP levels have been described in patients with acute coronary syndrome, TTP, heparin-induced thrombocytopenia (HIT), ITP with thrombotic complications, and in cardiopulmonary bypass surgery.

CD62P expression: P-selectin (CD62P) is present in the α-granules of resting platelets and is transferred to the plasma membrane surface of activated (degranulated) platelets, where it is readily detected by fluorescent anti-CD62P in flow cytometry (see Fig. 1).

These assays require only tiny volumes of blood ($\sim 50\ \mu$L), and results can be available within a few hours.

13. How can one diagnose and treat patients with HIT?

HIT is the most common acquired thrombocytopenia encountered in hospitalized patients. HIT with thrombosis (HITT) is a serious condition. Early detection of HIT is critical because delays in detection can result in thromboembolic complications with high mortality or gangrene of extremities requiring amputation.

In pathophysiology, anti-heparin antibodies interact with platelet factor 4 (PF4) and heparin to form an immune complex, which binds to Fc receptors of platelets, triggering platelet activation, aggregation, and adhesion to the vessel wall. The vessels are plugged by white clots consisting mainly of activated platelet aggregates.

Platelet counts decreasing by more than >50% after exposure to heparin should give suspicion of HIT. For patients not previously exposed to heparin, a week or more may pass before they develop HIT. In patients previously sensitized, HIT can develop in just one or a few days.

Serologic ELISA tests for heparin-associated antibodies are available. A positive test result occurs in approximately 30% of patients on heparin therapy but fewer than 1% actually develop HITT. Accordingly, the ELISA test is not highly specific for HIT or HITT. The serotonin release assay, or the flowcytometric assay of CD62P developed in our laboratory, appears more specific to HITT.

Heparin should be immediately stopped upon suspicion of HIT or HITT. Serologic tests can aid the decision to resume or stop heparin. If anticoagulation is indicated, derivatives of hirudin such as Leprudin™ may be used. Alternatively, the synthetic thrombin inhibitor, Agatroban™, developed expressly for this purpose, has proven useful in this situation.

14. How to control platelet activation?

Platelets are activated by numerous stimuli *via* multiple pathways; see Table 1. Accordingly, no single agent can suppress all platelet activation, but certain combinations of drugs can be highly effective in achieving this aim.

Cyclooxygenase/thromboxane A_2 (TXA_2) inhibitors: Asprin (ASA) is the most widely used antiplatelet therapy (and the most widely used nonsteroidal antiinflammatory drug). However, it suppresses only platelet activation induced by arachidonic acid or collagen and is ineffective against other agonists. It has been shown that at high doses, aspirin can inhibit both platelet TXA_2 and endothelial prostacyclin (PGI_2) synthesis. Therefore, low-dose aspirin is recommended for antiplatelet therapy.

ADP receptor antagonists: Plavix, a new antiplatelet drug, is quickly finding wide use. It inhibits ADP-induced platelet aggregation.

Dipyridamole, an older antiplatelet drug, inhibits platelet activation by increasing intracellular cyclic AMP (cAMP). However, conventional doses seldom achieve sufficient concentration to increase cAMP. Consequently, many have expressed doubts about its effectiveness *in vivo*.

GP IIb/IIIa inhibitors: Abciximab (Reopro) is now widely used in cardiology. It effectively blocks GP IIa/IIIa to inhibit platelet aggregation. Several other drugs with the same or similar targets are being developed.

Other new agents to control platelet activation are under development. These include inhibitors of platelet adhesion, platelet aggregation, and antagonists of thrombin receptors.

15. What do you do with patients with high platelet counts?

Platelet counts exceeding one million (i.e., thrombocytosis) can be associated with ACS. The main differential diagnosis is whether this is a primary thrombocythemia; associated with myeloproliferative disorders (MPDs); or a reactive disorder associated with iron deficiency, inflammation, or neoplasm. Patients with MPD often have thrombotic complications and may present with ACS or stroke related to high platelet counts. On the other hand, patients with reactive thrombocytosis are not as often associated with thrombosis, but high platelet counts may nevertheless contribute to thrombosis.

Accordingly, patients with thrombocytosis and signs of ischemic attacks should be treated aggressively to reduce platelet counts, by platelet pheresis or use of drugs such as anagrelide or hydroxyurea. If diagnosis of MPD is confirmed, appropriate therapy is indicated.

In patients with thrombocythemia, the platelets often clump in the blood sample tube, resulting in apparently normal platelet counts. Therefore, it is important to examine blood smears for the presence of platelet clumping. Another clue to high platelet counts is pseudohyperkalemia: because platelets release K^+ during clotting, serum K^+ increases if platelet levels are abormally high. For this test, plasma K^+ should be checked in freshly drawn blood with K-free anticoagulant.

16. How is endothelial dysfunction detected?

Endothelial cells (ECs) play a crucial role in thrombosis and inflammation. Therefore, reliable detection of EC activation or apoptosis has become an important goal. Existing methods include detection of circulating ECs (CECs) as a marker of endothelial injury; however, this approach is limited because CECs are scarce in the circulation, so an unacceptably large volume of blood is required. A second approach is detection of various molecules (e.g., cytokines, adhesins, secretoary products) known or believed to derive from stimulated ECs. Many publications based on such methods applied to CAD have appeared, but results have sometimes been conflicting and controversial, specificity has been questioned, and there is no consensus on the best marker.

It has recently been shown *in vitro* that stimulated EC release endothelial microparticles (EMPs) and a few laboratories have begun exploiting EMP assay for clinical detection of endothelial injury in various thrombotic and inflammatory conditions, especially CAD. EMP is significantly higher in patients with ACS than stable disease, and it is higher in patients with MI than UA, suggesting good specificity (i.e., correlation with severity of ischemia). In addition, EMP levels correlate well with the degree of risk associated with particular kinds of angiographic lesion.

Because our method is based on flow cytometry, EMP assay requires only a tiny blood sample (~50 μL), and results can be available within 1 to 2 hours. With further validation, EMP as-

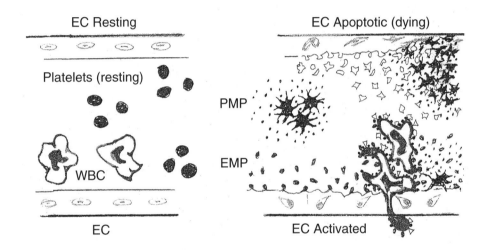

FIGURE 3. Overview of key events in thrombosis and inflammation.

This figure illustrates a few of the complex events and processes taking place at activated or injured endothelial cells (ECs), leading to thrombosis and inflammation.

Left, the normal quiescent state of flowing blood, with little interaction among resting EC, platelets, or leukocytes.

Top right, how injured EC quickly leads to platelet activation and leukocyte recruitment, leading to thrombosis.

Bottom right, similar events are associated with inflammation but with more emphasis on leukocyte recruitment, chemotaxis, and recruitment by cytokines, resulting in their extravasation (transendothelial migration) to surrounding tissues.

Injured endothelia expose or secrete adhesive molecules to the flowing blood (e.g., von Willebrand factor), inducing adhesion, activation, and aggregation of platelets. After they are activated, platelets release granules to recruit more platelets to form the platelet plug (white clot) at the site of EC injury (*top right*).

Activated platelets release platelet microparticles (PMPs) (*middle*), and both facilitate blood clotting, surrounding activated platelets to form fibrin and sealing off a platelet plug, resulting in formation of thrombus at the site of injury (*top*).

Injured or activated ECs also release microparticles (EMPs). EMPs released during EC activation or apoptosis appear to exist in several species, expressing different phenotypic profiles as judged by panels of monoclonal markers. Whereas EMPs preferentially bind to monocytes and activate them, PMPs preferentially bind to neutrophils and activate them.

Work is in progress to delineate the specific role (or roles) of microparticles in these complicated events. Meanwhile, assay of these microparticles is useful in detection of platelet activation (PMP) and endothelial dysfunction (EMP) in diverse thrombotic and inflammatory disorders.

say holds promise for routine clinical evaluation of endothelial injury in CAD and other diseases. Meanwhile, elevated EMP levels have already been reported in active phases of TTP and multiple sclerosis (MS): levels correlated with disease activity and normalized in remission. Elevated EMP levels were also noted in patients with severe malignant hypertension and preeclampsia.

By way of considering possible future advances, we recently found that the antigenic profiles of EMP differ in activation versus apoptosis (Fig. 3), holding the promise of being able to identify specific types of EC injury. Other laboratories have shown that ECs from different organs possess protein "address markers," suggesting the possibility of identifying the particular organ or type of vessel (e.g., venous, arterial; micro-, macro-) affected.

17. What are the major risk factors for thrombosis?

We have summarized the established risk factors in Table 2, classified according to heredity or acquired. Many of these are familiar to cardiologists but some are less well known, often overlooked, and deserve consideration when faced with patients who have idiopathic thrombosis. It is implicit that elevated cholesterol, triglycerides, and low-density lipoprotein (LDL) or ratio of high-density lipoprotein/LDL are included in atherosclerosis.

Table 2. Risk Factors for Thrombosis

HEREDITARY	ACQUIRED	
• Factor V Leiden	• Antiphospholipid antibody	• Atherosclerosis
• Prothrombin mutation G20210A	• Lupus anticoagulant	• Diabetes
• Deficiency of antithrombin III	• Elevated homocysteine	• Hypertension
• Deficiency of protein C or S	• Platelet hyperactivation	• Inflammation
• Deficiency of methlyenetetrahydrofolate reductase	• Thrombocytosis	• Cancer
	• HIT	• PNH
		• MPD

HIT = heparin-induced thrombocytopenia; MPD = myeloproliferative disorder; PNH = paroxysmal nocturnal hemoglobinuria.

18. What is the overall picture?

Blood clotting results from a complex interplay among several systems—chiefly, platelets, coagulation proteins, and endothelium—but is also affected by leukocytes, inflammatory cytokines, and other systems such as complement and hormones. Figure 3 summarizes some of these factors and their interactions.

BIBLIOGRAPHY

1. Boulanger CM, Scoazec A, Ebrahimian T, et al: Circulating microparticles from patients with myocardial infarctions cause endothelial dysfunction. Circulation 104:2649–2652, 2001.
2. Colman RW, Hirsh J, Marder VJ, et al. (eds): Hemostasis and Thrombosis, 4th ed. Philadelphia, Lippincott Williams & Wilkins, 2001.
3. Combes V, Simon AC, Grau GE, et al: In vitro generation of endothelial microparticles and possible prothrombotic activity in patients with lupus anticoagulant. J Clin Invest 104:93–102, 1999.
4. Horstman LL, Ahn YS: Platelet microparticles: a wide-angle perspective. Crit Rev Oncol/Hematol 30: 111–142, 1999.
5. Jimenez J, Jy W, Mauro L, et al: Elevated endothelial microparticles in thrombotic thrombocytopenic purpura (TTP): findings from brain and renal microvascular cell culture and patients with active disease. Br J Haematol 112:81–90, 2001.
6. Jy W, Mao WW, Horstman LL, et al: A flow cytometric assay of platelet activation marker P-selectin (CD62p) distinguishes heparin-induced thrombocytopenia (HIT) from HIT-with-thrombosis (HITT). Thromb Haemost 82:1255–1259, 1999.
7. Loscalzo J, Schafer AI (eds): Thrombosis and Hemorrhage, 2nd ed. Baltimore, Williams & Wilkins, 1998.
8. Mallat Z, Hugel B, Ohan J, et al: Shed membrane microparticles with procoagulant potential in human atherosclerotic plaques: A role for apoptosis in plaque thrombogenicity. Circulation 99:348–353, 1999.
9. Meroni PL, Raschi E, Testoni C, et al: Antiphospholipid antibodies and the endothelium. Rheum Dis Clin North Am 27:587–602, 2001.

9. RISK FACTORS AND PREVENTION

Maria P. Solano, M.D., and Ronald B. Goldberg, M.D.

RISK FACTORS AND PREVENTION

1. What are the risk factors for congestive heart disease (CHD)?

More that 100 risk factors for CHD have been described; however, not all of them have both biologic plausibility and strong epidemiologic evidence to support an independent association. CHD risk factors can be categorized as causative or major, conditional or novel, and predisposing (Table 1). The major risk factors account for approximately 50% of the variability in risk in high-risk populations. The conditional risk factors are those that have been correlated with CHD risk but their quantitative relationship to major coronary events remains to be defined. The predisposing risk factors are those that contribute to the development of causal and conditional risk factors.

The presence of multiple risk factors synergistically increases the risk of CHD risk. For example, in the National Health and Education Study (NHANES) I Follow-up, the presence of five risk factors (i.e., current cigarette smoking, hypertension [HTN], cholesterol > 240 mg/dL, diabetes, and being overweight) was assessed in 12,932 men and women. CHD risk tripled in the presence of three risk factors and increased fivefold with four or five risk factors. These results underscore the importance of adopting a multifactorial approach in risk reduction of CHD.

Table 1. Cardiovascular Risk Factors

Causative (major)
Cigarette smoking
Hypertension
Hypercholesterolemia
Low HDL cholesterol
Diabetes mellitus
Conditional (novel)
Triglycerides
Small LDL particles
Lp(a)
CRP
Homocysteine
PAI-1, fibrinogen
Predisposing
Being overweight or obese
Physical inactivity
Male gender
Family history of CHD
Socioeconomic factors
Behavioral factors
Insulin resistance

2. How is CHD risk assessed?

Several models have been formulated to identify patients at risk for CHD. The National Cholesterol Education Program–Adult Treatment Panel III (ATP III) approach for risk assessment starts by counting the presence of well-established risk factors (i.e., HTN, cigarette smoking, family history of premature CHD, low high-density lipoprotein [HDL] cholesterol levels [< 40 mg/dL], and age > 45 years for men and > 55 years for women). Persons with fewer than two risk factors are considered at low risk and those with two or more are at intermediate risk. Individuals with established CHD or with CHD risk equivalents constitute the high-risk group. A CHD risk equivalent is a condition that carries an absolute risk for developing new CHD equal to the risk of having recurrent CHD events in persons with established CHD. These conditions include diabetes mellitus, peripheral vascular disease, abdominal aortic aneurysm, and symptomatic carotid artery stenosis. Individuals with two or more risk factors should have their absolute 10-year risk of "hard CHD events" (myocardial infarction [MI] and CHD death) determined by the Framingham Risk Score in which age, gender, smoking history, blood pressure, (BP) total cholesterol, and HDL cholesterol are measured and entered into a risk calculation model. A 10-year risk of 20% or more moves a patient to the CHD risk equivalent category.

3. Is there a role for noninvasive cardiovascular testing in risk assessment?

In the Prevention Conference V, it was concluded that for patients in the intermediate risk group (global risk estimate 0.6–2% per year), further risk stratification with noninvasive measures of atherosclerosis burden might be valuable. Evidence suggests that ankle–brachial index, especially in persons older than age 60 years and in smokers, intima–media thickness (IMT) measured by carotid B-mode ultrasound in individuals older than age 50 years, and coronary calcium score determined by electron beam computed tomography (EBCT) could be useful in refining risk prediction in patients at intermediate risk of CHD. The relative risk of cardiovascular disease events found with an abnormal ABI, an abnormal IMT, or a calcium score of greater than 80 in prospective studies is similar to that seen in secondary prevention. Despite the cost limitation and lack of availability (for IMT and calcium score), these tests present an option to elevate the risk of individuals with multiple risk factors to a high-risk category.

4. What are the lipid targets in the different risk categories?

The primary lipid focus of the ATP III guidelines remains the low-density lipoprotein (LDL) cholesterol level. Target LDL cholesterol values continue to be less than 160 mg/dL for individuals with fewer than two risk factors, less than 130 mg/dL for those with two or more risk factors, and less than 100 mg/dL for patients with established CHD. For patients with CHD risk equivalents or with a 10-year risk of hard CHD events of 20% or more, the target is also less than 100mg/dL. The ATP III guidelines also expanded the indications for drug therapy and earlier therapy initiation. Non-HDL cholesterol (i.e., total cholesterol minus HDL cholesterol) was chosen as the secondary lipid target for patients with triglyceride levels greater than 200 mg/dL. Non-HDL cholesterol is closely correlated with apoliporotein B (apo B) and includes all atherogenic lipoproteins that contain apo B, namely, LDL, lipoprotein(a), intermediate-density lipoprotein (IDL) and very low density lipoprotein (VLDL). The goal for non-HDL cholesterol is 30 mg/dL higher than the LDL target. ATP III recognizes that the presence of conditional or emerging risk factors can have use in selected patients to guide the intensity of risk-reduction therapy; however, they do not categorically modify LDL cholesterol goals.

5. What is the metabolic syndrome?

The metabolic syndrome is the clustering of cardiovascular risk factors, including HTN, abdominal obesity, atherogenic dyslipidemia, and glucose intolerance. A prothrombotic and a proinflamatory state is also considered characteristic. Insulin resistance appears to be a common denominator of the syndrome. Two unifying definitions have been proposed. The first was published in 1998 by the World Health Organization (WHO); for individuals with normal glucose tolerance (NGT), at least two of the criteria listed below had to be fulfilled in addition to meeting criteria for insulin resistance. Insulin resistance can be assessed by the fasting insulin level or other parameters of insulin sensitivity with diagnostic values based on the population being studied. In patients with diabetes or impaired glucose tolerance, the metabolic syndrome is present if no two or more of the criteria are fulfilled. The criteria are hypertension (BP $>$ 160/90 mm Hg or antyhypertensive treatment, dyslipidemia (triglyceride $\geq$ 150 mg/dL or HDL $\leq$ 35 in men and $\leq$ 39 mg/dL in women), obesity (body mass index [BMI] $>$ 30 kg/m^2 or waist-to-hip ratio (WHR) $>$ 0.90 in men and $>$ 0.85 in women), and microalbuminuria ($>$ 20 µg/min).

The second definition was proposed by the NCEP ATP III in which the diagnosis of the metabolic syndrome can be made with at least three of five criteria namely, abdominal obesity (waist circumference > 40 inches in men and > 35 inches in women), elevated triglyceride levels (≥ 150 mg/dL), low HDL cholesterol (≤ 40 mg/dL in men, and ≤ 50 mg/dL in women), hypertension (BP ≥ 130/85), and abnormal fasting glucose (≥ 110 mg/dL).

6. What is the prevalence of the metabolic syndrome, and what is its associated cardiovascular risk?

The prevalence of the metabolic syndrome varies based on the definition used. For example, in the Botnia study in Finland and Sweden using the WHO criteria, about 10% of persons with NGT, 40% of those with IGT, and 85% of those with type 2 diabetes would have the metabolic syndrome. The prevalence was higher in men and increased with age. In subjects with the metabolic syndrome during 7 years of follow-up, there was a threefold increase risk of CHD, MI, and stroke and, consequently, increased mortality. In the United States, the prevalence of the metabolic syndrome as defined by ATP III based on data from the third NHANES (1988 to 1994) was 21.8%. The prevalence was age dependent, and the age-adjusted rates were similar in men and women. The age-adjusted prevalence was highest among Mexican Americans (31.9%). It is estimated that 47 million U.S. residents have the metabolic syndrome. Taken in aggregate, the presence of the metabolic syndrome accentuates the risk of CHD at any LDL level. The first strategy recommended by ATP III to treat the metabolic syndrome is to use lifestyle changes to reverse its "root causes" of being overweight or obese and being physically inactive. In addition, the other risk factors associated with the metabolic syndrome should be appropriately treated.

7. What is the value of measuring Lp(a)?

Lp(a) is a lipoprotein identical to LDL except for the addition of a large glycoprotein, apolipoprotein (a) [apo(a)], which is disulfide linked to apolipoprotein B-100. Plasma Lp(a) concentrations are largely genetically determined and are higher in African Americans than in whites. Some prospective studies have found Lp(a) to be an independent risk factor for CHD. Elevated Lp(a) levels appear to increase the risk of CHD, especially in the presence of concomitant high LDL cholesterol or low HDL cholesterol levels. An Lp(a) level of less than 30 mg/dL is considered desirable. Lp(a) measurement and treatment of Lp(a) excess are best reserved for persons with CHD and no other identifiable lipid disorder and for those with a strong family history of premature CHD. No clinical trial evidence currently supports a benefit from specific Lp(a)-lowering therapy, and the primary therapeutic target in individuals with high Lp(a) levels is LDL cholesterol lowering. Two statin trials, HATS and FATS, have suggested that statin treatment of hypercholesterolemia eliminates the CHD risk associated with increased Lp(a) levels. Among currently available lipid-lowering agents, only nicotinic acid at high doses (3–4 g/day) reduces Lp(a) levels by as much as 38%. Additionally, in postmenopausal women, hormone replacement therapy (HRT) can also reduce Lp(a) levels.

8. Should homocysteine levels be measured in high-risk patients?

Homocysteine (Hcy) is an intermediary amino acid formed during the metabolism of methionine. Many cross-sectional and case control studies have shown an association between elevated Hcy levels and increased risk for CHD, peripheral vascular disease (PVD), cerebrovascular disease, and thrombosis; however, not all prospective cohort studies have linked elevated Hcy levels with increased cardiovascular risk. Hcy levels also appear to correlate with the severity and extent of coronary atherosclerosis. Concentrations of Hcy can be reduced by pharmacologic dosages of folic acid (0.4–5.0 mg) and other B vitamins (B_6 and B_{12}), an inexpensive and safe intervention that makes Hcy an attractive therapeutic target in high-risk patients. Hcy-lowering therapy for 6 months with folic acid (1 mg), vitamin B_6 (10 mg), and vitamin B_{12} (0.4 mg) reduced the rate of restenosis and the need for revascularization of the target lesion after coronary angioplasty in a prospective, randomized trial of 209 patients. Several large randomized trials are underway evaluating whether lowering Hcy levels will reduce cardiovascular morbidity and mortality. At least until these results are available, we recommend measuring and lowering Hcy levels (target < 10 μmol/L) in patients with known cardiovascular disease and those who are at high risk.

9. What is the role of C-reactive protein (CRP) in CHD?

Growing evidence suggests that inflammation plays a role in the pathogenesis of athero-thrombosis. CRP is a nonspecific but sensitive marker of inflammation that has been associated with increased risk of cardiovascular disease. Highly sensitive CRP is a strong predictor of MI in adults with and without history of CHD and adds to the predictive value of total and HDL cholesterol. Therefore, CRP may be an adjuvant to lipid screening for risk stratification in primary prevention. CRP levels also appear to have important prognostic value in patients with acute coronary syndromes (ACS). Elevated serum CRP levels are predictive of short- and long-term cardiovascular events after unstable angina and MI. Likewise, increased pre-procedural CRP levels are associated with more cardiac events after percutaneous transluminal coronary angioplasty (PTCA) and stenting. CRP levels are higher in women than in men, particularly in women taking HRT. Statins, as well as fibrates, significantly reduce serum CRP levels.

10. Are HDL subfractions useful in predicting CHD?

HDL particles are heterogeneous and can be subdivided by ultracentrifugation into HDL2 and HDL3 subfractions or by apolipoprotein content into particles containing apo AI (LpA-I) only and particles containing both apoAI and apoAII (LpAI:A2). Although several studies have shown that HDL2 and LpAI are better predictors of CHD than total HDL cholesterol, HDL3, or LpAI:AII, other prospective studies have demonstrated a similar quantitative association of HDL3 and HDL2 (Physicians' Health Study) and of LpAI:AII and LpAI (PRIME Study) with CHD. At present, the clinical relevance of the different HDL subfractions is uncertain; therefore, routine measurement of HDL subfractions in CHD risk assessment is not recommended.

11. What is the role of small dense LDL in CHD?

Small dense LDL particles have been consistently associated in cross-sectional and prospective studies with increased risk of CHD. They are part of the "atherogenic dyslipidemia" also character-ized by higher levels of triglycerides, VLDL, IDL, and apo B and lower levels of HDL cholesterol and apoAI. Whether the small dense LDL phenotype predicts CHD independently of other risk factors has not been clearly established. However, a low binding affinity for the LDL receptor and low resistance to oxidative stress suggest a causal role for small dense LDL in the development of atherosclerosis. Therapeutic interventions leading to reduction in triglyceride levels below a threshold of approximately 133 mg/dL which promotes the formation of small dense LDL, increases LDL particle size. The use of niacin or fibrates can be considered as part of the lipid management plan in high-risk patients with small dense LDL phenotype, keeping in mind that LDL cholesterol remains the primary therapeutic target. Statins generally do not affect LDL particle size; however, they do significantly decrease the number of LDL particles, which is also important.

12. What clinical benefits of statin therapy were established from major lipid-lowering trials published before the new NCEP (ATP III) guidelines?

Statins have been shown to reduce morbidity and mortality associated with coronary artery disease. The Scandinavian Simvastatin Survival Study (4S), the Long-term Intervention with Pravastatin in Ischemic Disease (LIPID), and the Cholesterol and Recurrent Events Trial (CARE) trials used simvastatin (20–40 mg) and pravastatin (40 mg) to demonstrate that both hypercho-lesterolemic (4S, LIPID) and normocholesterolemic (CARE) individuals—mainly men—with CHD had a significant reduction in coronary events (all) or deaths (4S) compared with placebo, in the order of 25% to 35% (Fig 1).

The West of Scotland Coronary Prevention Study Group (WOSCOPS) and the Air Force Coronary Atherosclerosis Prevention Study (AFCAPS) trials using pravastatin (40 mg) and lo-vastatin (20–40 mg) demonstrated that men without CHD but with significant hyperchole-sterolemia (WOSCOPS) and men and women without CHD but with above average LDL cholesterol (AFCAPS) also had an approximate 25% reduction in the rates of initial cardiovascular events. These results support and strengthen the major NCEP recommendations.

Secondary analyses have shown that diabetic subjects with CHD benefit at least equally to nondiabetic individuals (4S, CARE), that women and older subjects (> age 60 years) benefit equally to the rest of the population (4S, CARE), and that healthy subjects with low HDL cholesterol levels benefit more than those with normal values (AFCAPS).

But we still do not know what the relative impact that the baseline and posttreatment LDL cholesterol values is or what the percent and absolute reduction of LDL cholesterol levels by statin treatment have on cardiovascular disease events rates.

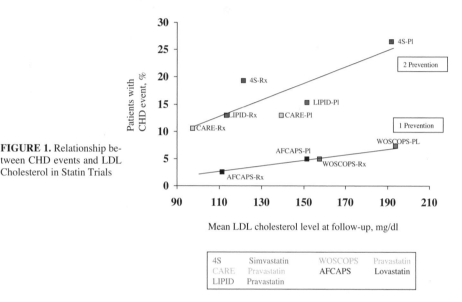

FIGURE 1. Relationship between CHD events and LDL Cholesterol in Statin Trials

4S	Simvastatin	WOSCOPS	Pravastatin
CARE	Pravastatin	AFCAPS	Lovastatin
LIPID	Pravastatin		

13. Do the results of the Heart Protection Study (HPS) require modification of NCEP guidelines?

The findings of the HPS suggest that this may be the case. The HPS was a large trial of the effects of 6 years of 40 mg of simvastatin and antioxidant therapy in a wide range of subjects at high risk of coronary disease death. A total of 20,536 men and women age 40 to 80 years and with total cholesterol levels of greater than 135 mg/dL were recruited. The subjects either had evidence of cardiovascular disease (i.e., CHD, cerebrovascular disease, or PVD) or were at increased risk because of diabetes or treated hypertension. Overall, the study showed that in this high-risk population with and without prior vascular disease, simvastatin produced a 17% reduction in cardiovascular mortality and lowered cardiovascular events by approximately 25% irrespective of history, age, gender, or baseline LDL cholesterol level. The implication is that simvastatin treatment is associated with the same relative reduction in events over a broad range of LDL cholesterol values and that this extends even to subjects with levels below 100 mg/dL.

14. Should statins be initiated early in patients with ACS?

Beyond LDL lowering, statins may decrease early cardiovascular events after ACS by potential favorable effects on platelet adhesion, plaque stability, inflammation, and endothelial function. One year mortality after an acute MI was lower in patients who were prescribed statins compared with those who were not in a cohort of approximately 20,000 patients from Sweden. Likewise, 30-day and 6-month mortality were reduced among patients treated with statins at the time of percutaneous coronary intervention in a cohort study of about 5000 patients from the Cleveland Clinic Foundation. In the Myocardial Ischemia with Aggressive Cholesterol Lowering

(MIRACL) study, early initiation of high-dose atorvastatin (80 mg) in patients with ACS (unstable angina and non–Q-wave MI) resulted in a 26% reduction in recurrent symptomatic ischemia requiring emergency hospitalization over the ensuing 16 weeks. In addition to the potential short-term benefits, initiation of lipid-lowering therapy in the hospital has the advantage of enhancing patient compliance and longer-term treatment use. Therefore, early initiation of statin therapy in patients with ACS may be warranted.

15. What is the risk of myopathy associated with statins?

The incidence of myalgias ($\leq 11\%$) in clinical trials of statin therapy was similar in the statin and placebo groups. However, in clinical practice, we find patients who develop myalgias of various severity and unclear significance without elevated creatine phosphokinase (CPK) levels after initiation of statin treatment that resolve upon discontinuation of the medication. Clinically significant myopathy, defined as an elevation in CPK levels greater than 10 times normal, occurred in fewer than 0.5% of statin-treated patients in clinical trials. The risk of significant myopathy and rhabdomyolysis is increased when patients have renal insufficiency or are concomitantly using certain medications, including cyclosporin, gemfibrozil, fenofibrate, erythromycin, clarythromycin, azole antifungals, and HIV protease inhibitors. Although described in early reports, rhabdomyolysis with the combination of niacin and statins appears to be rare. Statins should be used cautiously and at low doses when given in combination with fibrates to minimize the risk of myopathy. Monitoring serum CPK levels is not necessary; however, measuring a baseline CPK level before initiating statin therapy is helpful in clinical practice.

16. How should CHD patients with low HDL cholesterol be treated?

A well-established strong inverse correlation exists between HDL cholesterol levels and CHD risk. Evidence that increasing HDL cholesterol has a beneficial effect on CHD events comes from a large prospective study (VA HIT) showing a 24% reduction in the combined outcome of death from CHD, MI, or stroke with gemfibrozil in patients with CHD who had low HDL cholesterol (mean, 32 mg/dL) and below average LDL cholesterol (mean, 111 mg/dL) levels.

The primary target for CHD patients with low HDL cholesterol is an LDL cholesterol level less than 100 mg/dL; however, according to the latest NCEP guidelines, in high-risk individuals with LDL cholesterol values between 100 and 129 mg/dL and low HDL or high triglyceride levels, pharmacologic LDL-lowering therapy is not considered essential and the use of niacin or fibrates is regarded as an alternative. In this particular group of patients, combination therapy may be beneficial, as suggested by the HATS findings. In this study, despite a relatively small number of patients, the use of simvastain and niacin in CHD patients with HDL less than 35 mg/dL and LDL less than 140 mg/dL was associated with angiographic regression of coronary lesions and a 90% reduction in CHD events.

17. What is the effect of HRT in secondary prevention of CHD?

The impact of HRT on cardiovascular risk in postmenopausal women is uncertain. Multiple case control and observational epidemiologic studies suggest a role for estrogen alone or in combination with progestin in secondary prevention of CHD. However, this benefit was not confirmed in the Heart and Estrogen/Progestin Replacement Study (HERS), in which 2763 postmenopausal women with CHD were randomized to 0.625 mg of conjugated estrogen plus 2.5 mg of medroxy-progesterone acetate or placebo for 4 years. Overall, there was no difference in CHD events between HRT and placebo. Although CHD events were increased during the first year with a trend for MI to decrease during the latter years, this trend did not continue during additional years of follow-up (i.e., in HERS II). Furthermore, HRT increased the risk of venous thromboembolism and biliary tract surgery during the 6.8 years of follow-up. These results support the American Heart Association's recommendation that HRT should not be given to postmenopausl women with CHD for the express purpose of reducing CHD events. This recommendation now extends to postmenopausal women without CHD based on the results of the Women Health Initiative (WHI) showing an increased relative risk of CHD events in the women assigned to HRT (estrogen plus progestin).

18. Do antioxidants reduce the risk of CHD?

LDL oxidation and oxidative stress are believed to play a role in the development and progression of atherosclerosis. Thus, it has been hoped that antioxidant treatment will reduce the risk for CHD. Unfortunately, except for a reduction in nonfatal infarction with vitamin E supplementation seen in the Cambridge Heart Antioxidant Study (CHAOS), more recent large control trials using antioxidants mixtures (HATS and HPS) or vitamin E alone (Primary Prevention Project and HOPE) have failed to show a beneficial effect in reducing cardiovascular events. Furthermore, in HATS, the use of an antioxidant mixture (i.e., vitamin E, vitamin C, selenium, and beta carotene) blunted the HDL cholesterol–increasing effect of niacin and simvastatin therapy in patients with low HDL cholesterol. Although antioxidants most likely have a neutral effect in the population in general, they should not be used in patients with low HDL cholesterol.

BIBLIOGRAPHY

1. Brown BG, Zhao X, Chait A, Fisher LD, et al: Simvastatin and niacin, antioxidant vitamins, or the combination for the prevention of coronary disease. N Engl J Med 345: 1583–1592, 2001.
2. Executive Summary of the third report of the National Cholesterol Education Program (NCEP) expert panel on detection, evaluation, and treatment of high blood cholesterol in adults (Adult Treatment Panel III). JAMA 285:2486–2495, 2001.
3. Grady D, Herrington D, Bittner V, et al: Cardiovascular disease outcomes during 6.8 years of hormone therapy. Heart and Estrogen/Progestin Replacement Study Follow-up (HERS II). JAMA 288:49–57, 2002.
4. MRC/BHF Heart Protection Study of cholesterol lowering with simvastatin in 20,536 high-risk individuals: a randomised placebo-controlled trial. Lancet 360:7–22, 2002.
5. Rubins HB, Robins SJ, Collins D, et al: Gemfibrozil for the secondary prevention of coronary heart disease in men with low levels of high-density lipoprotein cholesterol. Veterans Affairs High-Density Lipoprotein Cholesterol Intervention Trial study Group. N Engl J Med 341:410–418, 1999.
6. Sacks FM, Pfeffer MA, Moye LA, et al: The effect of pravastatin on coronary events after myocardial infarction in patients with average cholesterol levels. Cholesterol and Recurrent Events Trial investigators. N Engl J Med 335:1001–1009, 1995.
7. Scandinavian Simvastatin Survival Study Group: Randomised trial of cholesterol lowering in 4444 patients with coronary heart disease: the Scandinavian Simvastatin Survival Study (4S). Lancet 344: 1383–1389, 1994.
8. Schnyder G, Roffi M, Pin R, et al: Decreased rate of coronary restenosis after lowering of plasma homocysteine levels. N Engl J Med 345:1593–1600, 2001.
9. Schwartz GG, Olsson AG, Ezekowitz MD, et al: Effects of atorvastatin in early recurrent ischemic events in acute coronary syndromes. The MIRACL Study: a randomized controlled trial. JAMA 285:1711–1718, 2001.
10. Smith SC, Greenland P, Grundy SM: Prevention Conference V. Beyond secondary prevention: identifying the high-risk patient for primary prevention. Executive summary. Circulation 101:111–116, 2000.

10. EPIDEMIOLOGY AND NONINVASIVE ASSESSMENT OF CORONARY ARTERY DISEASE

Vivek J. Goswami, M.D., and Robert A. O'Rourke, M.D.

1. What is the incidence of coronary artery disease (CAD) in the United States?

There are approximately 1,100,000 patients who experience an acute myocardial infarction (MI) each year in the U.S.; about one half of these (550,000) survive to reach hospitalization. Two population-based studies (from Olmsted County, MN, and Framingham, MA) examined the rates of MI in patients with symptoms of angina and reported similar annual rates of 3% to 3.5%, respectively. On this basis, it can be estimated that there are roughly 30 patients with stable angina for every patient with infarction that is hospitalized. As a result, the number of patients with stable angina can be estimated as 16,500,000 per year. This estimate does not include patients who do not seek medical attention for their chest pain or whose chest pain has a noncardiac cause.

2. How many percutaneous interventions (PCIs) are performed annually in the United States?

More than 500,000 PCI procedures are performed annually in the United States, and it has been estimated that more than 1,000,000 procedures are performed yearly worldwide. This figure now exceeds the number of coronary artery bypass graft (CABG) surgeries. New coronary devices have expanded the clinical and anatomic indications for revascularization initially limited by balloon catheter angioplasty. For example, stents reduce both the acute risk of major complications and late-term restenosis. The success of new coronary devices in meeting these goals is in part represented by the less frequent use of percutaneous transluminal coronary angioplasty (PTCA) alone ($< 20\%$) and the high ($> 80\%$) penetration of coronary stenting in the current practice of interventional cardiology.

3. What are the current success and complication rates of PCI?

Improvements in balloon technology coupled with the increased use of nonballoon devices, particularly stents and glycoprotein IIb/IIIa platelet receptor antagonists, have favorably influenced acute procedural outcome. This combined balloon-device-pharmacologic approach to coronary intervention in elective procedures has resulted in angiographic success rates of 96–99%, with Q-wave MI rates of 1–3%, emergency CABG rates of 0.2 to 3.0%, and unadjusted in hospital mortality rates of 0.5–1.4%.

4. Which anatomic lesions carry the highest risk?

Table 1. Lesion Classification System

Low risk
Discrete (length < 10 mm)
Concentric
Readily accessible
Nonangulated segment (< 45°)
Smooth contour
Little or no calcification
Less than totally occlusive
Not ostial in location
No major side branch involvement
Absence of thrombus

(continued)

Table 1. Lesion Classification System (Continued)

Moderate risk
Tubular (length 10 to 20 mm)
Eccentric
Moderate tortuosity of proximal segment
Moderately angulated segment ($> 45°$, $< 90°$)
Irregular contour
Moderate or heavy calcification
Total occlusions existing for < 3 months
Ostial in location
Bifurcation lesions requiring double guidewires
Some thrombus present

High risk
Diffuse (length > 20 mm)
Excessive tortuosity of proximal segment
Extremely angulated segments ($> 90°$)
Total occlusions existing for > 3 months or bridging collaterals
Inability to protect major side branches
Degenerated vein grafts with friable lesions

5. Describe the clinical risk factors associated with adverse events after PCI.

Table 2. Clinical Risk Factors Associated with In-Hospital Adverse Events

VARIABLES	DEFINITIONS
Age	Age > 65 years
Gender	Male or female
LVEF	Depressed LVEF, either calculated or estimated
Unstable angina	Progressive or new onset or occurs at rest accompanied by ECG changes, hypotension, or pulmonary congestion
Congestive heart failure	Hx of CHF before intervention
Recent MI	MI within previous 7 days
Urgency of procedure	*Elective:* Patient clinically stable; procedure routinely scheduled
	Urgent: Patient unstable; schedule before discharge
	Emergent ongoing ischemia: Ongoing ischemia, including rest angina despite maximal therapy
	Emergent salvage: Arrest with cardiopulmonary resuscitation immediately before entering laboratory
Cardiogenic shock	Hypoperfusion with SBP < 80 mmHg and central filling pressure > 20 mmHg or cardiac index < 1.8 L/min/m^2; also present if inotropes or IABP needed to maintain these values
Preprocedural IABP/CPS	IABP/CPS assisted device placed before intervention
Aortic valve disease	Aortic stenosis with valve area < 1.0 cm^2 or aortic regurgitation $> 2+$
Mitral regurgitation	Presence of mitral regurgitation $> 2+$
Diabetes mellitus	Clinical diagnosis of diabetes treated or not treated
Peripheral vascular disease	Presence of occlusive disease in the aorta, iliac, or femoral artery sufficient to cause symptoms
Stroke	History of stroke
Creatinine level	Creatinine > 2 mg/dL
Dialysis	Patient on dialysis
Cholesterol (reduced risk)	Measured cholesterol > 225 mg/dL
Same-vessel intervention (reduced risk)	Any previous intervention on same vessel
Type C lesion	High-risk lesion (see Table 1)
LMCA	Intervention involving all or part of LMCA
Vein graft intervention	Any intervention to SVG or IMA
Thrombus	Intraluminal filling defect, haziness, or contrast staining in artery before intervention

In patients with a higher-risk profile, consideration of alternative therapies, including CABG, formalized surgical standby, or periprocedural hemodynamic support, should be addressed before proceeding with PCI.

6. Should postprocedure chest pain be evaluated?

After PCI, chest pain may occur in as many as 50% of patients. Electrocardiographic (ECG) evidence of ischemia identifies those with significant risk for acute vessel closure. When angina pectoris or ischemic ECG changes occur after PCI, the decision to proceed with further interventional procedures, CABG surgery, or medical therapy should be individualized based on factors such as hemodynamic stability, amount of myocardium at risk, and the likelihood that the treatment will be successful.

7. List the contraindications to exercise testing.

- Acute phase of an unstable coronary syndrome
- Severe heart failure
- Active myocarditis or pericarditis
- High-grade atrioventricular block
- Severe aortic stenosis
- Uncontrolled hypertension
- ECG abnormalitites that preclude ECG interpretation (e.g., left bundle branch block [LBBB], Wolff-Parkinson-White [WPW] syndrome)
- Inability to exercise for any reason
- Uncontrolled arrhythmias
- Other uncontrolled severe illnesses, active endocarditis, or recent pulmonary embolus

8. What effects do LBBB, right bundle branch block (RBBB), and left ventricular hypertrophy (LVH) with repolarization abnormalities have on exercise stress testing interpretation?

Exercise-induced ST depression usually occurs with LBBB and has no association with ischemia. Even up to 1 cm of ST depression can occur in healthy normal subjects. There is no level of ST segment depression that confers diagnostic significance in LBBB. In addition, patients with LBBB should not undergo exercise testing with myocardial perfusion imaging (MPI) because of artifactual abnormal findings in the ventricular septum, despite no left anterior descending (LAD) lesions.

Exercise-induced ST depression usually occurs with RBBB in the anterior chest leads (V_1 through V_3) and is not associated with ischemia. However, in the left chest leads (V_5 and V_6) or inferior leads (II and aVF), its test characteristics are similar to those of a normal resting ECG. The presence of RBBB does not appear to reduce the sensitivity, specificity, or predictive value of the stress ECG for the diagnosis of ischemia.

LVH with repolarization abnormality is associated with a decreased specificity of exercise testing, but sensitivity is unaffected. Therefore, a standard exercise test may still be the first test, with referrals for additional tests only indicated in patients with an abnormal test result.

9. Is there a role for exercise testing after PCI?

Although restenosis remains the major limitation of PCI, symptom status is an unreliable index to development of restenosis with 25% of asymptomatic patients documented as having ischemia on exercise testing.

Because myocardial ischemia, whether painful or silent, worsens prognosis, *some* authorities have advocated routine testing. However, the American College of Cardiology/American Heart Association practice guidelines for exercise testing favor selective evaluation in patients considered to be at particularly high risk (e.g., patients with decreased left ventricular [LV] function, multivessel coronary artery disease [CAD], proximal left anterior descending disease, previous sudden death, diabetes mellitus, hazardous occupations, and suboptimal PCI results). The exercise ECG is an insensitive predictor of restenosis, with sensitivities ranging from 40% to 55%, significantly less than those obtainable with single photon emission computed tomography or exercise echocardiography. This lower sensitivity of the exercise ECG and its inability to localize disease limits its usefulness in patient management both before and after PCI. For these reasons, stress imaging is preferred to evaluate symptomatic patients after PCI. If the patient's exertional capacity is significantly limited, coronary angiography may be more expeditious to evaluate symptoms of typical angina. Exercise testing after discharge is helpful for activity counseling and exercise training as part of cardiac rehabilitation. Neither exercise testing nor radionuclide imaging is indicated for the routine, periodic monitoring of asymptomatic patients after PCI without specific indications.

10. What is the role of Holter monitoring in the evaluation of patients for CAD?

In patients with suspected CAD, transient ST segment depressions greater than 0.1mV for less than 30 seconds strongly correlate with myocardial perfusion scans that show regional ischemia and are rare in otherwise healthy individuals. In patients that are post-MI, the frequency of premature ventricular contractions (PVCs) increases for several weeks and then declines after 6 months. Persistently frequent or complex PVCs are independent markers for sudden death or an acute cardiac event.

11. Compare the various radiopharmaceuticals used in myocardial perfusion imaging (MPI).

Thallium 201, a potassium analog, is the most widely used and standard myocardial perfusion agent. It has a half-life of 73 hours and emits gamma rays from 68 to 80 kev. Thallium 201 has a linear relationship between blood flow to viable myocardium, and uptake is maintained during exercise up to very high levels of flow, giving it excellent physiologic properties for MPI.

Tc-99m sestamibi belongs to a class of compounds called *isonitriles* and is a complex organic compound that behaves physiologically as a monovalent compound. After its extraction from the blood, Tc-99m sestamibi is bound by mitochondria, and only a limited amount of myocardial washout occurs over time. Tc-99m sestamibi is similar to thallium 201 in its myocardial physiologic perfusion properties; however, it possesses improved imaging characteristics that result from the greater gamma photon energy emission (140 kev).

12. How should MPI be interpreted after PCI?

Serial tomographic imaging with Tc-99m sestamibi has been used at 18 to 48 hours after therapy to assess coronary artery patency. In this time frame, it will clearly identify patients who have both coronary artery patency and early evidence of myocardial salvage, but it will be unable to distinguish patients with persistent occlusion from patients with patent arteries without early evidence of myocardial salvage. Technetium-99m sestamibi imaging has yet to be tested earlier after reperfusion therapy (perhaps 4 to 6 hours) when additional revascularization might still be feasible. The use of nuclear testing very early after angioplasty is controversial. Some reports showed that the nuclear test may be falsely positive early after PCI. This may be attributable to stunned vasa vasorum in the coronary artery undergoing angioplasty, affecting vasodilator reserve, distal embolization of atheromatous material, and local vascular trauma.

13. In patients with multivessel coronary disease with persistent chest pain, why is it important to obtain MPI before revascularization?

In the setting of multivessel disease, it is often difficult to determine which lesion is responsible for a patient's angina by angiographic methods alone. MPI is useful in localizing the area of ischemia and thereby increasing the likelihood of the "culprit" lesion being revascularized.

14. What are the latest indications for radionuclide imaging after an elevated coronary artery calcium score (CACS) on electron beam computed tomography (EBCT)?

EBCT measures CACS to identify early coronary atherothrombotic lesions. Although some patients may benefit from nuclear stress testing after these elevated calcium scores, it would clearly not be cost effective for all patients with atherosclerosis on EBCT to go on and receive subsequent nuclear cardiology testing. In a recent study by He and colleagues, 370 men and women who had undergone EBCT were further evaluated by myocardial perfusion SPECT imaging. Only one of 100 patients with a calcium score less than 100 had an abnormal myocardial perfusion scan. In contrast, 12% of patients with calcium scores from 101 to 399 and 47% of patients with calcium scores greater than 400 had an abnormal myocardial perfusion SPECT. In general, when the EBCT score is greater than the 75th percentile for age and gender, stress nuclear imaging may be appropriate for purposes of risk stratification.

15. Which noninvasive procedure is most likely to demonstrate high-risk atherothrombotic plaque formation?

In vivo, high-resolution, multicontrast magnetic resonance imaging (MRI) is currently the most promising noninvasive technique for the assessment of high-risk plaques in carotid arteries. MRI is uniquely suited for serial, repeated examinations because it is a noninvasive diagnostic method. Motion artifacts caused by patient movement and swallowing sometimes complicate the adequate interpretation of the images. A modified technique that avoids the acquisition of data during motion is currently being refined. Assessment of coronary arteries using the same technique is as yet imperfect because of motion artifacts resulting from a beating heart; however, it will likely help to separate vulnerable from stable plaques and evaluate the patency of bypass grafts with further precision after additional modification of the method.

16. What is the best noninvasive test to assess LV function in the setting of CAD?

Overall, the left ventricular ejection fraction (LVEF) is one of the most powerful predictors of future myocardial events and sudden death in patients with CAD. Of the noninvasive studies, gated equilibrium blood pool imaging (multiple gated acquisition [MUGA] is the most accurate. In this study, an aliquot of the patient's red blood cells is labeled with sodium pertechnetate and reinjected for subsequent imaging in three static-image cardiac positions. The cardiac cycle is divided into 8–64 intervals, and data from multiple cardiac cycles are averaged to ensure adequate count statistics. The averaged data are then processed in an image format to simulate cardiac motion during the cardiac cycle. From this display, LV end-diastolic and end-systolic volumes are identified and used to calculate the LVEF. Also from the display, regional myocardial wall motion may be determined from each LV segment. MUGA provides a more accurate quantitative measure of LVEF than echo.

17. Why does single plane left ventricular angiography often give erroneous LVEF data?

The right anterior oblique (RAO) view shows the anterobasal, anterolateral, apical, diaphragmatic, and posterobasal segments of the LV cavity. In contrast, the left anterior oblique (LAO) view shows the lateral, posterolateral, apical septal, and basal septal segments. For this reason, biplane images of the ventriculogram are preferred (generally, 30° RAO and 60° LAO), which are more comprehensive and provide a much more accurate assessment of the posterior LV than the RAO view alone.

18. What is the role of noninvasive stress imaging before and after PCI?

The addition of echocardiographic imaging to exercise is particularly useful when the ECG changes of ischemia are obscured by baseline abnormalities (e.g., LV hypertrophy or resting repolarization changes). Imaging also provides information regarding the location of ischemic myocardium and the size of the territory at risk. Exercise or pharmacologic stress echocardiography provides greater diagnostic accuracy than exercise ECG alone; thus, these are useful procedures when the results of the latter test are equivocal or indeterminate. Patients unable to undergo exercise stress testing for reasons such as deconditioning, peripheral vascular disease, orthopedic disabilities, neurologic disease, or concomitant illness can often benefit from pharmacologic stress testing. Indications for these tests include establishing a diagnosis of CAD, determining myocardial viability before revascularization, assessing prognosis after MI or in chronic angina, and evaluating perioperative cardiac risk. In patients with multivessel disease, noninvasive stress imaging may be helpful in determining the "culprit" lesion. After PCI, stress echocardiographic techniques have been used to detect restenosis with diagnostic accuracies comparable to nuclear imaging. Sensitivity has been reported between 78% and 90%, and specificity approaches 93%.

19. Why does *contrast luminography* often show less than 50% coronary artery stenosis to areas with decreased myocardial perfusion by radionuclide imaging?

Traditional coronary angiography, or *contrast luminography,* helps to visualize the size of the lumen only. Actual plaque morphology and volume of hemodynamically significant lesions may be better visualized using methods such as intravascular ultrasound (IVUS). One of the advantages of this technique is its ability to precisely quantify the severity of coronary lesions. The tomographic orientation of ultrasound enables visualization of the full 360-degree circumference of the vessel wall, rather than a two-dimensional projection of the lumen. The tomographic perspective of ultrasound enables evaluation of vessels difficult to assess by angiographic techniques, including segments that are diffusely diseased, lesions at bifurcation sites, ostial stenosis, and highly eccentric plaques. Furthermore, IVUS imaging is superior to coronary angiography in the detection of coronary calcification.

20. What technique should supplement a coronary angiogram in patients with diabetes mellitus?

In patients with diabetes mellitus, coronary vessel involvement is usually extensive and diffuse compared with nondiabetic patients. Therefore, the calculation of the percentage diameter stenosis by coronary angiography is often underestimated because of diffuse disease of the reference vessel. The accurate assessment of the severity of CAD by angiography is further confounded by a phenomenon known as *coronary remodeling*. This process involves compensatory enlargement of the adventitia caused by outward growth of plaque, thus maintaining its initial coronary lumen size. Furthermore, coronary angiography does not reliably assess the physiologic or hemodynamic significance of an intermediate coronary stenosis. For these reasons, IVUS should be performed on any suspicious lesions to further define potential lesions amenable to PCI in patients with diabetes mellitus. Other invasive studies, such as fractional flow reserve (FFR), are detailed elsewhere in this text.

21. How can the diagnosis of endothelial dysfunction be made using noninvasive techniques?

Endothelial function can be evaluated invasively by investigating coronary artery response to acetylcholine or noninvasively by measuring vascular reactivity to increases in shear stress using brachial artery ultrasonography. Normally, acetylcholine stimulates the release of endothelium-derived NO, resulting in vascular relaxation. An impairment in this process is consistent with a NO-mediated defect in the endothelium-dependent vasodilation in response to acetycholine. Endothelium dysfunction in the brachial artery correlates with the presence of abnormal coronary vascular reactivity, which has been identified as a marker for atherothrombosis.

BIBLIOGRAPHY

1. Elveback LR, Connolly DC: Coronary heart disease in residents of Rochester, Minnesota. V: prognosis of patients with coronary heart disease based on initial manifestation. Mayo Clin Proc 60:305–311, 1985.
2. Forgione MA, Leopold JA, Loscalzo J: Roles of endothelial dysfunction in coronary artery disease. Curr Opin Cardiol 15:409–415, 2000.
3. Gibbons RJ, Balady GJ, Bricker JT, et al: 2002 Guideline update for exercise testing. Circulation 106: 1883–1892, 2002.
4. Gibbons RJ, Chatterjee K, Daley J, et al: ACC/AHA/ACP-ASIM guidelines for the management of patients with chronic stable angina. J Am Coll Cardiol 33:2092–2197, 1999.
5. Grundy SM, Pasternak R, Greenland P, et al: Assessment of cardiovascular risk by use of multiple-risk-factor assessment equations. J Am Coll Cardiol 34:1348–1359, 1999.
6. He ZX, Hedrick TD, Pratt CM, et al: Severity of coronary artery calcification by electron beam computed tomography predicts silent myocardial ischemia. Circulation 101: 244–251, 2000.
7. Kannel WB, Feinleib M: Natural history of angina pectoris in the Framingham study: prognosis and survival. Am J Cardiol 29:154–163, 1972.
8. O'Rourke RA, Brundage BH, Froelicher VF, et al: ACC/AHA expert consensus document on electron-beam computed tomography for the diagnosis and prognosis of coronary artery disease. J Am Coll Cardiol 36:326–340, 2000.
9. Pohost GM, O'Rourke RA, Berman DS, et al: Imaging in Cardiovascular Disease. Philadelphia, Lippincott Williams & Wilkins, 2000, pp 543–551.
10. Smith SC, Dove JT, Jacobs AK, et al: ACC/AHA guidelines for percutaneous coronary intervention (revision of the 1993 PTCA Guidelines). J Am Coll Cardiol 37:2215–2238, 2001.

11. CORONARY LESION CLASSIFICATION

Neerav Shah, M.D., and Eduardo de Marchena, M.D.

1. Why is it important to classify coronary lesions?

Lesion classification is important for many reasons. Most importantly, it is useful to help predict procedural success and in combination with clinical factors to predict complication rates.

2. What different classification types exist?

- Ambrose Criteria
- American Heart Association (AHA)/American College of Cardiology (ACC) Criteria
- Society of Coronary Angiography and Interventions (SCAI) Criteria
- ELLIS Classification for Coronary Lesions

3. Explain why the relationship between lesion characteristics and success has not remained constant.

Technology has vastly improved since the advent of coronary intervention. Newer balloons with their low profile, increased pushability, and ability to inflate to higher pressure without bursting has helped. The advent and improvement of coronary stents has also helped. Lastly use of clopidogrel (Plavix) and glycoprotein (GP) IIb/IIIa inhibitors and reduced need for antithrombotic therapy have reduced acute and subacute closures while reducing vascular bleeding complications.

4. What is the Ambrose classification?

Ambrose compared lesion morphology in stable and unstable coronary syndromes. He determined that lesion morphology was predictive of unstable angina. These lesions tended to be more eccentric than those associated with stable angina. Later, his classification system was modified. Type II eccentric lesions are now classified as complex or complicated eccentric lesions.

Concentric → Symmetric narrowing

Type I eccentric → Asymmetric narrowing with smooth borders and a broad neck

Type II eccentric → Asymmetric narrowing with a irregular borders, a narrow neck, or both

Multiple irregularities → Serial lesions or severe diffuse disease

5. What is the AHA/ACC's classification for coronary lesions?

Type A Lesions (High success > 85%, Low Risk)

Discrete (< 10 mm length)	Little or no calcification
Concentric	Not total occlusion
Readily accessible	Not ostial in location
Non-angulated segment < 45 degrees	No major side branch involved
Smooth contour	No thrombus

Type B Lesions (Moderate success 60% to 85%, Moderate Risk)

Tubular (10–20 mm length)	Ostial
Eccentric	Bifurcation lesions requiring double guidewires
Moderate tortuousity of proximal segment	Some thrombus present
Moderate angulation 45 to 90 degrees	Total occlusion < 3 months
Irregular contour	
Moderate to heavy calcification	

Type C Lesions (Low Success < 60% High Risk)

Diffuse (> 20 mm length)	Degenerated vein grafts with friable lesions
Excessive tortuousity of prox.	Segment
Total occlusion > 3 months	
Inability to protect major side branch	
Extreme angulation > 90 degrees	

6. Compare the initial success rate with the AHA/ACC classification to current practice.

	A	B	C
1987, %	>85	60–85	<60
1997, %	97	95	84

7. What is the Society of Coronary Angiography and Interventions (SCAI) classification for coronary lesions?

SCAI Type I (Highest Success; Lowest Risk)
Does not meet criteria for AHA/ACC type C lesion
Patent vessel
SCAI Type II (Type C → Patent)
Diffuse (> 20 mm length)
Excessive tortuosity of proximal segment
Extreme angulation > 90 degrees
Inability to protect major side branches
Degenerated vein grafts with friable lesions
Patent vessel
SCAI Type III
Does not meet criteria for AHA/ACC type C lesion
Occluded vessel
SCAI Type IV (Type C → Occluded)
Diffuse (> 20 mm length)
Excessive tortuosity of proximal segment
Extreme angulation > 90 degrees
Inability to protect major side branches
Degenerated vein grafts with friable lesions
Occluded vessel

8. What differentiates the AHA/ACC classification from the SCAI classification?

The SCAI classification evolved as a result of data from 41,071 interventions between 1993 and 1996. The two main differences were that it showed heterogeneity of procedural success between type B and type C lesions mainly based on vessel patency. This allowed simplification of the classification to C versus non-C and occluded versus patent arteries.

	Success Rate, %
Type A	97.2
Type B patent	96.5
Type B occluded	87.6
Type C patent	90.0
Type C occluded	75.0

9. From 1990 through 1992, the SCAI Registry showed that the lowest volume operators (< 25 interventions) had the highest complication rate. The second highest complication rate was found among the highest volume operators (> 200 interventions). Explain these results.

The skill of the operator obviously plays a role in complication rates. Thus, low-volume operators have the highest complication rate. The highest volume operators are doing a greater number of complex lesions and acute myocardial infarctions, (MIs) thus leading to a higher total complication rate. However, if the complication rate for a high-volume operator was stratified for lesion severity, there would be much less difference between lesion types than for a less skilled operator. The reason the low-volume operator complication rate is not higher is most likely the result of selecting simpler lesions, thus reducing the risk of major complications.

10. What is the Ellis classification for assessing acute procedural success during PCI?

Ellis et al. reviewed 4181 patients to analyze the risk associated with 27 different variables during the glycoprotein IIb/IIIa and stent era. Of these, he found that nine characteristics were helpful in predicting complications. He deemed these terms moderate risk characteristics and strong correlates.

Class I (low risk) → Absence of moderate-risk lesion characteristics
Class II (moderate risk) → One to two moderate-risk lesion characteristics
Class III (high risk) → Three or more moderate-risk lesion characteristics
Class IV (highest risk) → Any strong correlate characteristic

11. What are the moderate risk characteristics used by Ellis?

Length > 10 mm
Lumen irregularity
Large filling defect
Calcium and angulation greater than 45 degrees
Severe calcification
Saphenous vein graft (SVG) > 10 years old
Eccentricity

12. What are the strong correlates of risk as defined by Ellis?
They are nonchronic total occlusion and degenerated SVG.

13. Based on the Ellis classification data, what is the risk of death, MI, and emergent coronary artery bypass graft surgery of the different lesion classes?

Class I → 2.1%
Class II → 3.4%
Class III → 8.2%
Class IV → 12.7%

BIBLIOGRAPHY

1. Ambrose JA, Winters SL, et al. Angiographic morphology and the pathogenesis of unstable angina pectoris. J Am Coll Cardiol 5:609–616, 1985.
2. Ambrose JA, Israel DH: Angiography in unstable angina. Am J Cardiol 68 (Suppl B):78–83, 1991.
3. Ellis SG, Guetta V, Miller D, et al: Relation between lesion characteristics and risk with percutaneous coronary intervention in the stent and glycoprotein IIb/IIIa era: an analysis of results from 10,907 lesions and proposal for new classification scheme. Circulation 100:1971–1976, 1999.
4. Krone RJ, Laskey WK, Johnson C, et al. for the Registry Committee of the Society of Cardiac Angiography and Interventions: A simplified lesion classification for predicting the success and complications of coronary angioplasty. Am Cardiol 85:1179–1184, 2000.
5. Krone RJ: Classification of coronary lesions. Revista de la Federacion Argentina de Cardiologia 12/09/2001 review obtained via internet.
6. Ryan TJ, Faxon DP, Gunnar RM, et al: Guidelines for percutaneous transluminal coronary angioplasty: A report of the American College of Cardiology/American Heart Association Task Force on Assessment of Diagnostic and Therapeutic Cardiovascular Procedures (Subcommittee on Percutantion Transluminal Coronary Angioplasty). Circulation 78:486–502, 1984.
7. Zaacks SM, Allen JE, Calvin JE, et al: Value of the American College of Cardiology/American Heart Association stenosis morphology classification for coronary interventions in the late 1990's. Am J Cardiol 82:43–49, 1998.

III. Pharmacotherapy

12. HEPARIN AND THROMBIN INHIBITORS

Sameer Mehta, M.D., Samir Yebara, M.D., and Martha Reyes, M.D.

1. What is a direct thrombin inhibitor?

A direct thrombin inhibitor is a unique anticoagulant that binds directly to thrombin without requiring the cofactor antithrombin. It demonstrates efficacy in inhibiting both fibrin-bound and free circulating thrombin.

2. How is a direct thrombin inhibitor different from heparin?

Heparin acts as an anticoagulant by binding to antithrombin. It augments the rate at which antithrombin inactivates factor Xa and thrombin by binding to plasma proteins other than antithrombin. In contrast, direct thrombin inhibitors bind directly to thrombin without requiring the cofactor antithrombin.

3. What are the indications of direct thrombin indicators?

The classic indication for the use of direct thrombin inhibitors is in patients presenting with heparin-induced thrombocytopenia (HIT). In addition, bivalirudin is also approved as an alternative to heparin in patients undergoing PCI.

Anecdotal applications have also been used in patients undergoing coronary bypass surgery and for peripheral vascular disease (PVD).

4. Does bivalirudin provide any unique advantages for use in patients with PCI?

Antithrombotic agents appear to be the cornerstone of treatment for patients undergoing PCI. Platelet activation and thrombin result in significant ischemic complications during PCI. Although considerable progress has been made in decreasing these complications, the benefit is often offset by an increased incidence of bleeding. Direct thrombin agents may fill the void of agents used in PCI that accomplish a reduction in ischemic events without resulting in a concomitant increase in bleeding. In addition, bivalirudin possesses a very short half-life ~ 23 min). Beyond a potent direct thrombin inhibition, bivalirudin facilitates removal of the angioplasty sheaths and early ambulation. Data from numerous trials demonstrate the efficacy of bivalirudin in decreasing both the ischemic complications and the incidence of thrombocytopenia. Additionally, bleeding is significantly reduced.

5. What are the various direct thrombin inhibitors in use?

Presently available direct thrombin inhibitors include three parenteral agents: bivalirudin, hirudin, and argatroban. All of these agents bind directly to thrombin without the need of the cofactor antithrombin and are able to inhibit both circulating and clot-bound thrombin. The binding sites to thrombin are different: hirudin and bivalirudin are bivalent inhibitors that bind to thrombin at exocite 1 (the substrate recognition site) and at the active site (Fig. 1). Argatroban binds in a univalent fashion but only at the active site. Whereas hirudin and argatroban are indicated for use in HIT, only bivalirudin is indicated for use in patients with PCI.

6. What are the contraindications of direct thrombin inhibitors?

The contraindications are active internal bleeding; renal impairment (serum creatinine > 4.0 mg/dL); platelet count < 100,000/uL; and severe hypertension (blood pressure [BP] > 180/110 mmHg).

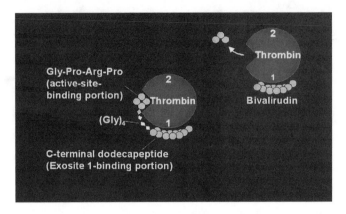

FIGURE 1. Bivalirudin: specific, reversible binding.

7. What studies have been done in relation to acute coronary syndromes (ACS) and PCI?
Numerous studies have been performed to evaluate the use of direct thrombin inhibitors, particularly bivalirudin, in the use of ACS and PCI. These include:

a. BAT (Bivalirudin Angioplasty Trial)
Study objective: To establish the safety of bivalirudin in patients undergoing PCI who are unable to tolerate heparin. This phase 3 study is to determine the safety of administration of bivalirudin in patients with HIT or HIT and thrombosis syndrome (HITTS) who are undergoing PCI. The significant results reported by Bittle et al. demonstrated the following:

- Bivalirudin was found to reduce the incidence of hemorrhagic complications by 62% compared with heparin during hospitalization after PCI. This effect was consistent across all patient subgroups.
- Bivalirudin resulted in a statistically significant 22% reduction in the combined clinical endpoint of death, myocardial infarction (MI), or revascularization within 7 days in the overall patient population.
- Bivalirudin resulted in a 51% reduction in ischemic events and a 73% reduction in major bleeding complication in the prespecified, separately randomized subset of patients with postinfarction angina.

b. REPLACE I
Study objective: To confirm the safety and efficacy of bivalirudin in the modern PCI setting, which includes stenting glycoprotein (GP) IIb/IIIa agents, and other antiplatelet therapies. This study demonstrates the efficacy of bivalirudin (0.75 mg/kg bolus followed by 1.75 mg/kg/h during the procedure) compared with heparin within the context of contemporary interventional practice ($n = 1056$), showing:

- A mean ACT of 304 seconds and 371 seconds were achieved among heparin- and bivalirudin-treated patients, respectively.
- Death and revascularization were reduced by 19% (6.9% to 5.6%) in the bivalirudin-treated patients at 48 hours. A 22% (3.4% to 2.8%) reduction in protocol defined major bleeding and a 19% (9.4% to 7.5%) reduction in the composite quadruple endpoint of death, MI, revascularization, and major bleeding at 48 hours were observed.
- Among patients receiving intravenous GP IIb/IIIa platelet receptor-blocking agents, bivalirudin demonstrated a 14% (10.3% to 8.8%) reduction in death, MI, and revascularization at 48 hours.

c. **CACHET A**

Study objective: To determine the coagulation profile and safety of bivalirudin when combined with abciximab in patients undergoing PCI. This study showed that administrations of full-dose bivalirudin (1 mg/kg bolus followed by 2.5 mg/kg/h for 4 hours) plus full-dose abciximab ($n = 30$), resulted in:

- Predictable and manageable anticoagulation with ACT of approximately 350 seconds
- Clinically meaningful inhibition of thrombin
- 80% to 90% inhibition of adenosine diphosphate (ADP)–induced platelet aggregation
- No excessive risk of hemorrhage or clinical ischemia

d. **CACHET B/C**

Study objective: To determine the safety of administration of reduced-dose bivalirudin with provisional abciximab. This study showed that administration of Angiomax (0.5–0.75 mg/kg bolus followed by 1.75 mg/kg/h during the procedure) with provisional administration of full dose abciximab ($n = 144$):

- Achieved and immediate ACT of approximately 280 to 230 seconds.
- Showed no apparent pharmacologic interaction with abciximab.
- Was associated with lower combined incidence of major adverse clinical outcomes, MI, revascularization, and major hemorrhage compared with heparin/abciximab ($n = 64$): (3.5% vs. 14.1%, P = 0.013).
- Among patients developing intraprocedural indications for provisional GP IIb/IIIa inhibitor use, a comparable ischemic event rate (5.9%) was observed.

8. Are there any significant ongoing trials with bivalirudin?

A larger trial is presently being conducted to validate the results of the REPLACE I trial. The REPLACE II trial is a large, multicenter, randomized, double-blind trial that is evaluating the safety and efficacy of bivalirudin (65 U/Kg heparin intravenous bolus) plus a GP IIb/IIIa inhibitor versus bivalirudin monotherapy (0.75 mg/kg bolus followed by a 1.75-mg/kg/h infusion [for ≤ 4 hours] with provisional GP IIb/IIIa therapy). Enrollment for REPLACE II is expected to be completed in late 2002.

9. What did the meta-analysis of bivalirudin data show?

A recent meta-analysis of 11 randomized clinical trials that compared direct thrombin inhibitors with heparin for treatment of ACS, including patients undergoing PCI, evaluated primary data from more than 35,000 patients. Compared with heparin, direct thrombin inhibitors produced a significant reduction in the combined endpoint of death and MI at the end of therapy (Fig. 2). Most of the benefit of direct thrombin inhibitors reflected a reduction in the endpoint of MI.

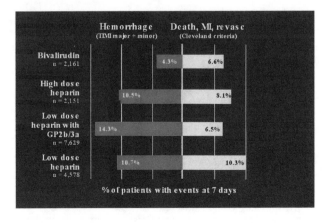

FIGURE 2. Cleveland Clinic meta-analysis of bivalirudin.

10. Are there any noncoronary applications of direct thrombin inhibitors?
Direct thrombin inhibitors are approved for treatment of patients with HIT. There is also increased use in peripheral interventions and in patients undergoing cardiac surgery as well as anecdotal reports of the use of these agents in patients with thrombotic venous disease and atrial fibrillation.

11. Can direct thrombin inhibitor be used in patients with acute MI?
Direct thrombin inhibitors have been extensively studied for their use in patients with acute MI. In a pilot angiographic phase II study (HERO I), 45 patients presenting within 6 hours of the onset of ST elevation MI were given 325 mg of aspirin and randomized to receive either bivalirudin or heparin as adjunctive therapy with streptokinase. Bivalirudin was administered in a dosage of 0.5 mg/kg/h for the first 12 hours and then 0.1 mg/kg/h. Heparin was administered in a dosage of 1000 IU/h and titrated to maintain the activated partial thromboplastin time (aPTT) at 2.0 to 2.5 time's control. At 90 minutes after treatment, thrombolysis in myocardial infarction (TIMI) grade 3 flow in the infarct artery was achieved in 67% of bivalirudin-treated patients versus 40% of heparin-treated patients. The duration of chest pain was shorter in the bivalirudin group, and the bleeding rates were similar (67%) in both treatment groups.

12. What is the future of direct thrombin inhibitors?
Direct thrombin inhibitors are a promising advance in antithrombin therapy. In particular, bivalirudin appears to have a favorable profile for PCI. Its predictable anticoagulant effect and short therapeutic half-life are attractive attributes for PCI. From early data, bivalirudin has demonstrated significant reduction in ischemic and bleeding complications. It is yet unclear if bivalirudin will prove to be monotherapy for PCI (inhibiting thrombin during the intrusion of the vasculature with PTCA hardware) or a complement to platelet receptor–blocking agents. Results of the REPLACE II trial will shed light on this aspect of bivalirudin use. Similarly, results from other ongoing trials will demonstrate the noncoronary applications of direct thrombin inhibitors.

13. What are the advantages of direct thrombin inhibitors?
Direct thrombin inhibitors have a few specific advantages, which are as follows:
- The ability to inhibit thrombin regardless of its location (fibrin-bound vs. soluble thrombin), a property of potential importance to patients with visible thrombi on angiography before stent placement
- Rapid return to hemostatic competence upon cessation of infusion (short plasma and biologic half-life)
- The ability to inhibit thrombin-mediated platelet aggregation
- The ability to achieve high levels of anticoagulation without causing platelet activation

14. What are the limitations of using heparin in ACS and PCI?
Despite remaining the traditional anticoagulant used in ACS and PCI, heparin has several limitations. Table 1 provides a list of these potential constraints, which have fuelled the search a better antithrombotic agent.

Table 1. Limitations of Heparin

1. Indirect thrombin inhibitor acting via antithrombin
2. Unable to inhibit clot-bound thrombin
3. Activity diminished by platelet factor-4
4. Nonlinear pharmacokinetics
5. Immunogenic potential
6. Clinically unpredictable dose response
7. Poor effect in acute disease
8. Narrow therapeutic window
9. "Rebound phenomenon" (thrombin generation)
10. Anticoagulant resistance

15. What are the features of HIT?

The incidence, time course, and clinical features of HIT and the more ominous heparin-associated thrombotic thrombocytopenia (HATT) are shown in Table 2. Platelet transfusion should be avoided in patients with HIT because of the risk of thrombotic complications.

Table 2. Heparin-induced Thrombocytopenia

	TYPE I	TYPE II (HATT)
Incidence	10%	Rare
Mechanism	Direct platelet aggregating effect of heparin	Autoantibody (IgG or IgM) directed against platelet factor IV–heparin complex
Onset	Early (1–5 days)	Late (> 5 days); may occur sooner if prior heparin exposure
Platelet count	50,000/mm^3–150,000 mm^3	< 50,000/mm^3
Duration	Transient; often improves even if heparin is continued	Requires discontinuation of *all* heparin; gradual recovery in platelet count over 1–5 days in most patients
Clinical course	Benign	Refractory venous and arterial thromboses and thromboembolism; may be fatal

BIBLIOGRAPHY

1. Bates SM, Weitz JI: Direct thrombin inhibitors for treatment of arterial thrombosis: potential differences between bivalirudin and Hirudin. Am J Cardiol 2(suppl B):12–18, 1998.
2. Bittl JA, Strony J, Brinker JA, et al: Treatment with bivalirudin (Hirulog) as compared with heparin during coronary angioplasty for unstable or post infarction angina. N Engl J Med 333:764–769, 1995.
3. Campbell KR, Mahaffey KW, Lewis BE, et al: Bivalirudin in patients with heparin-induced thrombocytopenia undergoing percutaneous coronar intervention. J Invasive Cardiol 12(suppl F):14–19, 2000.
4. Cannon CP, Maraganore JM, Loscalzo J, et al: Anticoagulant effects of hirulog, a novel thrombin inhibitor, in patients with coronary artery disease. Am J Cardiol 71:778–782, 1993.
5. Cannon CP, Weintraub WS, Demopoulos LA, et al: Comparison of early invasive and conservative strategies in patients with unstable coronary syndromes treated with the glycoprotein IIb/IIIa inhibitor tirofiban. N Engl J Med 344:1879–1887, 2001.
6. Fuchs J, Cannon CP, and the TIMI 7 Investigators: Hirulog in the treatment of unstable angina: results of the Thrombin Inhibition in Myocardial Ischaemia (TIMI) 7 Trial. Circulation 92:727–733.
7. Hirulog and Early Reperfusion or Occlusion (HERO)-2 Trial Investigators: Thrombin-specific anticoagulation with bivalirudin versus heparin in patients receiving fibrinolytic therapy for acute myocardial infarction: the HERO-2 randomized trial. Lancet 358:1855–1863, 2001.
8. Kong DF, Topol EJ, Bittl JA, et al: Clinical outcomes of bivalirudin for ischemic heart disease. Circulation 100:2049–2053, 1999.
9. Kottke-Marchant K, Lincoff AM, Kleiman N, et al: Direct thrombin inhibition by bivalirudin compared with abciximab, a GPIIb/IIIa antagonist, during percutaneous coronary intervention: favorable hemostatic profile compared to heparin/abciximab. Blood 94(suppl 1, part 1):623, 1999.
10. Lincoff AM, Bittl JA, Kleiman NS, et al: The REPLACE 1 Trial: a pilot study of bivalirudin versus heparin during percutaneous coronary intervention with stenting and GP IIb/IIIa blockade [abstract]. J Am Coll Cardiol 39(suppl A):16–17, 2002.
11. Maraganore JM, et al: Heparin variability and resistance: comparison with a direct thrombin inhibitor [abstract]. Circulation 86(suppl I):386, 1992.
12. Maraganore JM, Adelman BA: Hirulog: a direct thrombin inhibitor for management of acute coronary syndromes. Coron Artery Dis 7:438–448, 1996.
13. Topol EJ, Bonan R, Jewitt D, et al: Use of a direct antithrombin, hirulog, in place of heparin during coronary angioplasty. Circulation 87:1622–1629, 1993.
14. White HD, Aylward PE, Frey MJ, et al: Randomized, double-blind comparison of hirulog versus heparin in patients receiving streptokinase and aspirin for acute myocardial infarction (HERO). Circulation 96:2155–2161, 1997.

13. ASPIRIN AND THE THIENOPYRIDINES

Maria Isabel López, M.D.

1. What is the pathophysiologic basis for the use of antiplatelet agents in ischemic syndromes?

Constituents of blood do not normally interact with intact endothelium. Thrombosis superimposed on a disrupted atherosclerotic plaque is the main pathophysiologic event in acute ischemic syndromes. The response to plaque disruption involves both platelet activation and thrombin generation. Exposed subendothelial structures are highly thrombogenic (e.g., von Willebrand factor and collagen), and generation of thrombin leads to platelet aggregation with further thrombus growth.

Thrombin appears to be the most important platelet agonist generated at sites of vascular injury; other platelet "activators" are adenosine diphosphate (ADP) and thromboxane A_2 (TXA_2). These agonists provoke the expression of functional receptors for fibrinogen on the platelet surface known as glycoprotein (GP) IIb/IIIa receptors (most abundant receptor on platelets with 40 to 80.000 copies on each) as well as for other adhesive molecules. Because of its high concentration in plasma, fibrinogen is the preferred ligand for this receptors, which are the common final pathway in platelet aggregation.

Aspirin (ASA), through its permanent inactivation of prostaglandin (PG) H synthase 1 or cyclooxygenase (COX)–1, blocks the production of PGH_2, the immediate precursor of TXA_2. The thienopyridines (ticlopidine and clopidogrel) are direct inhibitors of ADP receptors on platelets.

2. Is the inhibition of prostacylin by ASA clinically important?

Human platelets and vascular endothelial cells process PGH_2 to produce TXA_2 and prostacyclin (PGI_2), respectively. TXA_2 induces platelet aggregation and vasoconstriction, and PGI_2 inhibits platelet aggregation and induces vasodilatation.

ASA is approximately 50 to 100 times more potent in inhibiting platelet COX-1 than monocyte COX-2. Vascular prostacyclin can derive from both COX-1 and COX-2; COX-2 is largely insensitive to ASA inhibition at conventional antiplatelet doses. This may account for the substantial residual COX-2–dependent PGI_2 biosynthesis *in vivo* at daily doses of ASA in the range of 30 to 100 mg, despite transient suppression of COX-1–dependent PGI release. Whereas vascular endothelial cells regenerate new COX and thus recover normal function, COX inhibition in platelets is irreversible.

Available data suggest that the potentially prothrombotic effects of PGI_2 inhibition are not clinically relevant and that the antithrombotic effects of TXA_2 inhibition predominate. Low-dose ASA or controlled-release preparations may result in somewhat preferential inhibition of platelet COX over endothelial COX.

3. Should ASA be used in patients without clinically apparent atherosclerotic coronary disease?

Approximately 25% of the reduction in the rate of death from coronary disease that has occurred during the past 30 years may be explained by the practice of primary prevention. In addition to the established risk factors of hypertension, smoking, hypercholesterolemia, diabetes, and sedentary lifestyle, the risk of coronary disease is known to be related to platelet activity and inflammation. ASA has both antiplatelet and antiinflammatory effects and has been tested for use in primary prevention.

In the 1970s, prospective cohort and case-control studies suggested that regular ASA use could reduce the risk of myocardial infarction (MI) and death from coronary causes. Since then, there have been five major randomized trials of ASA for the prevention of coronary events: the British Doctors' Trial, Physicians' Health Study, Thrombosis Prevention Trial, Hypertension Optimal Treatment Study, and Primary Prevention Project. With the exception of the British Doctors' Trial, all showed a reduction in the rates of cardiovascular events, mainly secondary to a reduction in the occurrence of MI. None of the trials showed a reduction in the risk of death from any cause or in the risk of stroke.

With the exception of the British Doctors' Trial, all the trials showed an increase in the risk of clinical hemorrhage with ASA use, with the gastrointestinal (GI) tract the most common site of major bleeding. It can be concluded from these trials that ASA reduces the risk of MI in men at risk who are older than age 50 years. It is important to note that most participants in the randomized trials of ASA were men; thus, it is unclear whether ASA therapy prevents MI in women. An ongoing study of 40,000 female health care professionals in the United States is comparing low-dose ASA (100 mg every other day) with placebo for the primary prevention of coronary disease.

For individual patients, the decision to initiate ASA therapy should be based on a careful assessment of absolute risk. The absolute risk of major coronary events should be calculated as the Framingham risk score (Table 1). Patients with an estimated risk of coronary events of 1.5 % per year or higher are, if no contraindications exist, good candidates for ASA prophylaxis, but those with a risk of 0.6 % per year or less are probably not. Among patients with an intermediate level of risk—that is, 0.7% to 1.4 % per year—other factors should be considered, including the preference of the patient; treatment should be considered more seriously if there is well-controlled hypertension with target organ damage, diabetes mellitus, or poor physical fitness.

Because the antithrombotic effect of ASA is achieved with doses as low as 30 mg/day and the GI toxicity appears to be dose related, the lowest dose of ASA shown effective should be used. The Second Joint Task Force of European and Other Societies on Coronary Prevention recommend 75 mg of ASA daily in patients with treated hypertension and in men who are at particularly high risk for coronary artery disease (CAD).

The absolute risk of vascular complications versus the risk of side effects determines the net benefit of antiplatelet prophylaxis.

Table 1. Framingham Scoring System for Calculating the 10-Year Risk of Major Coronary Events in Adults without Diabetes

Estimate of 10-Year Risk for Men (Framingham Point Scores)		Estimate of 10-Year Risk for Women (Framingham Point Scores)	
AGE	POINTS	AGE	POINTS
20–34	−9	20–34	−7
35–39	−4	35–39	−3
40–44	0	40–44	0
45–49	3	45–49	3
50–54	6	50–54	6
55–59	8	55–59	8
60–64	10	60–64	10
65–69	11	65–69	12
70–74	12	70–74	14
75–79	13	75–79	16

TOTAL CHOLESTEROL (mg/dl)	POINTS AGE					TOTAL CHOLESTEROL (mg/dl)	POINTS AGE				
	20–39	40–49	50–59	60–69	70–79		20–39	40–49	50–59	60–69	70–79
< 160	0	0	0	0	0	< 160	0	0	0	0	0
160–199	4	3	2	1	0	160–199	4	3	2	1	1
200–239	7	5	3	1	0	200–239	8	6	4	2	1
240–279	9	6	4	2	1	240–279	11	8	5	3	2
> 280	11	8	6	3	1	> 280	13	10	7	4	2

(continued)

Table 1. Framingham Scoring System for Calculating the 10-year Risk of Major Coronary Events in Adults without Diabetes (Continued)

Estimate of 10-Year Risk for Men (Framingham Point Scores)						Estimate of 10-Year Risk for Women (Framingham Point Scores)					
	POINTS						POINTS				
	AGE						AGE				
	20–39	40–49	50–59	60–69	70–79		20–39	40–49	50–59	60–69	70–79
Nonsmoker	0	0	0	0	0	Nonsmoker	0	0	0	0	0
Smoker	8	6	3	1	1	Smoker	9	7	4	2	1

HDL (mg/dl)	POINTS	HDL (mg/dl)	POINTS
> 60	−1	> 60	−1
50–59	0	50–59	0
40–49	1	40–49	1
< 40	2	< 40	2

SYSTOLIC BP (mmHg)	POINTS		SYSTOLIC BP (mmHg)	POINTS	
	IF UNTREATED	IF TREATED		IF UNTREATED	IF TREATED
< 120	0	0	< 120	0	0
120–129	0	1	120–129	1	3
130–139	1	2	130–139	2	4
140–159	1	2	140–159	3	5
> 160	2	3	> 160	4	6

	POINTS TOTAL	10-YEAR RISK %		POINTS TOTAL	10-YEAR RISK %
	< 0	< 1		< 9	< 1
	0	1		9	1
	1	1		10	1
	2	1		11	1
	3	1		12	1
	4	1		13	2
	5	2		14	2
	6	2		15	3
	7	3		16	4
	8	4		17	5
	9	5		18	6
	10	6		19	8
	11	8		20	11
	12	10		21	14
	13	12		22	17
	14	16		23	22
	15	20		24	27
10-year risk ____%	16	25	10-year risk ____%	> 25	>30
	> 17	> 30			

BP = blood pressure; HDL = high-density lipoprotein cholesterol. All age ranges are given in years. To convert values for cholesterol to millimoles per liter, multiply by 0.02586. Reprinted from the National Heart, Lung, and Blood Institute, May 2001.

4. What are the thienopyridines?

Ticlopidine and clopidogrel are structurally related compounds with platelet inhibitory properties. Clopidogrel differs structurally from ticlopidine by the addition of a carboxymethyl side group. They selectively inhibit ADP-induced platelet aggregation with no direct effects on arachidonic acid metabolism.

These drugs can also inhibit platelet aggregation induced by collagen and thrombin, but these effects are lost by increasing the agonist concentration and, therefore, are likely to reflect blockade of ADP-mediated amplification of the platelet response to other agonists. Both agents undergo hepatic transformation into active metabolites, which are primarily excreted renally. Maximal bioavailability occurs when they are taken after meals. The full antiplatelet action of ticlopidine is delayed for several days after commencement of therapy; by contrast, the full antiplatelet action of clopidogrel after a 300-mg bolus is evident after several hours.

5. How sensitive are platelets to the different oral "antiplatelet" agents?

Experimental studies in rats indicate that clopidogrel is 50 times more potent than ticlopidine and about 110-fold more active than ASA. However, recommended doses of clopidogrel achieve the same level of inhibition of ADP-induced platelet activation as ticlopidine. Platelets are exquisitely sensitive to ASA, and only 30 mg daily effectively eliminates the synthesis of TXA_2. All agents cause irreversible platelet inhibition that persists for 7 to 10 days after therapy is stopped. In the case of ASA, COX-1 inhibition is irreversible for the lifetime of the platelet because of the limited mRNA and protein synthesis in these anuclear cells; this time course corresponds to the lifespan of a circulating platelet. Synergy has been shown with concomitant use of ASA and thienopyridines, reflecting their different mechanisms of action.

ASA is a relatively weak antiplatelet agent because it provides insufficient blockade of the platelet activation that is induced by ADP, collagen, and low concentrations of thrombin, and it provides no inhibition of platelet adhesion. Instead, thienopyridines achieve moderate levels of platelet inhibition. By blocking the effects of ADP released from platelet-dense granules and inhibiting granule release, they also inhibit platelet aggregation induced by other agonists, including thromboxane analogues, platelet activating factor, collagen, and low concentrations of thrombin.

6. How fast do oral "antiplatelet" agents act?

ASA is rapidly absorbed from the upper GI tract, and measurable inhibition of platelet function is evident within 60 minutes; after an oral single dose of 100 mg, the serum concentration of TXB_2 (product of the hydrolysis of TXA_2) is decreased by 98%. These effects occur even before acetylsalicylic acid is detectable in the peripheral blood, owing to the exposure of platelets to ASA in the portal circulation.

Enteric coating significantly delays its absorption and peak plasma levels for up to 3 to 4 hours.

Thienopyridines require hepatic conversion to active metabolites through the cytochrome P450–1A enzyme system. Some prolongation of bleeding time begins immediately after oral administration of thienopyridines; significant inhibition is present after 2 to 3 days of therapy, and maximal inhibition, equivalent to 40% to 60% of ADP-induced platelet aggregation, takes 4 to 7 days to be achieved. Higher doses do not result in further platelet impairment, but loading doses appear to improve the speed of their antithrombotic activity

7. What is the current role of ASA in CAD?

Some of the strongest evidence available about the long-term prognostic effects of therapy in patients with CAD pertain to ASA.

The Second International Study of Infarct Survival (ISIS-2) unequivocally established the benefit of ASA in patients with acute MI. This trial randomized 17,187 patients to receive intravenous streptokinase, ASA 162.5 mg a day for 30 days, both, or neither. At the end of 5 weeks, patients receiving ASA alone had a highly significant 23% reduction in vascular mortality and a nearly 50% reduction in the risk of nonfatal reinfarction and nonfatal stroke. There was no increase in major bleeding complications, and the mortality benefit was maintained after a 10-year follow-up.

Among all clinical investigations with ASA, trials with unstable angina (UA) and non–ST segment elevation MI (NSTEMI) have most consistently documented a striking benefit of the drug, with a significant decrease in the incidence of death and nonfatal MI (despite differences in study design, such as time of entry after the acute phase, duration of follow up, and doses).

The VA Cooperative Study of ASA in men with unstable angina randomized 1266 patients to either 324 mg of ASA or placebo. The principal outcome was death or nonfatal MI, which was reduced from 10% to 5% over a 12-week follow-up period. Eighty-six percent of patients were followed up to 1 year, and a mortality reduction of 43% was found in the ASA-treated group. ASA should be initiated at a daily dose of 160 to 325 mg in patients with UA/NSEMI; the first dose should be chewed to rapidly establish a high blood level.

ASA is the standard therapy in patients undergoing percutaneous coronary intervention (PCI), and was the first oral antiplatelet agent shown to reduce ischemic events after PCI.

8. Does ASA therapy increase the conversion of an ischemic stroke into a hemorrhagic one?

There is biochemical evidence of episodic platelet activation during the first 48 hours after the onset of symptoms of an acute ischemic stroke and also of the suppression of *in vivo* TXA_2 biosynthesis in patients receiving low-dose ASA in this setting.

Two large, randomized trials of ASA use in the setting of acute, ischemic stroke (International Stroke Trial and Chinese Acute Stroke Trial) showed no significant increase in hemorrhagic stroke. Importantly, they demonstrated a significant decrease in the risk of recurrent stroke and in the combined incidence of death or nonfatal stroke. These results correspond to a reduction of 10 deaths or recurrent strokes per 1000 patients after 2 to 4 weeks of ASA therapy. Combined, these trials enrolled more than 40,000 patients within 48 hours of the onset of neurologic symptoms.

The ASA and Carotid Endarterectomy (ACE) trial unequivocally demonstrated that low doses of ASA (80–325 mg) are at least as effective as higher doses (500 to 1000 mg) in preventing stroke, MI, or death within 3 months of carotid endarterectomy.

9. How convenient is the familiar combination of ACE inhibitors with ASA or the thienopyridines?

Concomitant use of ASA and ACE inhibitors is frequent in patients with heart failure caused by CAD. Negative interaction between aspirin and enalapril has been reported, presumably through inhibition by ASA of ACE inhibitor–induced prostaglandin synthesis. ACE inhibitors inhibit the degradation of bradykinins, potent vasodilators, which are also known to enhance local production of vasodilatory prostaglandins.

A randomized, comparative trial of enalapril plus ASA (325 mg/day) or ticlopidine (500 mg daily) in patients with chronic heart failure showed a better reduction of systemic vascular resistance with the enalapril–ticlopidine association. Interestingly, the prostaglandin-independent action of ACE inhibition on the pulmonary vasculature was not altered, and total pulmonary resistance decreased significantly and equally in both groups.

A recent review of the literature suggests that whereas low-dose ASA ($\leq$ 100 mg/day) has very little interaction with the effects of ACE inhibitors, higher doses may attenuate the benefit of these agents in patients with hypertension and heart failure. In the Clopidogrel versus Aspirin in Patients at Risk of Ischemic Events (CAPRIE) trial, patients taking ASA plus ACE inhibitors were more likely to have hypertension, but the reduction in the primary endpoint (ischemic stroke, MI, vascular death) by clopidogrel over ASA was not affected by the concomitant use of ACE inhibitors.

The upcoming WATCH trial (Warfarin and Antiplatelet Therapy in Chronic Heart failure) will determine the optimal antithrombotic therapy for patients with chronic heart failure and will also examine the potential interaction between ASA and ACE inhibitors.

10. Do enteric coating or lower doses reduce the GI side effects of ASA?

The widely held belief that enteric-coated and buffered varieties of ASA are less likely to cause major upper GI bleeding than plain tablets was tested in a multicenter, case-control study. The relative risks (RRs) of upper GI bleeding for plain, enteric-coated, and buffered ASA at average daily doses of 325 mg/day or less were 2.6, 2.7, and 3.1, respectively. At doses greater than 325 mg, the RR was 5.8 for plain ASA and 7.0 for buffered ASA. Thus, it should not be assumed that these formulations are less likely to cause GI tract bleeding than plain ASA.

Even when administered at low doses, ASA can cause serious GI bleeding, as reported in studies using 30 to 50 mg daily. This is consistent with the mechanism of action made responsible for its GI side effects (i.e., inhibition of gastro-protective PG synthesis).

A case-control study found increased rates of GI bleeding with higher doses of ASA. A general change to lower doses (75 mg day) of ASA would not eliminate the risk but would reduce it by about 40% compared with 300 mg/day.

11. Should oral "antiplatelet agents" be used in patients undergoing coronary artery bypass surgery (CABG)?

CABG with saphenous vein graft (SVG) is associated with a 5% to 15% occlusion rate during the first postoperative month; this phenomenon is largely related to thrombosis at the anastomotic site caused by endothelial disruption and vessel damage. When given 6 hours after surgery, if no contraindications exist, ASA clearly decreases the rate of early thrombotic graft occlusion by about 50% and, if continued for 1 year, it further decreases the rate of occlusive events. Preoperative administration of ASA is associated with increased bleeding complications and offers no additional benefit in early graft patency compared with 6 hours postoperatively.

In the CURE trial (Clopidogrel in USA to prevent Recurrent events), patients who stopped clopidogrel less than 5 days before CABG experienced an increased risk of major bleeding complications by an absolute rate of 3.3%. A number of reports have documented an increased transfusion requirement and a four- to 10-fold increased risk of surgical reexploration for postoperative bleeding in patients who underwent CABG within 3 days of clopidogrel and ticlopidine administration.

If thienopyridines are used before CABG, the operation shoul be delayed at least 5 days — ideally, 7 days — to avoid serious bleeding complications.

12. What is the role of thienopyridines in patients with ischemic cerebrovascular disease?

The most common and most important vascular disease that affects both the brain and the heart is atherosclerosis. The most frequent cause of death in stroke patients is CAD.

The Ticlopidine ASA Stroke Study (TASS) randomized in a blinded fashion 3069 patients with a history of transient ischemic attack (TIA), amaurosis fugax, or minor stroke to receive 500 mg of ticlopidine or 1300 mg of ASA. In a follow-up of 2 to 6 years, there was a 12% decrease in the risk of nonfatal stroke or death of any cause with ticlopidine compared with ASA. The benefit was evident in the first year of therapy and persisted throughout the 6 years of the study.

In CAPRIE, clopidogrel was slightly superior to ASA in the prevention of vascular death, nonfatal or fatal stroke, and MI in treated patients. In the group of 6431 patients recruited with a history of a completed atherothrombotic stroke wihin the previous 6 months, the clopidogrel treated patients had an average annual event rate of 7.15% compared with 7.71% for those given ASA ($P = 0.26$).

In summary, randomized studies have shown that thienopyridines are equivalent, if not slightly superior, to ASA in the secondary prevention of cerebrovascular disease. The safety profile of these agents must be taken into account before recommending their long-term use.

Combined therapy may provide additional protection, mainly if ASA has been unsuccessful. The upcoming CHARISMA trial (Clopidogrel for High Atherothrombotic Risk and Ischemic Stabilization, Management and Avoidance) will investigate the role of clopidogrel plus standard therapy (including low doses of ASA) in more than 15,000 patients at high risk of atherothrombotic events or with evidence of atherosclerotic disease.

13. Are platelets from diabetic patients any different?

Numerous mechanisms have been purported to explain the exceptionally poor outcome of patients with diabetes mellitus (DM) and CAD. Diabetic patients have a propensity for adverse arterial remodeling, aggressive atherosclerosis, abnormal endothelial function, and platelet hyperactivity.

Diabetic platelets are larger, have a greater number of GP IIb/IIIa receptors and aggregate more readily to known agonists *in vitro* than platelets from nondiabetic patients. In an *ex vivo* model, a greater percentage of diabetic platelets were found to circulate in an activated state.

DM is associated with a risk of fatal CAD that is as high as the risk associated with a history of MI in patients without diabetes. Thus, it is not surprising that diabetic patients derive substantial benefit from ASA therapy. In the physicians' Health Study, ASA use reduced the risk of MI in patients with diabetes from 10% to 4% during 5 years of follow-up, and no interactions with treatments for diabetes were noted. ASA administration is requisite among diabetic patients with CAD and seems prudent in patients with DM type 2 at risk for CAD.

Thienopyridines may confer additional benefit among diabetic patients with macrovascular disease. In a CAPRIE substudy of 4000 diabetic patients randomized to clopidogrel versus ASA, a significant benefit was demonstrated for clopidogrel with an annual combined event rate of 15.6% versus 17.7% ($P = 0.042$).

14. What is the role of oral antiplatelet agents in chronic peripheral vascular disease?

Atherosclerosis is the cause of the vast majority of cases of chronic peripheral arterial occlusive disease. The arteries most frequently involved, in order of occurrence, are femoropopliteal-tibial, aortoiliac, carotid and vertebral, splanchnic and renal, and brachiocephalic.

In chronic disease, antithrombotic therapy is designed to prevent progression and thrombotic occlusion or to prevent thrombotic complications after vascular reconstruction and other interventions.

ASA therapy may modify the natural history of chronic lower extremity arterial insufficiency. Data from level I studies suggest that ASA delays the progression of established arterial occlusive disease as assessed by serial angiography and decreases the need for arterial reconstruction when used for primary prevention of adverse cardiovascular events in men.

Ticlopidine has also been evaluated in patients with intermittent claudication. In STIMS (Swedish Ticlopidine Multicentre Study), patients with claudication needed fewer vascular surgery procedures with 250 mg of ticlopidine per day versus placebo over a 7-year follow-up period.

The relative efficacy of clopidogrel compared with ASA in reducing the risk of a composite endpoint of ischemic stroke, MI, or vascular death was evaluated in the CAPRIE trial with more than 19,000 patients. The study population was composed of patients with recent ischemic stroke, recent MI, or symptomatic peripheral arterial disease. The overall incidence of composite endpoints was lower in the group treated with clopidogrel (5.32% per year) than with ASA (5.83%; $P = 0.043$).

It is important to note that a subgroup analysis revealed that virtually all of the benefit in the study associated with clopidogrel was observed in the group with symptomatic peripheral vascular disease, who as a group sustained fewer MIs and vascular-related deaths.

15. How do thienopyridines compare regarding major side effects?

Because of their structural similarity, thienopyridines share many side effects but differ regarding their frequency.

Similar to all antithrombotic agents, bleeding is common with thienopyridines. However, in the case of ticlopidine, the incidence of major hemorrhage in stent and stroke trials has been less than 2% and as low as 0.2% compared with either ASA or placebo. Clopidogrel is also infrequently associated with severe bleeding. In the large CAPRIE trial, major hemorrhage occurred in 1.4% of treated patients, not significantly different than the 1.6% observed with ASA.

Ticlopidine can result in neutropenia, a side effect that can be fatal. Neutropenia tipically occurs in the first few months after initiation of therapy, but it is seen infrequently in the first 2 to 3 weeks of therapy. It is, therefore, recommended that blood counts be checked every 2 weeks for at least the first 3 months of therapy. In most, but not all cases, the neutropenia resolves with cessation of drug administration within 1 to 3 weeks. In TASS, absolute neutrophil counts less than 1.200 cells occurred in 2.4%, and counts less than 450 cells occurred in 0.9% compared with 0% of patients receiving ASA.

Clopidogrel was developed because it did not show bone marrow toxicity in tissue cultures. In the CAPRIE trial, the incidence of severe neutropenia was only 0.1%, similar to the rate seen with ASA (0.17%).

Another serious and often fatal side effect of thienopyridines is thrombotic thrombocytopenic purpura (TTP). The estimated incidence of this complication with ticlopidine is one per 1600 to 5000 patients treated. In a review documenting 60 cases of ticlopidine-induced TTP world-wide, the associated mortality rate was 33%. Only two of the 60 cases occurred after less than 2 weeks of ticlopidine administration; this supports the relative safety of shorter therapy after coronary stent placement. In more than 3 million patients exposed to clopidogrel, TTP has been described in only 11. Some differences have been found in TTP induced by these agents. First, among ticlopidine-treated patients, 95% of the cases occurred between 2 weeks and 3 months of exposure; in clopidogrel-treated patients, all but one case occurred within 2 weeks of initiation of therapy. Second, TTP induced by ticlopidine responds better to plasma exchanges and has fewer relapses than clopidogrel-induced TTP.

16. What is the role of thienopyridines in acute coronary syndromes?

The use of antiplatelet therapy is based on the now well-established pathophysiology of the acute syndromes of CAD: UA, acute MI, and sudden death.

The Studio della Ticlopidina nell'Angina Instabile Group examined the role of ticlopidine in 6532 patients with UA. There was a 6.3% reduction in the combined endpoint of vascular death and nonfatal MI with 250 mg bid of ticlopidine compared with no antiplatelet therapy, similar to the benefit seen with ASA in UA. However, there was no placebo arm, and the study was performed on an open-label basis.

The Clopidogrel in unstable angina to prevent Recurrent ischemic events (CURE) study compared the concomitant use of clopidogrel plus ASA versus placebo plus ASA in 12,562 patients with unstable angina. Clopidogrel 300 mg loading dose followed by 75 mg/day was given for a mean period of 9 months. ASA 75 to 325 mg was started or continued simultaneously with the study drug. The first primary outcome—a composite of death from cardiovascular causes, nonfatal MI, or stroke—occurred in 9.3% of the patients in the clopidogrel group and 11.4% of the patients in the placebo group. There were significantly more patients with major bleeding in the clopidogrel group than in the placebo group, but there were not significantly more patients with episodes of life-threatening bleeding or hemorrhagic strokes.

The ongoing CHARISMA trial will further clarify the role of combined antiplatelet therapy in patients at high risk of atherothrombotic events.

Currently, ticlopidine and clopidogrel are indicated in patients with acute coronary syndromes who are unable to tolerate ASA because of either hypersensitivity or major GI contraindications, principally recent significant bleeding from a peptic ulcer or gastritis. Care must be taken during the acute phase with these drugs because of the delay required to achieve a full antiplatelet effect; loading doses may improve the antithrombotic effects of these agents. In general, clopidogrel is preferred because of its more favorable safety profile.

17. Is there any role for thienopyridines in angioplasty?

Periprocedural complications of angioplasty (including death, MI, and vessel occlusion) are caused by arterial thrombus formation at the site of vessel injury. These complications have been reduced, but not eliminated, by the use of conventional platelet inhibitors such as ASA.

In a study comparing ticlopidine (750 mg/day) or the combination of ASA (650 mg/day) plus dipyridamole (75 mg/day) with placebo, the frequency of immediate complications after angioplasty was similar in the patients treated with ticlopidine and with ASA plus dipyridamole (2% and 5%, respectively).

Whenever possible, thienopyridines should be given at least 24 hours before the procedure to achieve better platelet inhibition.

18. Which thienopyridine should be used for stent placement?

The development of improved stent implantation techniques and the use of ticlopidine and ASA has decreased the occurrence of stent thrombosis, with reported rates of 0.6% in the Intracoronary Stenting and Antithrombotic regimen (ISAR) trial and 0.5% in the Stent Anticoagulation Restenosis Study (STARS).

Ticlopidine and clopidogrel have been directly compared in a randomized manner. In Muller et al., clopidogrel without a loading dose was better tolerated than ticlopidine. However, there were more cardiac events in patients treated with clopidogrel (3.1% vs. 1.7%; $P = 0.24$), raising the question of clopidogrel efficacy.

In the Clopidogrel ASA Stent International Cooperative Study (CLASSICS), clopidogrel had a favorable safety profile at 28 days with a lower combined incidence of major bleeding, neutropenia, thrombocytopenia, or early discontinuation. The 30-day rates of major adverse cardiac events were similar between the two agents, at 0.9% with ticlopidine (250 mg bid without a loading dose) and 1.2% with clopidogrel (using a loading dose of 300 mg).

A third trial with loading doses of both agents (500 mg for ticlopidine and 300 mg for clopidogrel) and a treatment period for ticlopidine of 14 days in order to decrease side effects showed that drug intolerance was greater with ticlopidine even during a shortened 2-week treatment period. The occurrence of acute closure and subacute stent thrombosis, as well as the combined 30-day major adverse cardiac events, were essentially equal for the two arms.

The safety profile of clopidogrel favors its use over that of ticlopidine (associated with ASA) after intracoronary stenting.

BIBLIOGRAPHY

 1. Awtry EH, Loscalzo J: Aspirin. Circulation 101:1206, 2000.
 2. Bennet CL, Weinberg PD, Rozenberg-Ben-Dror K: Thrombotic thrombocytopenic purpura associated with ticlopidine. Ann Intern Med 128:541–544, 1998.
 3. CAPRIE Steering Committee: A randomized, blinded, trial of clopidogrel versus aspirin in patients at risk of ischaemic events (CAPRIE). Lancet 348:1329–39, 1996.
 4. Clopidogrel in Unstable Angina to Prevent Recurrent Events Trial Investigators: Effects of clopidogrel in addition to aspirin in patients with acute coronary syndromes without ST-segment elevation. N Engl J Med 345:494–502, 2001.
 5. Gorelick PB, Born GVR, D'Agostino RB: Aspirin revisited in light of the introduction of clopidogrel. Stroke 30:1716–1721, 1999.
 6. Herbert JM, Savi P, Maffrand JP: Biochemical and pharmacological properties of clopidogrel: a new ADP receptor antagonist. Eur Heart J 1(suppl A):31–40, 1999.
 7. Lauer MS: Aspirin for primary prevention of coronary events. N Engl J Med 346:1468–1474, 2002.
 8. Marso SP: Optimizing the diabetic formulary: beyond aspirin and insulin. J Am Coll Cardiol 40:652–661, 2002.
 9. Sharis PJ, Cannon CP, Loscalzo J: The antiplatelet effects of ticlopidine and clopidogrel. Ann Intern Med 129:394–405, 1998.
10. Sixth ACCP Consensus Conference on Antithrombotic Therapy. Chest 119(suppl):1–336, 2001.

14. GLYCOPROTEIN IIB/IIIA RECEPTOR INHIBITORS

Marco Roffi, M.D., and Debabrata Mukherjee, M.D.

1. What is the mechanism of action of the platelet glycoprotein (GP) IIb/IIIa receptor inhibitors?

These agents block the fibrinogen receptor GP IIb/IIIa located on the platelet membrane surface and consequently inhibit platelet aggregation. The first agent developed was abciximab (ReoPro), a monoclonal antibody directed against the fibrinogen recognition region of the GP IIb/IIIa receptor. Approved non-antibody GP IIb/IIIa inhibitors include tirofiban (Aggrastat) and eptifibatide (Integrilin). These agents are administered intravenously.

2. Should all patients undergoing percutaneous coronary intervention (PCI) receive GP IIb/IIIa inhibitors?

Prospective randomized studies with abciximab, eptifibatide, and tirofiban have demonstrated the efficacy and relative safety of intravenous (IV) platelet GP IIb/IIIa inhibitors therapy in patients undergoing PCI. All patients, including low-risk patients, benefit from GP IIb/IIIa integrin blockade, although the magnitude of benefit is higher in high-risk patients. These agents are cost effective in patients undergoing PCI, with costs per death or myocardial infarction (MI) prevented ranging from $13,000 to $23,000 with abciximab; $30,000 with eptifibatide; and $37,000 for tirofiban. An argument can be made that all patients undergoing PCI should receive adjunctive GP IIb/IIIa inhibitors unless there is a contraindication.

3. Are there differences among the GP IIb/IIIa inhibitors currently approved for use in PCI?

All three individual agents—abciximab, eptifibatide, and tirofiban—have been shown to be effective in reducing major adverse cardiac events (MACE) when used as an adjunct to PCI. The TARGET trial compared tirofiban and abciximab among patients undergoing PCI and demonstrated that tirofiban provided significantly less protection from major ischemic events based on individual and composite endpoints of death, nonfatal MI, or urgent target-vessel revascularization. There has been no randomized data comparing eptifibatide with abciximab. Based on the TARGET substudies, it appears reasonable to use abciximab in patients with acute coronary syndromes (ACS) undergoing PCI and use either eptifibatide or tirofiban in patients undergoing elective percutaneous revascularization.

4. What is the optimal activated clotting time (ACT) for PCI with adjunctive GP IIb/IIIa inhibitors?

The American College of Cardiology/American Heart Association guidelines recommend that in patients who do not receive GP IIb/IIIa inhibitors, the optimal ACT is 250 to 300 seconds with the Hemotec device and 300 to 350 s with the Hemochron device. Typically, the Hemochron device gives ACT values 30 to 50 seconds higher than the Hemotec at all unfractionated heparin concentrations. Weight-adjusted bolus heparin ($\leq$ 70–100 IU/kg) is recommended to avoid excess anticoagulation. Early sheath removal when the ACT falls to less than 150 to 180 s is also recommended to reduce access site bleeding complications. When an adjunctive GP IIb/IIIa inhibitor is used, heparin bolus should be reduced to 50 to 70 IU/kg or more in order to achieve a target ACT of 200 seconds using either the Hemotec or Hemochron device.

5. Do women receive equivalent clinical benefit with GP IIb/IIIa inhibitors for PCI?

Initial small studies had provided conflicting reports on the effectiveness of GP IIb/IIIa inhibitors in women undergoing PCI. A pooled analysis of the EPIC, EPILOG, and EPISTENT trials demonstrated no gender difference in protection from major adverse outcomes with GP IIb/IIIa inhibition with abciximab. Although women had higher rates of both major and minor bleeding events with abciximab compared with men, major bleeding in women was similar with and without abciximab. Similarly, eptifibatide has been demonstrated to be effective in preventing ischemic complications of PCI in women. Thus, these agents appear equally effective for both genders.

6. Is there additional benefit of GP IIb/IIIa inhibition in patients treated with aspirin and clopidogrel before PCI?

The TOPSTAR trial was a single-center, double-blind, randomized, prospective trial to evaluate whether additional administration of a GP IIb/IIIa receptor antagonist might be beneficial in patients undergoing elective PCI already pretreated with aspirin and clopidogrel. This study demonstrated that administration of the GP IIb/IIIa receptor antagonist leads to a reduced incidence of postinterventional troponin release in elective, non-acute PCI. This suggests patients an incremental benefit with adjunctive GP IIb/IIIa inhibition despite pretreatment with aspirin and clopidogrel.

7. What is the role of point-of-care platelet inhibition testing with GP IIb/IIIa inhibitors in patients undergoing PCI?

The GOLD study demonstrated that the degree of inhibition of platelet function through treatment with a GP IIb/IIIa antagonist can be measured with a rapid, point-of-care assay and significantly correlates with the risk of ischemic adverse events in patients undergoing PCI. By multivariate analysis, platelet function inhibition of 95% at 10 minutes after the start of therapy was associated with a significant decrease in the incidence of major adverse cardiac events (odds ratio, 0.46; 95% confidence interval 0.22–0.96; $P = 0.04$). However, point-of-care testing of the degree of platelet inhibition has not been widely incorporated in interventional cardiology practice.

8. What are the recommended dosages of the GP IIb/IIIa inhibitors used in PCI?

The recommended dosages for the individual agents are:

AGENT	BOLUS	INFUSION
Abciximab	0.25 mg/kg IV	0.125 µg/kg/min (maximum 10 µg/min) for 12 hours
Eptifibatide (creatinine < 2.0 mg/dL)	180 µg/kg double bolus	2.0 µg/kg/min infusion for 12–24 hours
Eptifibatide (creatinine > 2.0 mg/dL)	135 µg/kg double bolus	0.5 µg/kg/min infusion for 12–24 hours
Tirofiban (creatinine clearance > 30 mL/min)	10 µg/kg	0.15 µg/kg/min infusion for 20–24 hours
Tirofiban (creatinine clearance < 30 mL/min)	5 µg/kg	0.075 µg/kg/min infusion for 20–24 hours

9. What are the contraindications for use of GP IIb/IIIa inhibitors in PCI?

The contraindications of GP IIb/IIIa inhibitors include 1) hypersensitivity to the agent; 2) active internal bleeding or history of bleeding within the previous 6 weeks; 3) a history of intracranial hemorrhage, intracranial neoplasm, arteriovenous malformation, or aneurysm; 4) a history of thrombocytopenia with prior exposure to the agent; 5) history of stroke within 2 years or any history of hemorrhagic stroke; 6) severe hypertension (systolic blood pressure > 180 mmHg or diastolic blood pressure > 110 mmHg); 7) thrombocytopenia with platelet count < 100,000/mL; 8) acute pericarditis; 9) anticoagulation within the past 7 days unless INR < 1.2; and 10) history of vasculitis. Eptifibatide should not be used if the serum creatinine level is greater than 4.0 mg/dL.

10. What is the benefit of GP IIb/IIIa integrin blockade in the medical management of patients with non–ST segment elevation ACS?

The benefit of GP IIb/IIIa inhibitors in this setting has been less consistent than as for PCI. Accordingly, a meta-analysis of all major placebo-controlled GP IIb/IIIa ACS trials including almost 30,000 patients demonstrated a statistically significant but moderate (9%) relative reduction in death or MI at 30 days. To put this result in perspective, the combination of aspirin and clopidogrel compared to aspirin alone in the CURE trial was associated with a 21% reduction of cardiovascular death, MI, or stroke at 30 days. Therefore, GP IIb/IIIa inhibitors are not recommended for patients with ACS not deemed to be candidate for revascularization unless high-risk features such as troponin positivity or diabetes are present.

11. Do any subgroups derive particular benefit from GP IIb/IIIa inhibitors for non–ST elevation ACS?

Among patients with ACS treated medically, those who derive most benefit from GP IIb/IIIa inhibitors are diabetics and the troponin-positive patients. In a meta-analysis of the diabetic cohorts enrolled in the six large-scale GP IIb/IIIa ACS trials, the allocation to these potent platelet inhibitors was associated with a highly statistically significant 26% mortality reduction at 30 days. The survival benefit was even greater among diabetic patients who underwent PCI. Among troponin-positive patients, whereas a marked benefit of tirofiban was detected in substudies of PRISM and PRISM PLUS, no benefit of abciximab was observed in GUSTO IV.

12. What is the benefit of GP IIb/IIIa integrin blockade among patients with non–ST segment elevation ACS undergoing PCI?

Only one placebo controlled study (CAPTURE) focused on the use of these potent platelet inhibitors in patients with ACS undergoing PCI. An 18 to 24-hour infusion of abciximab before coronary revascularization, which was continued for 1 hour after PCI, was associated with a significant reduction in death, MI, or urgent revascularization (11.3% vs. 15.9%; $P = 0.012$) among 1265 patients with refractory ischemia. The enhanced efficacy of these agents in the setting of ACS PCI is also suggested from a meta-analysis of GP IIb/IIIa ACS trials showing an enhanced efficacy (26% reduction in 30-day death or MI) among patients undergoing PCI while taking GP IIb/IIIa inhibitors compared with a nonsignificant 5% event reduction for patients solely medically managed. Importantly, the TACTICS study showed for the first time a lack of "early hazard" among patients undergoing early percutaneous revascularization, suggesting a strong protective effect of GP IIb/IIIa inhibitors in this setting.

13. What about oral GP IIb/IIIa inhibitors?

Four large scale clinical trials that included more than 30,000 patients have addressed the use of oral GP IIb/IIIa inhibitors either after PCI or in the medical management of ACS. A meta-analysis of these studies showed a statistically increase in mortality associated with active treatment. The development of this class of antiplatelet agents has not been further pursued.

14. What is the role of GP IIb/IIIa inhibitors in acute MI?

A strategy of low-dose fibrinolytic plus abciximab was tested in two large-scale AMI trials. In the GUSTO V trial, half-dose r-PA plus full-dose abciximab was equivalent to full-dose r-PA in terms of mortality but was associated with a reduction in re-infarction, recurrent ischemia, and AMI complications such as sustained ventricular tachycardia, ventricular fibrillation, or ventricular septal defect. This alternative treatment may be suited for younger patients, those with high-risk MI such as anterior location, and patients who are being considered for acute transfer for a cardiac catheterization laboratory. Similar results, namely a significant reduction in in-hospital reinfarction and refractory ischemia rates as well as in the need for urgent intervention, was observed in the comparison of half-dose TNK-t-PA and full-dose abciximab versus full-dose TNK-t-PA in the ASSENT 3 trial. In both trials, the combination of half-dose lytic and abciximab was associated with more bleeding but no increased intracranial hemorrhage. With respect to patients undergoing stent based PCI for AMI, the use of abciximab was associated with a significant event reduction in the ADMIRAL trial but not in the stent arm of the CADILLAC trial.

BIBLIOGRAPHY

1. Adgey AA. An overview of the results of clinical trials with glycoprotein IIb/IIIa inhibitors. Am Heart J 135(Suppl):43–55, 1998.
2. Bonz AW, Lengenfelder B, Strotmann J, et al: Effect of additional temporary glycoprotein IIb/IIIa receptor inhibition on troponin release in elective percutaneous coronary interventions after pretreatment with aspirin and clopidogrel (TOPSTAR trial). J Am Coll Cardiol 40:662–668, 2002.
3. Chew DP, Bhatt DL, Sapp S, et al: Increased mortality with oral platelet glycoprotein IIb/IIIa antagonists: a meta-analysis of phase III multicenter randomized trials. Circulation 103:201–206, 2001.
4. Cho L, Topol EJ, Balog C, et al: Clinical benefit of glycoprotein IIb/IIIa blockade with abciximab is independent of gender: pooled analysis from EPIC, EPILOG and EPISTENT trials. J Am Coll Cardiol 36:381–386, 2000.
5. Hillegass WB, Newman AR, Raco DL: Economic issues in glycoprotein IIb/IIIa receptor therapy. Am Heart J 138:(Suppl)24–32, 1999.
6. Roffi M, Chew D, Mukherjee D, et al: Platelet glycoprotein IIb/IIIa inhibition in acute coronary syndromes: gradient of benefit related to the revascularization strategy. Eur Heart J 23:1441–1448, 2002.
7. Roffi M, Chew DP, Mukherjee D, et al: Platelet glycoprotein IIb/IIIa inhibitors reduce mortality in diabetic patients with non-ST-segment-elevation acute coronary syndromes. Circulation 104:2767–2771, 2001.
8. Smith SC, Dove JT, Jacobs AK, et al: ACC/AHA guidelines of percutaneous coronary interventions. J Am Coll Cardiol 37:2215–2239, 2001.
9. Steinhubl SR, Talley JD, Braden GA, et al: Point-of-care measured platelet inhibition correlates with a reduced risk of an adverse cardiac event after percutaneous coronary intervention: results of the GOLD (AU-Assessing Ultegra) Multicenter Study. Circulation 103:2572–2578, 2001.
10. Topol EJ, Byzova TV, Plow EF: Platelet GPIIb-IIIa blockers. Lancet 353:227–231, 1999.
11. Topol EJ, Moliterno DJ, Herrmann HC, et al: Comparison of two platelet glycoprotein IIb/IIIa inhibitors, tirofiban and abciximab, for the prevention of ischemic events with percutaneous coronary revascularization. N Engl J Med 344:1888–1894, 2001.

15. RADIOCONTRAST MEDIA REACTIONS AND CONSCIOUS SEDATION

Christian Fierro-Renoy, M.D.

1. Does radiocontrast media (RCM) cause anaphylaxis?

No. Anaphylactic reactions typically involve IgE-mediated mast cell activation. Although there have been some reports of patients exhibiting anti-RCM IgE antibodies, most patients do not. RCM causes activation of mast cells via an unknown mechanism with a clinical picture similar to anaphylaxis and shock; for this reason, they have been called anaphylactoid reactions. A more appropriate name would be RCM immediate allergic reactions.

2. What is the mechanism of anaphylactoid reactions to RCM?

Immediate or anaphylactoid reactions have been associated with mast cell activation because histamine and other substances, products of the degranulation of these cells, have been found in high concentrations in the plasma and urine of patients experiencing these reactions. Leukotriene D4, prostaglandin D2, and serum tryptase have also been found in high concentrations, sometimes 100 times above normal, in the plasma of patients experiencing anaphylactoid reactions to RCM. Similarly, the worse the reaction, the higher the concentrations of this substances. High complement levels have also been observed

3. Name the types of reactions to RCM.

The most accepted classification regarding the types of reactions known to occur with RCM is the classification by the 1998 American College of Radiology that separates reactions into anaphylactoid, non-anaphylactoid, and combined (Table 1).

Table 1. Types of Reactions to Radiocontrast Material

Anaphylactoid
Nonanaphylactoid
Renovascular injury
Vasovagal
Idiopathic
Neurotoxicity
Arrhythmias
Cardiac depression
Combined

4. Describe some signs and symptoms that should not be confused with RCM reactions.

High osmolar agents can cause marked osmotic effects such as nausea and retching. Hemodynamic signs include a temporary decrease in blood pressure (BP) with compensatory tachycardia, transitory decrease in chronotropy, and cardiogenic pulmonary edema. Noncardiogenic pulmonary edema has also been described. Although infrequent, salivary gland enlargement also occurs.

5. What is the incidence of fatal and nonfatal reactions to RCM?

Mortality rates from high osmolar RCM have been estimated to occur in one of 75,000 procedures; the incidence of fatal reactions to low osmolar RCM has been estimated at one of 100,000. There appears to be no relationship between the volume injected and the complication rates.

From 1978 to 1994, the United States Food and Drug Administration tabulated 26,000 reports of adverse reactions to radiocontrast materials (an estimated 170,000.000 procedures were performed, probably underreporting) and identified 920 deaths, an incidence of one in 184,782. The estimated incidence of nonfatal reactions was one in 64,418.

Interestingly, this report found no relationship between the osmolality of the RCM used and the incidence of urticaria, angioedema, or hypotension, in contrast to other reports that demonstrate fewer immediate reactions to lower osmolality materials.

6. Is there a grading system to assess the severity of immediate generalized reactions to RCM?

Yes. The grading system proposed by Ring and Messmer states:

Grade 1 refers to cutaneous reactions such as urticaria and angioedema BP, but no systemic symptoms.

Grade 2 includes cutaneous lesions, mild dyspnea, decreased BP, and abdominal pain.

Grade 3 occurs when the systolic BP decreases below 60 mmHg and cyanosis or bronchospasm occurs.

Grade 4 ensues when cardiac or respiratory arrest is present.

Another grading system proposed by the Committee on Drugs and Contrast Media of the American College of Radiology states:

Mild reactions include nausea, vomiting, cough, warmth, headache, dizziness, shaking, itching, flushing, chills, rash or hives, and anxiety

Moderate reactions include tachycardia or bradycardia, hypertension, pronounced cutaneous reaction, hypotension, bronchospasm, wheezing, and laryngeal edema

Severe reactions include life-threatening laryngeal edema, profound hypotension, unresponsiveness, cardiopulmonary arrest, and convulsions

7. If a person has experienced an anaphylactoid reaction to RCM, what is the likelihood of a subsequent reaction when re-exposed?

If a patient with a history of an anaphylactoid reaction to higher osmolality RCM is challenged again with a high osmolality agent, without pretreatment, the incidence of a reaction is 16% to 44%; however, if the patient receives a lower osmolality RCM without pretreatment, the incidence of a repeated reaction is 4% to 5%. When prednisone and diphenhydramine are used, the risk lowers to 1%. In this context, it appears that low osmolality agents are safer.

8. Which is the recommended protocol to prepare patients who have had reactions to RCM?

In 191 high-risk patients who were treated with a protocol that included prednisone 50 mg PO (orally) administered 13, 7, and 1 hour before the procedure together with diphenhydramine 50 mg PO or intravenous (IV) 1 hour before the procedure, the incidence of adverse reactions was 1%. If the procedure was mandatory, hydrocortisone 200 mg IV was administered immediately and then every 4 hours until the procedure was performed. Most centers also add an H_2 blocker to their protocols. It is important to remember that a high index of suspicion has to be maintained and the appropriate medications should be readily available.

9. Is there a time frame between the challenge with RCM and the appearance of anaphylactoid reactions?

Yes. In several studies, it has been demonstrated that anaphylactoid reactions begin minutes after the first injection in the majority of patients and virtually all occur within the first 20 minutes. Some reactions can occur immediately.

10. Are there patients who have never been challenged with RCM who are at increased risk of developing immediate reactions?

Yes. Although there has been debate for years over this matter, expert consensus advises that patients with a history of asthma who are not receiving treatment; who have allergies to food, including seafood; or who have experienced severe allergic reactions to drugs are at increased risk of developing anaphylactoid reactions.

CONSCIOUS SEDATION

11. What is conscious sedation?

Conscious sedation is one of the stages of nondissociative sedation. Used since 1995, this term has been replaced. The 2001 revised JCAHO sedation care standards replaced the term with moderate sedation/analgesia (MSA). This stage is a "drug-induced depression of consciousness during which patients respond purposefully to verbal commands, either alone or accompanied by light tactile stimulation. Reflex withdrawal from a painful stimulus is not considered a purposeful response. No interventions are required to maintain a patent airway, and spontaneous ventilation is adequate, cardiovascular function is usually maintained."

Nondissociative sedation exists as a continuum that starts with anxiolysis or minimal sedation that progresses to moderate sedation, deep sedation, and finally general anesthesia. For this reason, a high index of awareness has to be maintained to avoid deeper stages of sedation in which respiratory and cardiovascular function are depressed. At the same time, reversal drugs and emergency cardiorespiratory equipment must be readily available.

12. What are the benefits of MSA?

It has been extensively documented that MSA allows patients to tolerate unpleasant procedures by relieving anxiety, discomfort, pain, and shame. In uncooperative patients, it may expedite procedures that require that the patient remain still. This is especially important in cardiac catheterization laboratories, where procedures can be lengthy and concentration by the operator is paramount.

MSA is not the only way to effectively relieve anxiety. In our laboratory, we tested virtual reality glassess during diagnostic cardiac catheterization, which proved to be as effective as MSA in decreasing anxiety level.

13. Is it really necessary for patients to fast before MSA?

Although there is insufficient literature regarding this issue, expert consensus recommends that patients undergoing MSA should not drink fluids or eat solid food for a sufficient time to allow gastric emptying. This means 6 to 8 hours for solids and 2 to 3 hours for fluids.

14. What is the primary cause of morbidity and mortality associated with MSA?

The primary cause of morbidity associated with MSA is drug-induced respiratory depression. It has been observed that respiratory monitoring is essential because of the fact that moderate sedation can turn into deep sedation and general anesthesia if proper care is not taken.

In the cardiac catheterization laboratory and because of radiation exposure concerns, an automated apnea monitoring may decrease risks. The Task Force of the Society of Anesthesiologists cautions that impedance plethysmography may fail to detect airway obstruction. In the same way, early detection of hypoxemia by pulse oximetry decreases complications, and it is widely accepted that it is easier to detect hypoxemia with this method than with physical examination alone.

15. What other monitoring is required for MSA?

Sedatives and analgesics may blunt the autonomic response to hypovolemia, so constant monitoring of BP and heart rate is important. In cardiac patients, electrocardiographic monitoring is mandatory.

16. Should MSA for cardiologic procedures be performed by an anesthesiologist?

No. In a well-conducted study, sedation was administered for cardioversion and electrophysiologic (EP) study by an anesthesiologist in one group and a cardiologist in another group. In this study, anesthesiologists used propofol and the electrophysiologist used midazolam and morphine. The results in quality of sedation and complications were comparable. However, it was more cost effective when a cardiologist gave MSA.

17. The most frequently administered drugs used for MSA are midazolam and fentanyl. Do these drugs have any effect on the electrophysiology of the heart?

No. These drugs are used together because they produce better sedation than either drug alone. One study investigated the EP effects in BP, heart rate, respiratory rate, oxygen saturation, atrioventricular and ventricular conduction times, accessory pathway conduction, sinus node function, and inducibility of tachycardia. There were no significant changes in all the EP variables compared with placebo. However, there were mild decreases in mean arterial pressure and respiratory rate.

BIBLIOGRAPHY

1. Comittee on Drugs and Contrast Media: Manual on Contrast Media, 4th ed. Philadelphia, American College of Radiology, 1998, pp 1–46.
2. Goldner B, Baker J, Accordino A, et al: Electrical cardioversion of atrial fibrillation or flutter with consciuos sedation in the age of cost containment. Am Heart J 136:961–961, 1998.
3. Greenberg PA, Patterson R: The prevention of inmediate generalized reactions to Radiocontrast Material in high-risk patients. J Allergy Clin Immunol 87:867–872, 1991.
4. Greenberg PA: Systemic reactions to radiocontrast material. Immunol Allerg Clin North Am 21:4, 2001.
5. Joint Commision on Accreditation of Health Care Organizations 2001: Sedation and Anesthesia Care Standards. http://www.JCAHO.org/standards frm html.
6. Laroche D, Aimore-Gustin I, Dubois F, et al: Mechanism of severe, inmediate reactions to iodinated contrast material. Radiology 209:183–190, 1998.
7. Lasser EC, Lyon SG, Berry CC: Reports on contrast media reactions: analysis of data from reports to the U.S. Food and Drug Administration. Radiology 203:605–610, 1997.
8. Practice Guidelines for Sedation and Analgesia by Non-Anesthesiologists. A Report by the American Society of Anesthesiologists Task Force on Sedation and Analgesia by Non-Anesthesiologists. Anesthesiology 84:459–471, 1996.
9. Siegle RL, Halvonsen RA, Dillon J, et al: The use of iohexol in patients with previous reactions to ionic contrast material: a multicenter clinical trial. Invest Radiol 26:411–415, 1991.
10. Spring DB, Bettman MA, Barkon HE: Deaths related to iodinated contrast media reported spontaneously to the U.S. Dood and Drug Administration, 1978–1994: effect of the availability of low osmolality contrast media. Radiology 204:333–337, 1997.

16. CORONARY VASODILATORS AND VASOACTIVE DRUGS

Jeffrey Scott Fenster, M.D., and Mauricio Velez, M.D.

1. What is the significance of coronary vasodilators and vasoactive drugs?

The vascular endothelium controls the tone of blood vessels, mainly through the production of vasodilator mediators. Located between the vascular lumen and the smooth muscle cells (SMCs) of the vessel wall, the monolayer of endothelial cells is able to respond to stimuli from autonomic and sensory nerves, circulating hormones, coagulation derivatives, and platelet products; sense mechanical forces within the lumen; and regulate vascular tone through the production of a variety of factors. The endothelium produces both potent vasodilators, such as the endothelium-derived relaxing factor (EDRF or nitric oxide [NO]), prostacyclin, and endothelium-derived hyperpolarizing factor (EDHF), and vasocontrictors, such as endothelin-1. Endothelium-derived vasoactive factors are of great interest because the endothelial vasodilator function is attenuated in most vascular diseases. It may even become completely abolished in advanced disease stages. This endothelial impairment may then lead to disturbances in coronary blood flow, can contribute to the pathogenesis of myocardial ischemia, and is a central feature in the evolution of atherosclerosis and thrombosis. The tendency to inappropriate vasoconstriction that characterizes atherosclerosis is related to vasodilator dysfunction of the endothelium, permitting unopposed constriction of vascular smooth muscle. Responses to endothelium-dependent stimuli that produce vasodilation of normal human coronary arteries have been found to be markedly impaired in patients with both early and advanced atherosclerosis.

Furthermore, a number of vasoactive substances are clinically useful in diagnostic procedures (e.g., testing for coronary vasospasm), and in evaluating the influence of an epicardial coronary stenosis on myocardial blood flow. Other substances (e.g., nitrovasodilators) are fundamental in the treatment of patients with coronary artery disease, given the direct vasodilator effect they have on the coronary circulation.

2. Classify the coronary vasoactive drugs by their mechanism of action.

Table 1. Coronary Vasoactive Substances by Their Effect and Mechanism of Action

VASODILATORS			VASOCONSTRICTORS
METABOLIC MEDIATORS	ENDOTHELIUM-DEPENDENT	ENDOTHELIUM-INDEPENDENT	ENDOTHELIUM-DEPENDENT
Adenosine	Endothelium-derived relaxing factor-NO	Nitrovasodilators	Endothelin
Nitric oxide	Acetylcholine		
	Serotonin		
	Bradykinin		
	Adenosine diphosphate		
	Thrombin		
	Endothelium-derived hyperpolarizing factor		
	Prostacyclin		

3. What is EDRF? What effects does it have on the coronary vasculature?

EDRF is the NO radical. This molecule is a major modulator of vascular tone. It is released in response to various stimuli, including hypoxia, shear stress, and multiple vasoactive substances, causing vasodilation at times of increased coronary flow to prevent endothelial damage. Endothelial cells constitutively express an NO synthase that generates NO from L-arginine. Mutations in this enzyme are associated with an impaired production of NO and are clinically manifested by propensity to coronary vasospasm, hypertension, and myocardial infarction (MI). This genetic aberration helps to prove the importance of NO in the clinical setting.

Moreover, endothelium-derived vasodilators have angiogenic and smooth muscle modulator properties, exert a profound regulatory influence on the thrombolytic and proliferative functions of the endothelium, and possess antiinflammatory activity.

4. Which stimulants induce production of NO by the endothelial cell? What is the mechanism of NO synthesis? How does nitric oxide induce vasodilation?

Acetylcholine (Ach), serotonin (Ser), thrombin (Thr), bradykinin (BK), adenosine diphosphate (ADP), and changes in shear stress are all stimuli that elicit the production of NO by the endothelium, resulting in vasodilation.

L-arginine is the substrate from which NO is made. Endothelial NO synthase is modulated by increases in intracellular calcium and binding with calmodulin. Endothelial NO synthase is an NADPH-dependent oxygenase that requires tetrahydrobiopterin (BH_4), FAD, and FMN to convert L-arginine into NO. L-citrulline is produced as a byproduct of NO synthesis and can be recycled to produce L-arginine.

After NO is made, it diffuses out of the endothelial cells to interact with the vascular SMCs in the vessel wall, where it increases the activity of guanylate cyclase. This enzyme mediates the reaction that converts guanosine triphosphate (GTP) to cyclic guanosine monophospate (cGMP). The elevation of intracellular levels of cGMP induces a decrease in cytoplasmic calcium, inhibition of the contractile machinery and, consequently, vasodilation.

5. What is EDHF? How does it support the vasodilating function of NO?

Inhibition of both NO and prostacyclin does not abolish endothelium-dependent vasodilation. This finding led to believe that another factor was implicated in supporting the activity of NO and prostacyclin.

EDHF is released after stimuli that normally would stimulate the production of NO and prostacyclin, such as acetylcholine, bradykinin, and shear stress. However, a prerequisite for the production of EDHF is the absence of NO because the latter apparently exerts powerful inhibition on the metabolic pathway that leads to EDHF. As long as NO is present in appropriate amounts, it will be responsible for maintaining vasodilation. It is only when circumstances affect NO synthesis that levels of EDHF increase by upregulation and the hyperpolarizing factor takes over the main role in maintaining endothelium-dependent vasodilation.

After a stimulus that induces its production, EDHF diffuses to vascular SMCs and activates calcium-dependent potassium channels, resulting in hyperpolarization. The effect of this hyperpolarization is relaxation of the vascular SMCs.

6. What is the role of prostacyclin in the coronary circulation?

Vasodilator prostaglandins are important in the control of coronary blood flow and metabolic vasodilation. Prostacyclin (PGI_2) is a potent vasodilator produced by the activity of endothelial cyclooxygenase. It appears that PGI_2 is not a major determinant of resting coronary blood flow through vasodilation in intact blood vessels. However, under pathological circumstances that impair endothelial vasodilator function, such as in patients with coronary risk factors, PGI_2 is fundamental in maintaining resting conduit and resistance vessel tone, and it also contributes to metabolic and flow-mediated vasodilation.

Prostacyclin receptors are coupled to adenylate cyclase to increase the intracellular levels of cAMP in the vascular SMC. This, in turn, causes hyperpolarization of the cell membrane and increases the extrusion of calcium from the cytoplasm. These two mechanisms result in inhibition of muscular contraction.

7. What is endothelin?

Endothelin is a powerful vasoconstrictor peptide that exists in three isoforms: ET1, ET2, and ET3. ET1 is the predominant isopeptide released by endothelial cells, and it is likely to have the most important physiologic role in the regulation of vascular tone. Thrombin, interleukin-1, platelet products, vasopressin, angiotensin II, and catecholamines can induce the secretion of ET1. However, NO inhibits the synthesis of endothelin.

ET1 binds two types of receptors in the heart, ETa and ETb. The former has high affinity for ET1, and it is selectively expressed in vascular smooth muscle cells. The latter has equal affinity for all three isoforms of endothelin and is present in SMCs as well as endothelial cells.

ET-mediated vasoconstriction has a slow onset because substances that stimulate its release do so by initiating the transcription of endothelin messenger RNA. Contrasting the rapidity of onset and inactivation typical of the vasodilator action of NO, which usually occurs in seconds, the effects of endothelin can last from minutes to hours.

8. What conditions favor the development of endothelial dysfunction? Are there any interventions that can improve endothelial vasodilator function in individuals with impaired NO production?

The loss of endothelium-dependent vasodilation occurs early in atherosclerosis, even before its detection by angiography. Hypercholesterolemia, cigarette smoking, and insulin-dependent diabetes mellitus (IDDM) are proven risk factors for atherosclerosis and are also known to impair endothelial function, a key factor in the development of early atherogenesis. The mechanisms by which these three risk factors result in endothelial dysfunction are not completely understood. Apparently, the loss of NO bioavailability may be related to a decrease in the concentrations of L-arginine and to reduced synthesis and accelerated breakdown of NO.

Evidence suggests that high levels of low-density lipoprotein (LDL), especially in its oxidized form, have direct injurious effects on the vascular endothelium. Medical treatment aimed at an aggressive reduction of LDL cholesterol results in significant improvements in endothelium-dependent vasomotor responses. Epidemiologic studies also provide evidence that vasomotor function is subject to modification by specific antioxidants, such as vitamin E. Other strategies effective in restoring endothelium-dependent vasodilation include the use of angiotensin-converting enzyme inhibitors, and the oral administration of L-arginine.

9. What impact does serotonin have on coronary arteries with normal and damaged endothelium?

Serotonin is released from aggregating platelets in the blood vessel lumen. It binds to 5-hydroxytryptamine 1 (5-HT1) receptors on the endothelial cell surface to stimulate the release of NO and PGI_2. It also binds to 5-HT2 receptors on vascular SMCs to induce vasoconstriction.

When the endothelium is intact, the concentration of the endothelium-dependent vasodilators increases in response to several physiologic stimuli, including serotonin. When platelets aggregate in the vicinity of normal endothelial cells, the release of serotonin by the platelets results in endothelium-dependant vasodilation, favoring the removal of platelet aggregates and thrombus. If the endothelium is damaged, absent or dysfunctional (e.g., in atherosclerosis), the local concentrations of these endothelium-dependent vasodilators are markedly decreased. As a result, vasoconstriction occurs because the direct serotoninergic activation of the 5HT-2 receptors on vascular SMCs is not countered by endothelium-dependent vasodilation.

10. Which vasoactive drug is most commonly used to assess endothelial vasodilator function in humans?

Acetylcholine is the classical pharmacologic stimulant used to assess endothelial vasodilator function. This agent has a primary endothelium-independent contractive action on vascular SMCs, and an opposite endothelium-mediated vasodilatory effect. The latter is predominant in normal conditions and at physiologic concentrations.

Acetylcholine acts via muscarinic membrane receptors, with signal transduction through G proteins, to stimulate the synthesis of the endothelium-derived relaxing factor, NO. It also induces the release of EDHF, which counteracts the direct vasoconstrictor effects of acetylcholine via its muscarinic receptors on the vascular SMCs.

The observed vasodilation or vasoconstriction after acetylcholine is the net effect of the conflicting action of this substance on endothelial cells and SMCs. Vasodilation in response to acetylcholine indicates preserved endothelial vasodilator function. Acetylcholine causes vasoconstriction in atherosclerotic arteries because of its unopposed contractive effect on vascular SMCs, signaling the presence of a dysfunctional endothelium incapable of synthesizing NO.

11. What is the dosage of acetylcholine required to assess coronary vasospasm? What are the possible adverse complications of provocation testing with acetylcholine?

Coronary vasospasm is diagnosed through coronary angiography. Sueda et al. studied 715 patients, to whom they administered acetylcholine injections over 20 seconds in incremental dosages of 10, 50, and 80 μg into the right coronary artery (RCA) and 10, 20, 100 μg into the left coronary artery (LCA), with at least 3-minute intervals between injections. Seven patients (0.98%) developed ventricular tachycardia, five of whom developed it when acetylcholine was injected into the RCA. Two patients (0.28%) developed severe hemodynamic instability, loss of consciousness, and shock. Cardiac tamponade occurred in one patient (0.14%) after insertion of a 6-Fr temporary pacemaker in the right ventricular apex. The authors concluded that the complications were not directly caused by the acetylcholine infusion but instead were caused by the myocardial ischemia resulting from the acetylcholine-induced coronary vasospasm.

12. What is fractional flow reserve (FFR)? What is its clinical significance?

FFR is the maximum achievable blood flow in the presence of a stenosis divided by maximum flow in that same distribution as it would be if the supplying artery were normal. It represents the fraction of maximum coronary or myocardial blood flow that is preserved despite the presence of epicardial stenosis. It is a lesion-specific index of stenosis severity that can be calculated by simultaneous measurement of mean arterial, distal coronary, and central venous pressure, during pharmacologic vasodilation, commonly achieved with the use of adenosine.

Because the functional capacity of patients with angina pectoris is directly related to the maximum achievable blood flow from the myocardium, FFR indicates the functional significance of an epicardial coronary lesion for the patient. An abnormally low value of FFR is associated with inducible ischemia.

13. What features would an ideal coronary vasodilator have to study flow reserve in humans? List some examples of vasodilators and their associated characteristics.

An ideal coronary vasodilator for studying coronary flow reserve would rapidly produce maximal coronary vasodilation (hyperemia), be short acting to permit repeated measurements, would not alter systemic hemodynamics, and would not have significant side effects. Some examples of vasodilators and their characteristics include:

- **Dipyridamole:** This agent produces maximal coronary vasodilation, but its disadvantage is its long duration of effect (> 30 minutes), which makes the repeated assessment of the coronary hyperemic response impossible during a single procedure.
- **Papaverine:** Wilson and White showed that a selective intracoronary infusion of papaverine resulted in a maximal hyperemic response, in most cases after 12 mg, but has been associated with prolongation of the QT interval and torsades de pointes.
- **Adenosine:** Kern and colleagues have shown that a continuous intravenous infusion of 140 mg/kg/min induces maximal coronary vasodilation, it is short acting, and it can be used multiple times in the same procedure. Adenosine side effects may be associated with burning, flushing, and angina-like sensation in the chest or neck. These reactions are not severe and disappear rapidly.

14. How does adenosine cause coronary vasodilation?

Adenosine is a potent vasodilator that participates in the control of coronary circulation. This molecule qualifies as a metabolic regulator of coronary blood flow because its production increases during periods of high myocardial oxygen consumption, especially when NO activity alone is not able to restore adequate flow and oxygen delivery to the myocardium.

Adenosine is formed by degradation of adenine nucleotides under conditions in which ATP utilization exceeds the capacity of myocardial cells to resynthesize high-energy phosphate compounds, a process dependent on oxidative phosphorylation in the myocardial mitochondria (i.e. ischemia). This results in the production of adenosine monophosphate (AMP), and the enzyme 5-nucleotidase is responsible for the formation of adenosine from AMP.

The myocytes of coronary resistance vessels have adenosine receptors (A2) on their cell membranes. When combined with adenosine, the plasma membrane-bound receptor protein causes an increase in adenylate cyclase activity and a subsequent increase in intracellular cyclic AMP (cAMP), resulting in vasodilation. A supplemental mechanism of action of adenosine consists of a presynaptic inhibition of norepinephrine release from sympathetic nerve terminals. Studies have demonstrated that adenosine reduces, but does not fully override, coronary vasoconstriction during neural sympathetic stimulation.

15. What are the dosages of adenosine to test for fractional flow reserve?

Coronary hyperemia is induced by an intracoronary injection of adenosine. Usual dosing is 18 to 24 μg in the RCA and 24 to 36 μg in the LCA.

16. How does insulin induce vasodilation in the peripheral vasculature? How does it affect the coronary circulation?

Insulin induces vasodilation through an endothelium-dependent mechanism by activating L-arginine transport and NO synthase. In vascular SMCs, insulin increases cAMP and cGMP concentrations.

17. What is sodium nitroprusside? What are its pharmacologic characteristics?

Sodium nitroprusside is a nitrovasodilator. It is administered by intravenous infusion and metabolized in the blood vessels to its active metabolite, NO. NO diffuses to the vascular SMCs, activates guanylate cyclase, and leads to the formation of cyclic GMP (cGMP). An increase in cGMP causes a decrease in the levels of intracellular calcium and ends in vasodilation.

Sodium nitroprusside dilates both arterioles and venules, and the hemodynamic response to its administration results from a combination of venous pooling and reduced arterial impedance. It is indicated in the management of hypertensive emergencies and acute heart failure. This drug has also been shown to be effective in treating the "no-reflow" phenomenon.

The short-term side effects from nitroprusside are caused by excessive vasodilation, with hypotension being the main concern. Less commonly, toxicity may result from conversion of nitroprusside to cyanide and thiocyanate. The risk of thiocyanate toxicity increases when sodium nitroprusside is infused continuously for more than 24 to 48 hours, especially if renal function is impaired.

18. What are the signs and symptoms of thiocyanate toxicity?

Common signs from thiocyanate toxicity include anorexia, nausea, fatigue, disorientation, and toxic psychosis. The plasma concentration of thiocyanate should be monitored during prolonged infusions of nitroprusside and should not be allowed to exceed 0.1 mg/mL. Rarely, excessive concentrations of thiocyanate may cause hypothyroidism by inhibiting iodine uptake by the thyroid gland. In patients with renal failure, thiocyanate can be removed by dialysis.

19. What is the "no-reflow" phenomenon? How frequent is it?

No-reflow is defined as a failure to reperfuse myocardial tissue in the absence of epicardial coronary obstruction, which is further defined as a reduction in antegrade flow ($<$ 1, as defined by the Thrombolysis in Myocardial Infarction [TIMI] trial) not attributable to abrupt vessel closure, high-grade stenosis, or spasm of the original target lesions.

This phenomenon complicates approximately 2% to 10% of all percutaneous transluminal coronary interventions (PTCIs). Higher rates of no-reflow occur in settings of acute MI, vein graft interventions, and with the use of atherectomy devices.

20. Which vasodilators have been used to treat the "no-reflow" phenomenon? What are their usual dosages?

    a. Intracoronary nitroprusside (50–1000 μg). A study performed by Myers et al. showed that in a PTCI that resulted in no-reflow, nitroprusside (median dose 200 μg) was found to result in rapid and highly significant improvement in both angiographic flow and blood flow velocity.

    b. Intracoronary nitroglycerin (100–200 μg) and intracoronary verapamil (100–200 μg). A trial comparing intracoronary verapamil with intracoronary nitroglycerin in degenerated vein grafts showed that intracoronary verapamil (100–500 μg) was superior to nitroglycerin. Treatment with intracoronary verapamil was successful in improving no-reflow in all cases, with normalization in 88% of cases.

BIBLIOGRAPHY

1. Abbo KM, Dooris M, Glazier S, et al: Features and outcome of no-reflow after percutaneous coronary intervention. Am J Cardiol 75:778–782, 1995.
2. Anderson TJ, Meredith IT, Yeung AC, et al: The effect of cholesterol-lowering and antioxidant therapy on endothelium-dependent coronary vasomotion. N Engl J Med 332:488–493, 1995.
3. Baim D, Grossman W: Coronary angiography. In Baim D, Grossman W (eds): Grossman's Cardiac Catheterization, Angiography, and Intervention, 6th ed. Philadelphia, Lippincott, Williams & Wilkins, 2000, pp 247–253.
4. Diaz MN, Frei B, Vita JA, et al: Antioxidants and atherosclerotic heart disease. N Engl J Med 337: 408–416, 1997.
5. Duffy S, Castle S, Harper R, et al: Contribution of vasodilator prostanoids and nitric oxide to resting flow, metabolic vasodilation, and flow-mediated dilation in human coronary circulation. Circulation 100: 1951–1957, 1999.
6. Ganz P, Ganz W: Coronary blood flow and myocardial ischemia. In Braunwald E, Zipes DP, Libby P (eds): Braunwald: Heart Disease. A Textbook of Cardiovascular Medicine, 6th ed. St. Louis, W.B. Saunders, 2001, pp 1090–1097.
7. Halcox J, Nour K, Zalos G, Quyyumi A: Coronary vasodilation and improvement in endothelial dysfunction with endothelin ETa receptor blockade. Circ Res 89:969–976, 2001.
8. Hillegass W, Dean N, Laurence L, et al: Treatment of no-reflow and impaired flow with the nitric oxide donor nitroprusside following percutaneous coronary interventions: initial human clinical experience. J Am Coll Cardiol 37:1335–1343, 2001.
9. Hillis D, Lange R: Serotonin and acute ischemic heart disease. N Engl J Med 324:688–690, 1991.
10. Ignarro LJ, Cirino G, Casini A, et al: Nitric oxide as a signaling molecule in the vascular system: An overview. J Cardiovasc Pharmacol 34:879–886, 1999.
11. Kaplan B, Benzuly K, Kinn J, et al: Treatment of no-reflow in degenerated saphenous vein graft interventions: comparison of intracoronary verapamil and nitroglycerin. Cathet Cardiovasc Diagn 39:113–118, 1996.
12. Kinlay S, Selwyn AP, Delagrange D, et al: Biological mechanisms for the clinical success of lipid-lowering in coronary artery disease and the use of surrogate end-points. Curr Opin Lipidol 7: 389–397, 1996.
13. Minamino T, Kitakaze M, Matsumura Y, et al: Impact of coronary risk factors on contribution of nitric oxide and adenosine to metabolic coronary vasodilation in humans. J Am Coll Cardiol 31:1274–1279, 1998.
14. Mombouli JV, Vanhoutte P: Endothelial dysfunction: From physiology to therapy. J Mol Cell Cardiol 31:61–74, 1999.
15. Nakayama M, Yasue H, Yoshimura M, et al: T-786 to C mutation in the 5'-flanking region of the endothelial nitric oxide synthase gene is associated with coronary spasm. Circulation 99:2864–2870, 1999.
16. Oates J, Brown NJ: Antihypertensive agents and the drug therapy of hypertension. In Hardman J, Limbird L (eds): Goodman and Gilman's: The Pharmacological Basis of Therapeutics, 10th ed. New York, McGraw-Hill, 2001, pp 888–891.

17. Ooi H, Colucci W: Pharmacological treatment of heart failure. In Hardman J, Limbird L (eds): Goodman and Gilman's: The Pharmacological Basis of Therapeutics, 10th edition. New York, McGraw-Hill, 2001, pp 906–911.

18. Pijls NHJ, Van Gelder B, Van der Voort P, et al: Fractional flow reserve: A useful index to evaluate the influence of an epicardial coronary stenosis on myocardial blood flow. Circulation 92:3183–3193, 1995.

19. Quilley J, Fulton D, McGiff JC: Hyperpolarizing factors. Biochem Pharmachol 54:1059–1070, 1997.

20. Ross R: Atherosclerosis—an inflammatory disease. N Engl J Med 340:115–126, 1999.

21. Schalchinger V, Britten M, Zeiher A: Prognostic impact of coronary vasodilator dysfunction on adverse long-term outcome of coronary heart disease. Circulation 101:1899–1906, 2000.

22. Sueda S, Saeki H, Otani T, et al: Major complications during spasm provocation test with an intracoronary injection of acetylcholine. Am J Cardiol 85:391–394, 2000.

23. Sundell J, Nuutila P, Laine H, et al: Dose-dependent vasodilating effects of insulin on adenosine-stimulated myocardial blood flow. Diabetes 51:1125–1130, 2002.

24. Thorne S, Mullen MJ, Clarkson P, et al: Early endothelial dysfunction in adults at risk from atherosclerosis: Different responses to L-arginine. J Am Coll Cardiol 32:110–116, 1998.

25. Van Der Voot P, Van Hagen E, Hendrix G, et al: Comparison of intravenous adenosine to intracoronary papaverine for calculation of pressure-derived fractional flow reserve. Cathet Cardiovasc Diagn 39:120–125, 1996.

26. Wilson R, Wyche K, Christensen B, et al: Effects of adenosine on human coronary arterial circulation. Circulation 82:1595–1606, 1990.

IV. Percutaneous Coronary Intervention Tools

17. ANGIOPLASTY GUIDE CATHETER, BALLOON, AND GUIDEWIRE SELECTION AND TECHNIQUES

Craig A. Thompson, M.D., and Igor F. Palacios, M.D.

1. What are the operator's primary considerations during guiding catheter selection for PCI?

The primary considerations for guiding catheter selection are: **fit, support, device delivery, and visualization.**

Fit	• What is the angulation of the vessel engaged?
	• Which guide will likely be aligned coaxial with the vessel?
	• Will engagement obstruct anterograde flow? Do I need a catheter with sideholes?
	• Will the guide tip destabilize an ostial/proximal lesion in the vessel?
	• What are the size and shape of the aortic root?
Support	• Do I need more support to negotiate complex vascular anatomy (calcification, tortuosity, etc.)?
	• Will I deliver large or stiff devices?
Device delivery	• Will the inner lumen accommodate the caliber of devices I plan, or may need, to use?
	• Is atherectomy (e.g., rotational or directional), thrombectomy (Angiojet, TEC), or brachytherapy planned?
Visualization	• Is the inner lumen diameter sufficient to allow dye injection and angiography when the device is in place?

2. What are the major differences between over-the-wire (OTW) and monorail (rapid exchange, RX) balloon catheter systems?

Monorail balloon catheters have a limited lumen tract (usually 1–20 cm) located at the distal tip for coaxial tracking over the guidewire "rail." This is conducive for single-operator interventions because a single individual can control the wire and balloon/stent simultaneously. As the name *rapid-exchange* implies, once the device is used, it may be rapidly withdrawn and exchanged for supplemental devices as necessary. Optimally, standard guidewires (175 cm) are used with this approach to facilitate less awkward transition of devices when withdrawn from the sheath. Compared with over-the-wire balloons, monorails often have a lower profile, which may be advantageous. Disadvantages of RX systems include inability to exchange or reshape guidewires once lesions are crossed (exception: some manufacturers have external magnetic devices that maintain guidewire position for exchange if necessary), and reduced pushability and trackability compared with OTW systems.

Over-the-wire balloon catheters have a central lumen throughout their entire length as their guidewire "rail." These systems typically require two operators and an exchange length (~270, 300 cm) guidewire. As stated above, guidewire modification or exchange, pushability, and trackability are generally better at the expense of occasionally larger balloon/stent crossing profiles.

3. What is the utility of a polymer tip (PT) coating on a coronary guidewire?

Polymer-tipped guidewires can be the best friend and, occasionally, the worst enemy of the interventional cardiologist. A PT coating on a guidewire tip decreases the frictional coefficient and may facilitate guidewire placement through complex lesion and total occlusion subsets. One potential pitfall of polymer tips is that they may occasionally burrow beneath and destabilize plaques, or exit the vessel altogether with less tactile feedback to the operator. In addition, polymer tips are less likely to maintain pre-formed or operator-determined curvature throughout the procedure.

4. What is the primary determinant of successful passage of devices through complex, tortuous, calcified anatomy?

Guide selection. Proper guiding catheter selection to ensure strong support, coaxial alignment, and visualization/pressure monitoring during the case is key. Often, stronger, stiffer guidewires may "straighten" the vessel and increase the bias and likelihood of the device being advanced into vessel angles, plaques, and calcified segments rather than coaxially through the lumen. Optimal guidewire selection and low profile devices often cannot overcome inadequate guide support in these situations.

5. What are the components of a coronary guidewire?

Guidewires generally consist of three components: a central "core" composed of stainless steel or nitinol, a distal flexible spring coil of platinum or tungsten, and a coating such as silicone, PTFE, or other hydrophilic substances. Single-core constructions usually provide a smoother transition and enhanced torque response and less prolapse than dual-core designs.

6. How does the operator select the appropriate guidewire(s) for PCI?

The operator must consider the primary performance characteristics of the guidewire anticipated to be required for successful PCI: flexibility, torque control, steerability, support, and visibility. We must recognize that a single guidewire does not share equivalency with other wires with respect to these features. Guidewires with increased torque control, steerability, and support have less flexibility and may straighten the vessel. High-torque designs may be less traumatic and have greater torque control but be suboptimal support for device passage. The authors of this chapter generally use high-torque floppy guidewires to minimize trauma in most cases and exchange for stronger support wires as necessary using exchange with balloon or infusion catheters. We generally reserve polymer tipped wires for inability to cross lesions or anticipated complexity.

7. How does compliance characteristics affect balloon catheter selection?

Angioplasty balloons are broadly divided into compliant and noncompliant subtypes. The compliance refers to the ability of the balloon to increase its diameter above nominal at progressively higher pressures. Compliant balloons tend to have increased compliance with repetitive inflations and may be more prone to deform longitudinally during inflation. Typically, compliant balloons are best used for stand-alone balloon angioplasty or pre-dilation for stent or other device placement. Non-compliant balloons may be used for stent post-dilation or for angioplasty/pre-dilation of recalcitrant lesion subsets (e.g., calcification).

8. What is the role of fixed-wire balloon systems?

Fixed-wire balloons are currently used less frequently given the success and requirement for adjunctive PTCA or device utilization in complex lesion subsets. Fixed-wire balloons typically have lower profile than their OTW or RX counterparts and may have niche utility when conventional balloons/devices are unable to cross lesions or during side-branch retrieval when guiding lumen diameter limits OTW/RX double balloon technique.

9. What is the "buddy wire" technique?

The "buddy wire" is a secondary wire that is placed across a lesion alongside the primary coronary guidewire. This serves well in situations where balloons/devices cannot be advanced through complex anatomy by facilitating a coaxial deflection point thereby orienting the balloon/device toward the lumen rather than preferentially into a plaque or the vessel wall.

10. Is the operator committed to an RX system if a standard length wire is used to cross a lesion?

Not necessarily. Many manufacturer's guidewires are compatible with a "docking" wire extension or an external magnet device (which is positioned with the proximal end of the guide catheter outside the body), which may allow for change to over-the-wire technique.

11. What guidewires and techniques should be considered when device passage is difficult through tortuous, calcified, or other complex anatomy (given optimal guide support)?

The buddy wire, or a secondary wire placed alongside the first, may be of great value. Exchange for a "wiggle wire" can be helpful as well. The wiggle wire has a corkscrew appearance at its distal aspect and tends to lift stents/devices away from plaque or the vessel wall. Over-the-wire systems will improve pushability compared with their RX counterparts (perhaps at the expense for device profile). The second operator may perform small tugs on the guidewire as the device is advanced by the primary operator. This tends to displace force anterograde, facilitating forward mobilization of the device. Occasionally, adjunctive angioplasty at the site of device immobility may improve cross-sectional area of an angiographically unimpressive lesion that is impeding progress. Exchange for stronger support wires is often helpful, except in situations of proximal tortuosity where the stiffness of the wire increases bias.

12. What techniques are helpful when post-dilation balloon catheters are unable to enter a as a result of incomplete stent strut expansion?

One may consider dilating the balloon (very low pressure) outside the body and re-performing negative suction preparation. This flattens, or "pancakes," the balloon catheter and may facilitate advancement into the stent. In addition, a second guidewire may be used to cross the stent with a secondary balloon (or a fixed-wire balloon) advanced proximal to the stent. The post-dilation balloon may be readvanced using the "balloon deflection" technique to enter the stent.

13. How does one recross a newly stented lesion without placing the guidewire between the stent struts and vessel wall?

A nice technique for this is to preload the guidewire on a balloon catheter or introducer and create an exaggerated ($\sim$180 degree) small J-bend on its distal tip. This J-tip is generally too large to fall behind the stent struts and may pass through the lumen with ease. If the operator is unable to use this technique, emphasis should be on spinning the guidewire tip to displace its motion forward (as opposed to advancing the wire in a static orientation) as the stent is entered. Beware if subsequent balloons or devices do not pass easily through the stent; you may be under a strut! IVUS may be helpful for clarification.

14. What is the next step after crossing a chronic total occlusion (CTO) with a guidewire?

We exclusively use OTW balloons for CTO (though we often preload a standard length wire for greater control). When the lesion is crossed, the operator should ensure that the distal tip is freely mobile, and presumably in the true lumen. Contrast angiography is then performed. The balloon catheter is advanced distal to the CTO with emphasis on the tactile feedback on how easily it passes the CTO. Excessive resistance may suggest entry into a dissection channel rather than the true lumen (if this is the case, balloon advancement may extend the dissection and be unpleasant for all involved). When the balloon crosses the lesion, the wire is withdrawn, and contrast is injected through the balloon lumen to assure intraluminal position. An exchange length wire may then be placed and the CTO predilated with the balloon catheter.

15. How does one select balloon sizes for "kissing balloon" angioplasty at bifurcation lesions?
We generally select the sidebranch balloon first based on estimated optimal sizing. Then the main vessel balloon is selected estimating the cumulative diameter of the balloons at the site of overlap in the main vessel, recognizing that compliance properties will not provide strict additive sizing of the balloons (the overlapping balloon segments are less than the additive sizes, e.g., two 2.5-mm balloons will not be 5 mm in the vessel body). We try to match compliance characteristics of the balloons. If the balloon overlap is within an endolumenal stent, we are less concerned with minor discrepancies in cumulative oversizing.

BIBLIOGRAPHY

1. Abernethy WB 3rd, Choo JK, Oesterle SN, Jang IK: Balloon deflection technique: A method to facilitate entry of a balloon catheter into a deployed stent. Catheter Cardiovasc Inter 51(3):312–313, 2000.
2. Baim DS: Coronary angioplasty. In Baim DS, Grossman W (eds): Cardiac Catheterization, Angiography, and Intervention, 5th ed. Baltimore, Williams & Wilkins, 1996, pp 537–580.
3. Bruek M, Scheinert D, Flachkampf FA, et al: Sequential vs. kissing balloon angioplasty for stenting of bifurcation coronary lesions. Catheter Cardiovasc Interv 55(4):461–466, 2002.
4. Safian RD, Freed M: Coronary intervention: Preparation, equipment, and technique. In Freed M, Grines C, Safian RD (eds): The New Manual of Interventional Cardiology. Birmingham, MI, Physicians' Press, 1998, pp 1–35.
5. Selig MB: Lesion protection during fixed-wire balloon angioplasty: Use of the "buddy wire" technique and access catheters. Cathet Cardiovasc Diagn 25(4):331–335, 1992.

18. CORONARY STENTS

Nilesh J. Goswami, M.D., and Steven R. Bailey, M.D.

1. Who invented the coronary artery stent?

In 1964, Dotter and Judkins devised the concept of implanting coiled stents into peripheral artery walls during percutaneous angioplasty. The Gianturco-Roubin (G-R) stent was the first stent to be approved by the Food and Drug Administration, but it was indicated only for acute or threatened closure during coronary intervention with balloon angioplasty. Julio Palmaz designed the first coronary stent for elective implantation as a single tube with several rows of staggered rectangles forming diamond-shaped cells when expanded. This design was modified by Richard Schatz, who included a 1-mm articulation between two longer rigid segments to improve flexibility and deliverability. The result was the Palmaz-Schatz stent (Cordis Corporation, Miami Lakes, FL) for use in the coronary arteries in patients with discrete *de novo* lesions in large diameter vessels.

2. What are the major characteristics of stents?

- *Biocompatibility* is the ability of a stent to oppose thrombosis and corrosion.
- *Conformability* is to the ability of a stent to "flex" after deployment.
- *Deliverability* describes the capacity with which a stent can be positioned across the lesion. The deliverability refers to several characteristics of the stent, including trackability over the wire.
- *Flexibility* is to the ability to maneuver the unexpanded stent through tortuous bends in the vessel.
- *Radial strength* is a component of strength and resistance to recoil of the artery. This characteristic is determined primarily by the stent design and strut thickness, which is inversely proportional to the flexibility.
- *Scaffolding* is the ability of a stent to cover and compress a lesion. Insufficient scaffolding may result in prolapse of a part of the lesion through the stent struts, which may subsequently lead to stent thrombosis or restenosis. The key variables that establish scaffolding are radial strength and surface area of the stent. An increase in surface area of a stent in an effort to increase scaffolding can result in an increased risk of thrombosis with the added disadvantages of decreased flexibility.
- *Side branch access or preservation* is the ability to wire and dilate the side branches through the stent after it has been deployed. This characteristic is determined by the stent cell design and size.
- *Visibility* is the ability to see the stent under fluoroscopy and is crucial for determining placement of therapies for restenosis or placing overlapping stents.
- *Shortening* is the decrease in the length of the stent after it is deployed.

3. What are the advantages of stenting over balloon angioplasty (POBA)?

The main advantage of stenting is that a larger vessel lumen can be achieved compared with balloon angioplasty alone. In addition, dissection planes can be sealed, which improves acute procedural outcomes. Stenting, in selected lesion subsets, reduces target vessel revascularization and restenosis.

4. How are stents deployed?

There are two types of stent delivery systems: balloon expandable and self-expanding.

5. What are the indications for stenting?

Current indications include 1) preventing restenosis; 2) improving the results of initial treatment, that results in a high-risk angiographic or intravascular ultrasound (IVUS) appearance (thrombus, dissection, intramural hematoma); 3) correcting suboptimal balloon angioplasty results; and 4) treating patients with acute or threatened closure. The stents can be used in all native coronary arteries and saphenous vein bypass grafts (SVGs) of appropriate size, including left anterior descending stenoses and chronic total occlusions.

6. Are there any contraindications to stenting?

Poor distal run-off is a contraindication to stenting because it results in slow flow and substantially increases the risk of stent thrombosis.

The presence of extensive thrombus has also traditionally been a contraindication to stenting, in these cases, thrombectomy is usually preferred before stent deployment.

Finally, a lesion that cannot be dilated should not be stented.

7. What is the major limitation of stenting?

Restenosis.

8. List the clinical markers for increased likelihood of in-stent restenosis?

1) Diabetes, 2) vessels < 3.25 mm in diameter, 3) lesions > 15 mm, 4) in-stent stenosis; 5) ostial or bifurcation lesions, 6) small body mass, and 7) female gender have all been identified to increase the risk of restenosis.

9. Does debulking before stent implantation decrease restenosis?

Both the AMIGO (Atherectomy and Multilink Stenting Improves Gain and Outcome) trial of directional atherectomy before stent implantation and the SPORT (Stenting Post Rotational Atherectomy Trial) trial of rotational atherectomy before stent implantation failed to demonstrate decreased restenosis compared to stent implantation alone.

10. Define provisional stenting and direct or primary stenting.

Provisional stenting is the use of stenting only if the results of balloon angioplasty or atherectomy are suboptimal. Direct or primary stenting involves the high-pressure deployment of stents directly to the lesion without predilatation or atherectomy.

11. Does the adjunctive use of IVUS improve stent results?

The AVID (Angiography vs. Intravascular Ultrasound-Directed Coronary Stent Placement) trial demonstrated that although IVUS did not improve the outcome in all lesions, it did improve outcome in SVGs, vessels less than 3.25 mm in diameter, and vessels with more than 70% stenosis. This suggests that IVUS is very important in all complex lesion subsets.

12. Should patients undergoing mechanical revascularization during acute myocardial infarction (MI) receive stents?

The Controlled Abciximab and Device Investigation to Lower Late Angioplasty Complications (CADILLAC) trial randomized 2665 patients presenting with acute ST elevation MI to one of four treatment arms. These included balloon angioplasty with or without a glycoprotein (GP) IIb/IIIa antagonist (abciximab) and stenting with or without abciximab. The primary endpoint was MACE (major adverse clinical events, including death, re-infarction, target vessel revascularization, or disabling stroke) at 6 months. In contrast to previous MI trials evaluating stenting, thrombolysis in myocardial infarction 3 flow rates were excellent in all groups, including those with stents. Approximately 20% of patients in the balloon angioplasty arms had a primary adverse event compared with only 10.9% in the stent arms. Thus, despite earlier evidence that stents are not beneficial in acute MI, the results of this large, randomized study indicate that use of stents improves outcomes. As a result, most operators currently deploy stents to improve results in patients undergoing PCI during MI.

13. From what materials are stents manufactured?

Coronary stents are most commonly constructed from stainless steel, but many other compounds have been used in stents. These include 1) nitinol (a combination of nickel and titanium);

2) biodegradable, bioresorbable material, including polylactide compounds; 3) PTFE-covered stents; 4) tantalum; 5) and cobalt and platinum.

14. Does the thickness of the stent's strut influence restenosis rates?

Thicker struts result in more intense formation of neointimal hyperplasia, which results in higher restenosis rates.

15. What are the various types of stent designs?

More than 30 different types of stents have been implanted into the coronary arteries. The basic architecture can be divided into several groups: slotted tube, modular, coiled wire, and hybrid. Slotted tube and modular stents are currently the most commonly implanted stents. Among these designs, there are various "cell" designs and sizes. These may be important in situations in which side branch access is needed (Fig. 1).

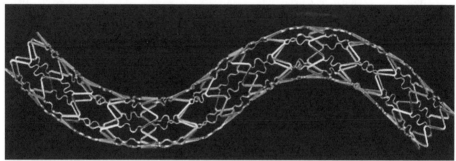

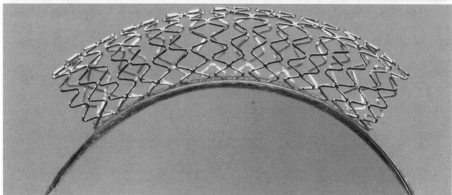

FIGURE 1. *Top,* Slotted tube stent design represented by the Express stent from Boston Scientific/SCIMED (Maple Grove, MN) versus *bottom,* modular stent design of the S7 stent by Medtronic AVE (Minneapolis, MN). (Reproduced permission from Serruys PW, Rensing B: Handbook of Coronary Stents, 4th ed. London, Martin Dunitz, 2002.)

16. What sizes (length and diameter) of coronary stents are available?

Stent diameters range from 2.25 to 6 mm in diameter and 8 to 38 mm in length.

17. What are the most common techniques used to stent bifurcations?

There are various approaches to the complex bifurcation lesion. The first is stenting of the larger caliber vessel and salvage of the smaller branch with balloon angioplasty through the stent struts. Another technique involves stenting of one vessel and then stenting of the sidebranch through the struts of the initial stent (*T stent technique*). A third technique is *kissing stents,* which results in simultaneous deployment of two stents in each branch with *double-barrel* stents side by side in the proximal vessel. Culotte stenting is similar to *T* stenting; however, the second stent (placed through the side struts of the first) is positioned distal in the side branch. Rarely, the *crushed T stent* technique is used. In this situation, a stent is placed in the side branch with the proximal portion of the stent positioned in the main vessel. Then the second stent is deployed in the main vessel. The inflation of this stent in the main vessel crushes the proximal portion of the initial stent, resulting in one lumen. Multiple variations of the above techniques have been used. Finally, the SIRIUS (A multicenter, double blind study of the SIRolImUS-coated Bx Velocity Balloon Expandable Stent in the Treatment of Patients with de novo Coronary Artery Lesions) Bifurcation trial is evaluating the use of sirolimus eluting stents in this patient subset.

18. What are the potential complications of stenting?

Complications of stenting include 1) incomplete expansion, resulting in subacute thrombosis or restenosis; 2) side branch occlusion; 3) coronary artery perforation; 4) infective endarteritis; 5) coronary artery dissection; 6) intramural hematoma; and 7) stent embolization.

19. What types of stent coatings have shown potential for reduction of restenosis?

Most recently, sirolimus (Rapamycin) and paclitaxel have been shown to significantly reduce restenosis rates compared with bare metal stents. (Fig. 2) The SIRIUS trial enrolled 1100 patients and randomized them to sirolimus coated Bx Velocity (Cordis, Johnson & Johnson) stents versus bare metal Bx Velocity stents. At 8 months' follow-up, the restenosis rates in the drug-eluting stent arm had a restenosis rate of 3.2% versus 35.0% in the bare metal stent group. Similarly, the TAXUS II (prospective randomized evaluation of the slow-rate release and moderate-rate release polymer-based taxol-eluting stents in patients with *de novo* coronary lesions) trial showed improvement in restenosis using paclitaxel drug-eluting stents (for the slow paclitaxel release cohort: restenosis rate of 2.3% vs. 20.2% in the bare metal stent group; in the moderate release cohort, 4.7% vs. 20.2% in the bare metal group).

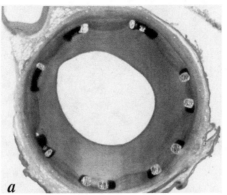 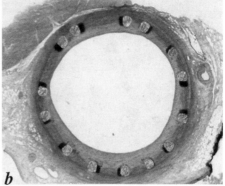

FIGURE 2. Cross-sections of porcine arteries after placement of **(A)** bare metal and **(B)** sirolimus-coated stents. A significant reduction of neointimal hyperplasia is seen with sirolimus-eluting stents resulting in clinically lower restenosis rates. (Reproduced with permission from Serruys PW, Rensing B: Handbook of Coronary Stents, 4th ed. London, Martin Dunitz, 2002.)

20. In which clinical subsets is the use of stents controversial?

The use of stents in ostial lesions, small vessels, and bifurcation lesions remains controversial with respect to the superiority of stents over balloon angioplasty. Recent randomized trials suggest that stenting may be superior to percutaneous transluminal coronary angioplasty, but this remains controversial.

BIBLIOGRAPHY

1. AVID Investigators: Angiography versus intravascular ultrasound directed stent placement [abstract]. Circulation 92(suppl 1):1–546, 1995.
2. Holmes D, Hirshfeld J, Faxon D, et al: ACC expert consensus document of coronary artery stents. JACC 32:1471–82, 1998.
3. Kastrati A, Mehilli J, Dirschinger J, et al: Intracoronary stenting and angiographic results: Strut thickness effect on restenosis outcome (ISAR-STEREO) trial. Circulation 103:2816–2821, 2001.
4. Serruys PW, Rensing B: Handbook of Coronary Stents, 4th ed. London, Martin Dunitz, 2002.
5. SIRIUS: A multicenter, randomized, double-blind study of the Sirolimus eluting stent in de novo native coronary lesions. Preliminary results presented by Jeffrey Moses at the Transcatheter Cardiovascular Therapeutics 2002. Results are available at http://www.tctmd.com.
6. Smith SC, Dove JT, Jacobs AK, et al: ACC/AHA Guidelines for Percutaneous Coronary Intervention (Revision of the 1993 PTCA Guidelines): A report of the American College of Cardiology/American Heart Association Task Force on Practice Guidelines (Committee to Revise the 1993 Guidelines for Percutaneous Transluminal Coronary Angioplasty). J Am Coll Cardiol 37:2239i–lxvi, 2001.
7. Stone GW, Grines C, Cox DA, et al: A prospective, multicenter, international randomized trial comparing four reperfusion strategies in acute myocardial infarction: Principal report of the Controlled Abxicimab and Device Investigation to Lower Late Angioplasty Complications (CADILLAC) Trial. J Am Coll Cardiol 37(suppl A):1–648, 2001.
8. TAXUS II: Slow and moderate release formulations. Preliminary results presented by Antonio Colombo at the Transcatheter Cardiovascular Therapeutics 2002. Results are available at http://www.tctmd.com.

19. ROTATIONAL ATHEROABLATION AND DIRECTIONAL CORONARY ATHERECTOMY

Alan Schob, M.D., and Oscar C. Muñoz, M.D.

ROTATIONAL ATHERECTOMY

1. Why rotational atherectomy?

Heavily calcified and fibrotic lesions have historically responded poorly to PTCA. Ineffectual dilatation, dissections, and high restenosis rates have been associated with balloon angioplasty in this lesion subset. Rotational atherectomy (RA) directly attacks this problem by abrading or sanding hard fibrotic and calcific atheromas as described below. Millions of microscopic particles are generated, which pass through the coronary circulation to be removed by the reticulendothelial system (see below). The ERBAC trial compared balloon angioplasty, laser angioplasty, and RA. The patients who underwent rotational atherectomy had a higher rate of procedural success than those who underwent excimer laser angioplasty or conventional balloon angioplasty (89% versus 77% and 80%, respectively; p = .0019).

2. What are the angiographic indications for RA?

Complex, calcified type B2 and C lesions (ACC/AHA classification), ostial stenoses, bifurcation lesions, total occlusions (if a guidewire can be successfully passed), and debulking of plaque prior to stent placement are the most common indications. The applicability of RA for in-stent restenosis is addressed in question 17. Aorto-ostial stenoses (e.g., protected left main) are good candidates for RA, especially prior to stent placement, owing to the dense fibrotic and calcific nature of these lesions. If the risk of side branch occlusion is thought to be high prior to intervention, debulking of either the side branch or both the side branch and parent vessel can result in a high success rate and low incidence of side branch occlusion.

3. What are the components of the Rotablator (Scimed) system, and how does it work?

At the business end of the system is an elliptically shaped burr, which is coated on its leading edge with 30–50 micron diamond chips. A reusable console controls the speed of rotation of the burr. The burr is welded to a flexible drive shaft through which passes a steerable, movable 0.009-inch stainless steel guidewire. The drive shaft is enclosed in a flexible sheath. This sheath protects the arterial wall from the rotating drive and simultaneously permits the pressurized infusion of a heparinized saline solution that lubricates and cools the drive shaft and burr. A compressed-air turbine rotates the drive shaft at 140,000–200,000 rpm. Burrs are available in diameters of 1.25, 1.5, 1.75, 2.0, 2.15, 2.25, and 2.5 mm.

4. How is RA performed?

To perform an atherectomy, the Rotablator guidewire is advanced distal to the target lesion. Depressing the foot pedal initiates the turbine, which spins the burr. The console controls the speed, which is usually in the range of 140,000–160,000 rpm. The rotating burr is slowly advanced through the lesion. A saline flush through the catheter serves to lubricate and reduce heat and friction. Nitroglycerin, heparin, and a calcium blocker are usually administered through the burr catheter to minimize vasospasm. As the burr is advanced to and across the stenosis, attention is given to deceleration of rotational speed. Excessive deceleration drops in rpm > 5000 below the platform speed have been shown to increase the risk of complications such as spasm, slow or no flow, and consequent myocardial infarction. The generation of heat associated with large drops in rpm (>5000) is also a likely inducement to restenosis. A pacemaker may be inserted prior to atherectomy to prevent significant bradycardia.

5. What is the mechanism of ablation, and does RA damage adjacent tissues?

Differential cutting describes the preferential ablation of hard, fibrotic, and calcific plaque. During rotational atherectomy, elastic non-atherosclerotic tissue is pushed away or deflected from the spinning burr. With the absence of elastic elements in the diseased segments, the fibrotic calcified plaque is unable to be deflected and thus selectively ablated. This is analogous to the effect of a fingernail file on the flesh of a finger compared with its effect on a fingernail. Endothelial segments adjacent to the treated stenosis may be denuded, leading to vasospasm. Experimental animal studies have shown that RA smoothes and polishes the treated areas with removal of only 10–30% of the internal elastic lamina without causing dissection or damage to the media.

6. What is guidewire bias, and how does the choice of guidewire effect bias?

In tortuous vessels, the relatively stiff Rotablator guidewires tend to straighten the vessel. This places the point of attack of the burr on the lesser curvature of the vessel. Both a floppy guidewire and an extra-support guidewire are available. The floppy guidewire tends to minimize guidewire bias but may fail to control the travel of the burr around tight bends, leading to uncontrolled cutting on the greater curvature of the vessel. This phenomenon is not seen with the extra-support guidewire. The extra-support guidewire may straighten out curved vessel segments and cause deep, uncontrolled cuts or dissection in the lesser curvature of the vessel. Appropriately placed hand made bends placed in extra-support wires can help accurately direct the burr to ablate eccentric or angled lesions when guidewire bias away from the lesion is noted.

7. What is the optimal burr to artery ratio?

The luminal diameter following rotablation exceeds the largest burr diameter by 1.19-fold. A 0.7 to 0.8 burr-to-artery ratio for optimal and safe debulking is recommended. In the step technique, a series of gradually larger burrs (usually gradations of 0.5 mm), up to the maximal determined size, are advanced through the lesion. It is advised to start with the smallest effective burr, usually 1.25–1.75 mm. This technique ensures the safest approach with minimization of complications such as no-flow or slow-flow.

8. What are the contraindications to RA?

Angiographic evidence of thrombus and very long lesions (> 25 mm) are contraindicated. Relative contraindications include very angulated lesions and extreme tortuosity, which increase the likelihood of perforation. Degenerated saphenous vein grafts are also contraindicated, although hard fibrotic ostial stenoses have been successfully attempted.

9. Are the particles generated by RA a matter of concern?

During high-speed (140,000–200,000 rpm) RA, only 1.5–2% of the particles generated are larger than 10 μm. With larger burrs (>2.0), some of the particles are bigger. However, the majority of debris is smaller than 15 μm (too small to obstruct the capillary bed) and is cleared by the reticuloendothelial system in the liver, spleen, and lungs. Low speed (<75,000 rpm) RA can generate larger particles that could be a matter of concern.

10. Which strategy, aggressive debulking vs. moderate debulking with adjunctive PTCA, is preferable?

The STRATAS study showed that an aggressive debulking (burr-to-artery ratio of 0.7 to 0.9) followed by no or low-pressure (<1 atm) balloon inflation was not superior to moderate debulking (burr-to-artery ratio < 0.75) followed by balloon angioplasty with conventional inflation pressure (>4 atm). Both strategies had similar angiographic success (90% versus 90.3%), no significant differences in complications (death, MI, or CABG), or in percent restenosis at follow-up.

11. Is RA an effective therapy for in-stent restenosis (ISR)?

Although registry data demonstrate that RA is a safe therapy for ISR, two randomized trials and one non-randomized trial have led to conflicting reports with regards to long-term results. The recently published results of the multicenter Angioplasty Versus Rotational Atherectomy for Treatment of Diffuse In-Stent Restenosis Trial (ARTIST) suggest that balloon angioplasty is a more effective treatment than the combination of RA with adjunctive low pressure (<6 atm) inflation (n = 298). Mean net gain in minimal lumen diameter (MLD) was 0.67 mm and 0.45 mm for PTCA and RA, respectively (p = 0.0019). Angiographically determined restenosis rates (≥50%) were 51% for PTCA and 65% for RA (p = 0.039). Interim results for a single center study (ROSTER) comparing the two strategies demonstrated a benefit for RA over PTCA: MLD 2.8 ± 0.2 mm vs. 2.5 ± 0.3 mm (p = 0.03) and clinical restenosis rates of 20% vs. 43% (p = 0.01), respectively (n = 150).

Until the definitive results of the ROSTER trial are published and can be evaluated, it would seem that RA should not be considered primary therapy for diffuse in-stent restenosis. Preliminary studies suggest it may have some utility in debulking prior to brachytherapy.

12. What are the potential complications of RA?
The periprocedural complications of RA differ to some extent from those seen with balloon angioplasty. Spasm at the site of atherectomy can largely be prevented by the use of intracoronary vasodilators prior and during the procedure. Slow-reflow phenomenon occurs in approximately 1.2–7.6% of the patients. It is more frequent in long, calcified lesions and usually responds to intracoronary nitrates or intracoronary calcium channel blockers. Transient AV block may occur as a result of passage of microparticulate debris or microcavitation bubbles through the vessels perfusing the AV node, SA node, or infranodal conducting tissue. Angiographic complications include dissection in 10–13%, abrupt closure in 1.8–11.2%, and perforation in 0.4–1.5%. Clinical complications are, in general, similar to the ones reported for balloon angioplasty: Q wave MI in 1.3%, urgent coronary artery bypass grafting (CABG) in 1.96%, elevated CK-MB (more than two times normal) in 6% of cases, and death in 0.9% of patients.

DIRECTIONAL CORONARY ATHERECTOMY (DCA)

13. What is directional coronary atherectomy (DCA)?
DCA utilizes a rotating cutting blade to cut and retrieve plaque material. There is a metal chamber, which is open on one side and has a balloon on its opposite side (Fig. 1). After appropriate placement at the site of obstruction, the balloon is inflated. This forces plaque into the cutting cham-

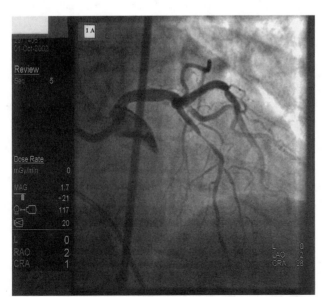

FIGURE 1. Rotoablator-stent. **A,** Coronary angiogram reveals a high grade stenosis of the mid left anterior descending coronary artery. (*continued*)

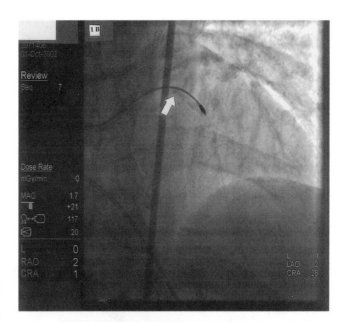

FIGURE 1. (*continued*) **B,** Under fluoroscopy, heavy calcification of the target vessel is seen (arrow) being crossed with a rotoablator burr. **C,** Final result after rotablation and stent deployment.

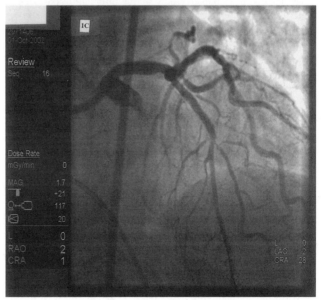

ber. The cutting blade passes through the chamber, excising the plaque and pushing it into a nosecone chamber at the distal end of the catheter for later retrieval. The cutter inside the housing is attached to a flexible drive shaft. A battery-operated motor drive unit that is held by the operator causes the cutting blade to turn at a rate of 2000 rpm. The prototype is the Simpson AtheroCath (Guidant, Santa Clara, CA).

14. How does DCA compare with percutaneous transluminal balloon angioplasty (PTCA)?

In CAVEAT, a large randomized trial comparing DCA with PTCA, DCA was associated with a higher incidence of death and myocardial infarction than balloon angioplasty. Restenosis rates were high in both treatment groups. There was a statistically nonsignificant trend favoring DCA. The Balloon vs. Optimal Atherectomy Trial (BOAT) was conducted with the hypothesis that maximal debulking with adjunctive PTCA would yield improved clinical results compared with PTCA alone. Although restenosis rates were significantly lower (31.4% versus 39.8%; p = 0.16) for the DCA group, late follow-up demonstrated that the risks of death, MI, and target vessel revascularization were similar for DCA and PTCA. In summary, there appears to be no distinct advantage for DCA over PTCA. DCA can be considered a safe alternative to PTCA, especially when lesion specifics are unfavorable for PTCA.

15. What are the complications associated with DCA?

Most complications that occur are similar to those encountered with PTCA. These include dissection with abrupt closure, thrombosis, distal embolization with slow or no-reflow, vasospasm, and side branch occlusion. The incidence of perforation is higher than that found in PTCA.

16. What is the present role for DCA?

DCA is particularly useful in ostial lesions of the right coronary artery or saphenous venous grafts in which PTCA is frequently limited by lesion rigidity and elastic recoil provided by a thick-walled aorta. Both DCA and rotational atherectomy have been used successfully in bifurcation lesions, which are often complicated by the shifting of plaque into the branch vessel. Atherectomy of the main vessel followed by atherectomy or sequential PTCA of the branch is the usual approach. The use of atherectomy in true bifurcations has been shown to improve long-term as well as acute outcomes compared with PTCA alone. DCA has been used successfully in focal lesions of non-degenerated vein grafts; however, there was no difference seen in angiographic restenosis, target lesion revascularization, or event-free survival compared with PTCA in CAVEAT II. Stenoses of the left main coronary artery are well suited for DCA, but most operators prefer stents. DCA should not be used in vessels that contain a large clot burden, owing to the risk of acute closure.

17. Is there a role for DCA in in-stent restenosis?

There have been no randomized trials of this form of debulking compared with conventional therapy. A small series of 45 patients treated with DCA for diffuse in-stent (Palmaz-Schatz) restenosis showed a target lesion revascularization rate of 28.3% at a mean follow-up of 10 ± 4.6 months. Higher rates of CK-MB spillage as well as the possibility of stent damage due to catheter rigidity have limited its application in this regard. A, new more flexible cutting catheter (Flexicut) has shown some early promise in treating this condition with a low incidence of enzyme spillage. More definitive data in this regard are necessary before application of this technique can be recommended.

18. Does debulking with DCA prior to stent implantation improve outcome?

Both the Stenting after Optimal Lesion Debulking (SOLD) and the AtheroLink registries have evaluated the feasibility of DCA prior to stent placement. Both studies have found remarkably low angiographic restenosis rates, 11% and 10.8%, respectively. Combined periprocedure infarct rates (Q-wave and non-Q-wave) were 14.1% and 3%, respectively. The Atherectomy before Multilink Stent Improves Lumen Gain and Clinical Outcomes Study (AMIGO) will help determine whether plaque debulking prior to stenting can reduce restenosis.

19. How does DCA compare with stenting?

There have been few studies directly comparing the two therapies. One intriguing single center study randomized 122 patients to either intravascular ultrasound (IVUS) guided DCA or Palmaz-Schatz stenting. Procedural success and post-procedure lumen diameter were similar in both groups. Angiographic restenosis at 6 months was 32.8% for the stent group and 15.8% for the DCA group (p = 0.032). Target vessel failure defined as either target vessel revascularization or death at 1 year tended to be lower in the DCA group (33.9% vs. 18.3%; p = 0.056). IVUS data suggested the difference in restenosis was primarily due to more profound intimal proliferation in the stent group. This study suggested that angiographic outcome and perhaps clinical outcome with DCA may be better than Palmaz-Schatz stenting. The drawbacks of routinely using this technique are greater technical expertise required for DCA and IVUS, need for multiple passes of the IVUS catheter to evaluate results of DCA, greater procedure and fluoroscopy time, and higher risk of perforation associated with maximal debulking. It is unlikely that DCA will ever supplant stenting, owing to the ease of the later technique.

BIBLIOGRAPHY

1. Baim DS, Cutlip DE, Sharma SK, et al: Final results of the Balloon vs. Optimal Atherectomy Trial (BOAT). Circulation 97:322–331, 1998.
2. Bertrand ME, Van Belle E: Rotational atherectomy. In Topol EJ (ed): Textbook of Interventional Cardiology, 3rd ed. Philadelphia, WB Saunders, 1999, pp 523–532.
3. Dauerman HL, Higgins PJ, Sparano AM, et al: Mechanical debulking versus balloon angioplasty for the treatment of true bifurcation lesions. J Am Coll Cardiol. 32(7):1845–52, 1998.
4. Etsuo T, Satoru S, Nobuhisa A, et al: Final results of the stent versus directional coronary atherectomy randomized trial (START). J Am Coll Cardiol 34(4):1050–1057, 1999.
5. Hopp HW, Baer FM, Ozbek C, et al: A synergistic approach to optimal stenting: directional atherectomy prior to coronary artery stent implantation—the AtheroLink Registry. AtheroLink Study Group. J Am Coll Cardiol 36(6):1853–1859, 2000.
6. Kiesz RS, Rozek MM, Ebersole DG, et al: Novel approach to rotational atherectomy results in low restenosis rates in long, calcified lesions: Long-term results of the San Antonio Rotablator Study (SARS). Cath Cardiovasc Intervent 48:48–53, 1999.
7. Kuntz RE, Baim DS: Coronary atherectomy, atheroablation, and thrombectomy. In Baim DS, Grossman W (eds): Grossman's Cardiac Catheterization, Angiography, and Intervention, 6th ed. Philadelphia, Lippincott Williams & Wilkins, 2002, pp 601–636.
8. Mahdi NA, Pathan AZ, Harrell L, et al: Directional coronary atherectomy for the treatment of Palmaz-Schatz in-stent restenosis. AM J Cardiol 82(11):1345–1351, 1998.
9. Moussa I, Moses J, Di Mario C, et al: Stenting after optimal lesion debulking (SOLD) registry. Angiographic and clinical outcome. Circulation 98(16):1604–1609, 1998.
10. Reifart N, Vandormael M, Krajcar M, et al: Randomized comparison of angioplasty of complex coronary lesions at a single center. Excimer Laser, Rotational Atherectomy, and Balloon Angioplasty Comparison (ERBAC) Study. Circulation 96:91–98, 1997.
11. Reisman M, Safian, RD: Rotablator atherectomy. In Safian RD, Freed MS (eds): The Manual of Interventional Cardiology, 3d ed. Royal Oak, Physician's Press, 2001, pp 617–639.
12. Sharma SK, Kini A, King T, et al: Randomized trial of rotational atherectomy versus balloon angioplasty for in-stent restenosis (ROSTER): Interim analysis of 150 cases (abstr). Eur Heart J 20:281A, 1999.
13. Teirstein PS, Warth DC, Haq N, et al: High-speed rotational coronary atherectomy for patients with diffuse coronary artery disease. J Am Coll Cardiol 18:1694–1701, 1991.
14. Thomas WJ, Cowley MJ, Vetrovec GW, et al: Effectiveness of rotational atherectomy in aortocoronary saphenous vein grafts. Am J Cardiol 86:88–91, 2002.
15. Topol E, Leya F, Pinkerton C, et al: A comparison of directional atherectomy with coronary angioplasty in patients with coronary artery disease. N Engl J Med 329:221–227, 1993.
16. vom Dahl J, Dietz U, Haager PK, et al: Rotational atherectomy does not reduce recurrent in-stent restenosis. Results of the angioplasty versus rotational atherectomy for treatment of diffuse in-stent restenosis trial (ARTIST). Circulation. 105:583–588, 2002.
17. Whitlow PL, Bass TA, Kipperman RM, et al: Results of the study to determine rotoablator and transluminal angioplasty strategy (STRATAS). Am J Cardiol 87:699–705, 2001.

20. THROMBECTOMY DEVICES AND LASERS

On Topaz, M.D.

1. What is the thrombolytic ceiling phenomenon?

Thrombolytic therapy is an established pharmacologic modality that reduces morbidity and mortality in patients with acute myocardial infarction (MI). The principle action of pharmacologic thrombolysis is lysis of a fibrin clot. Indeed, early restoration of antegrade thrombolysis in myocardial infarction (TIMI) 3 coronary flow is associated with improved survival and clinical outcomes. The term *thrombolytic ceiling* describes a clinical phenomenon related to the outcome of administration of reteplase, alteplase, tissue plasminogen activator (t-PA), and streptokinase. These agents succeed in restoring optimal antegrade coronary flow in only 50% to 60% of treated patients. Even triple combination mutant (TNK) t-PA, which has a slower plasma clearance, a greater fibrin specificity, and is 80-fold more resistant to plasminogen activation inhibitor-1 (PAI-1), is unable to "break through" the "angiographic ceiling." A similar phenomenon of partial response to pharmacotherapy can be observed in patients with unstable angina; therefore, its existence carries clinical implications that affect the management of the entire spectrum of acute coronary syndromes (ACS).

2. What are the causes of the thrombolytic ceiling phenomenon?

Pharmacologic therapy for ACS may fail to achieve its reperfusion goals in several scenarios. First, the lytic action of these agents may expose thrombin and enhance its activity. This accelerates formation of more thrombin and promotes increased aggregation of platelets. Then a platelet-rich thrombus can resist thrombolytic therapy and glycoprotein (GP) IIb/IIIa receptor antagonists because of abnormally increased platelet resistance and contractibility as well as increased presence of platelet PAI, a potent inhibitor of fibrinolysis. Furthermore, if the occlusive lesion is mainly composed of atheromatous plaque, fibrotic tissue, or smooth muscle cells, then only a small portion of the cross-sectional area of the target thrombus is exposed to the drug's activity. Other factors accountable for the "thrombolytic ceiling" include older clot age, fibrin fibers' resistance, and clot retraction and organization. Thus, in patients sustaining the phenomenon of "thrombolytic ceiling," restoration of adequate antegrade coronary flow necessitates the application of a mechanical force for thrombus removal (i.e., a thrombectomy device).

3. Which thrombectomy devices are available for PCI?

Mechanical devices for debulking and thrombolysis of obstructive coronary thrombi include ultrasound sonication, AngioJet, TEC, X-Sizer, RESCUE thrombectomy system, lasers, and (to a limited extent) directional coronary atherectomy (DCA). Balloon angioplasty and stents can be used, at times, for successful treatment of a thrombotic lesion; however, their mechanism of action involves platelet shift and thrombus displacement rather than actual debulking. Similarly, cutting balloons slice the target plaque and its associated thrombus and, therefore, are prone to distal embolization and inadequate clot clearance from the target vessel.

4. Describe the technical characteristics of thrombectomy devices.

Ultrasound: The device (Acolysis System, Angiosonics, Inc.) uses a 125-cm probe connected at its proximal and to a piezoelectric transducer. The last 18-cm of the probe is a three-wire flexible segment with a 1.6-mm tip. This design enables the use of a solid metal probe for optimal ultrasound transmission while maintaining flexibility. Ultrasonic energy (42 Hz; 18 W) generated at the transducer is transmitted as longitudinal vibration of the probe and directs the energy into the coronary artery. The effects of therapeutic ultrasound on the thrombus are attributed to mechanical contact, cavitation, formation of intracellular microcurrents and micro-streaming, and thermal phenomenon. The device has a rapid-exchange design and is compatible with 7-Fr percutaneous transluminal coronary angioplasty (PTCA) guiding catheter and 0.014-inch guidewire.

AngioJet: The rheolytic thrombectomy device known as AngioJet (Possis Medical, Minneapolis, MN) is based on technology that removes thrombus from blood vessels by means of the Bernoulli principle. The catheter is sized 5, 6, or 8 Fr. It consists of a 140-cm dual-lumen shaft that connects at its proximal end to a drive unit console. The smaller of the two lumen shafts contains a stainless steel hypotube that transports pressurized saline from the pump of the device unit to the catheter tip. The larger central lumen exhausts the effluent material from the catheter to an external collection chamber and provides a passage for the guidewire. When activated, high-speed saline jets energize from six holes, each of 50-μ diameter, in a showerhead-like ring tip aimed at the evacuation lumen of the catheter. The catheter tip is placed proximal to the target thrombus and passed slowly across the thrombus at a rate of 1 to 2 mm/sec. Prophylactic temporary pacing is a considerable limitation. Pacing is often necessary to overcome serious heart blocks during the activation of the AngioJet.

TEC (transluminal extraction catheter): The TEC device (IVT, San Diego, CA) combines thrombectomy, aspiration, and atherectomy capabilities. It consists of a conical cutting head with two stainless steel blades attached to the distal end of a flexible, hollow torque tube. The proximal end of the catheter attaches to a battery-powered handheld motor drive unit and to a vacuum bottle for aspiration of excised material. The motor unit activates cutting blade rotation (750 rpm) and aspiration and a lever controls advancement and retraction of the cutter. A special 0.014-inch steel guidewire for TEC has a terminal 0.021-inch ball to prevent advancement of the cutter beyond the guidewire tip and to prevent wire tip entrapment. The cutters are available in sizes from 5.5 to 7.5 Fr (1.8–2.5 mm). Guiding catheters sized 8 to 10Fr with a variety of shapes are available from the TEC manufacturer or other companies. For a 2.5-mm cutter, a 10-Fr guiding catheter is necessary, and for the smallest cutter (1.8 mm) an 8-Fr guiding catheter is adequate.

X-Sizer: The device (Endicor, San Clemante, CA) is designed to extract thrombus and soft atherosclerotic material. It consists of a helical cutter assembly and a dual-lumen catheter. The cutter tip sizes are 2.0 and 2.3 mm, and it can be applied with 8- and 9-Fr guiding catheters over extra support guidewire. It appears that the only practical difference between the X-Sizer and TEC is the rate of cutter spinning (2100 vs. 750 rpm, respectively).

RESCUE Thrombectomy System: This new percutaneous device is an aspiration and thrombectomy tool (Boston Scientific, Redmond, WA) with a collection bottle for aspirated thrombi. The catheter is compatible with a 7-Fr guiding catheter. It is expected that the design of the system will assist in easy manipulation and achieve improved coronary thrombectomy.

5. What are the current indications for thrombectomy devices?

These devices can be used in a variety of ACS. In unstable angina, they can be applied for treatment of thrombus-containing lesions. In acute MI, they are used as primary PCI tool if standard techniques are deemed unsuitable. Also, they are indicated in cases of "thrombolytic ceiling," which require a mechanical force for thrombus debulking in order to overcome thrombus resistance. These modalities are useful as well in management of patients with contraindications to either pharmacologic thrombolysis or platelet glycoprotein (GP) IIb/IIIa receptor inhibitors. The presence of complex underlying plaque or depressed left ventricular function should not deter experienced interventionalists, and these devices can actually perform emergency revascularization efficiently and safely in severely compromised patients such as those in cardiogenic shock.

6. Are GP IIb/IIIa receptor antagonists contraindicated with thrombectomy devices?

GP IIb/IIIa inhibitors reduce recurrent ischemic events in patients undergoing PCI. They have also been shown to reduce subsequent adverse coronary events. The mechanism accountable for the decrease in frequency of ischemic events is inhibition of crosslinking of platelets by fibrinogen. Of note, the benefit of the platelet IIb/IIIa inhibitors remains clinically unproven for lesions with *angiographic* thrombus. A recent publication containing pooled data from six large clinical trials confirmed that these agents have no positive impact on clinical outcomes in PCI for *angiographic* thrombus-containing lesions. An angiographic subanalysis of the PRISM-PLUS trial demonstrated that the presence of *angiographic thrombus,* despite treatment with a IIb/IIIa antagonist, was a predictor of major adverse coronary events such as MI, repeat revascularization, 30-day mortality, and composite endpoints. According to the RAPPORT study, final TIMI flow is predicted to be less than grade 3 when abciximab is used in the presence of an angiographic thrombus. Hence, a thrombectomy device can potentially enhance the effect of GP IIb/IIIa receptor antagonists and increase the grade of TIMI flow in the target vessel. Sullebarger et al. compared PCI of saphenous vein grafts using TEC and abciximab versus combined treatment of TEC and heparin. All patients treated with combination of TEC and abciximab had successful, complete revascularization without any complications. In only 50% of patients treated with TEC and heparin, a complete success was achieved, and in 30%, distal embolization occurred. Thus, an approach combining mechanical thrombectomy device with pharamacologic agent such as GP IIb/IIIa receptor antagonist may be safe and highly effective.

7. What is power thrombectomy?

Power thrombectomy is a new term describing a revascularization strategy incorporating a mechanical device for removal of occlusive coronary thrombi in conjunction with or after administration of pharmacologic thrombolytic agents or platelet GP IIb/IIIa inhibitors or both. The goals of power thrombectomy are to achieve enhanced vessel patency; improve antegrade coronary flow; and, consequently, gain greater myocardial preservation than that achieved by pharmacotherapy alone.

8. Is adjunctive medical treatment for thrombectomy devices different than for balloons and stents?

Basically, medications are the same as those for PTCA. All patients should receive aspirin (325 mg/day at least 1 day before the procedure), heparin to achieve and maintain activated clotting time (ACT) $\geq$ 250 seconds during the procedure, and intracoronary nitroglycerin 100 to 200 μg intracoronary injection before activation of the device. Intracoronary verapamil 100 μg/min up to 1.0 to 1.5 mg is often administered for prophylactic or cessation of no reflow. Many interventionalists begin Plavix PO 300 mg the day before the procedure or during the PCI.

9. What are the principles governing the formation of laser energy?

Albert Einstein was the first scientist to postulate and explain the principles of a physical phenomenon he termed LASER (light amplification by stimulated emission of radiation). Lasers generate intense, monochromatic, coherent light beams that are delivered to small areas of biologic tissue with great precision through optic fibers. Lasers are categorized by their wavelength and mode of pulse generation. The first cardiovascular lasers were continuous-wave sources distinguished by weak power (e.g., argon lasers) and significant heat production at the target lesion. In the mid 1980s, Grundfest et al. pioneered the delivery of pulsed-wave photoacoustic energy with second-generation laser devices, the excimer cold laser (xenon chloride active medium, energy emitted at the ultraviolet zone of the electromagnetic spectrum with a 308 nm wavelength). This device successfully vaporates atherosclerotic plaques with limited irradiation of thermal energy to the surrounding arterial wall. To debulke an atherosclerotic plaque or thrombus, a process of absorption of the laser energy within the plaque must occur. The excimer laser, which is currently the only laser approved by the Food and Drug Administration for treatment of coronary artery disease (CAD), relies on energy absorption in the nonaqueous constituents of the atherosclerotic plaque, such as proteins and nucleic acids. Absorption of laser energy within a plaque, thrombus, or myocardium accounts for photomechanical (i.e., buildup of pressure and propagation of acoustic pressure waves), photochemical (i.e., breaking of chemical bonds), and photothermal (i.e., increase in material temperature) interactions that are manifested by vaporization and removal of the irradiated target tissue. If the laser catheter is maneuvered in a fashion that violates efficient and safe laser techniques, the photoacoustic energy will not be absorbed; instead, it will be reflected, scattered, or transmitted either with no effect at all on the tissue or by creating adverse effects such as thrombosis, acute vessel closure, spasm, dissection, or perforation. This frequently occurs when operators advance the laser catheter rapidly, reaching an advancement speed of 0.5 mm/sec or faster, thus exceeding the actual penetration depth for excimer laser, which is

only 35 to 50 μ. Choice of laser catheter size is important as well because, in contrast to the practice with balloons and stents, the laser's size should be matched to the severity of the target lesion
(i.e., the more *severe* the stenosis, the *smaller* catheter size).

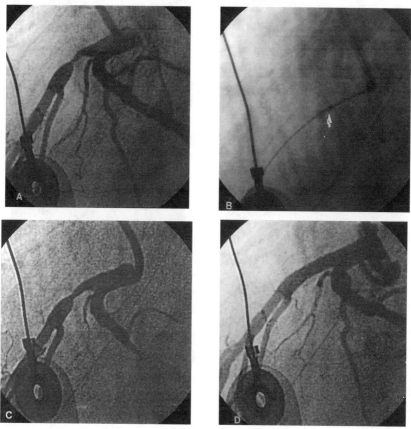

FIGURE 1. Application of excimer laser in a patient with severe unstable angina. *A*, Lateral-cranial view;
95% stenosis of proximal left anterior descending coronary artery. *B*, 0.9-mm rapid exchange Vitesse excimer
laser catheter (*tip marked*) (Spectranetics, Colorado Springs, CO) at the target lesion. This is currently the
smallest debulking device available. *C*, Angiographic demonstration of laser-induced pilot recanalization.
D, Final view after adjunct stenting.

10. What processes does laser energy initiate within the atherosclerotic plaque?

During pulsed-wave laser emission, several processes occur within the target plaque. Powerful, high-frequency acoustic compression is generated; then it transforms into shock waves that
propagate through the plaque. If uncontrolled, these acoustic waves can cause dissections and perforations, although they can assist in fragmentation of calcified athroma. Then the plaque is transformed into an expanded vapor bubble, which essentially is the byproduct of debulking.

11. What are the current clinical indications for excimer laser angioplasty?

Currently, excimer laser angioplasty is indicated for treatment of complex atherosclerotic lesions that deemed "non ideal" for standard balloon angioplasty. The clinical conditions in which
excimer laser has been demonstrated as an efficient and safe technology include unstable angina,
acute MI, and peripheral atherosclerotic occlusive vascular disease. Of note, this laser is used suc-

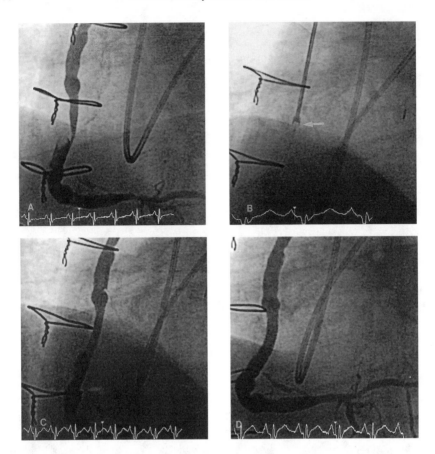

FIGURE 2. Application of TEC in a patient s/p coronary artery bypass graft surgery with acute inferior wall MI and cardiogenic shock. *A,* A critical eccentric thrombotic lesion in a saphenous vein graft to distal RCA. Another lesion is noted at the anastamosis. *B,* A 2.0-mm TEC catheter (*tip marked*) (IVT, San Diego, CA) at the target lesion. Large amount of thrombotic material was aspirated. *C,* Angiography after TEC. *D,* Final results after stenting. The lesion at the anastamosis of the saphenous vein (SV) graft was dilated with balloon and stenting

cessfully in heart transplant recipients who develop severe, focal, atherosclerotic allograft disease. This laser is also approved for pacemaker lead removal by electrophysiology practice.

Indications and Contraindications: Excimer Laser Angioplasty

TARGET LESION INDICATION	CONTRAINDICATIONS
Complex eccentric and concentric plaques	Target vessel smaller than catheter size
Thrombotic lesions: coronary and peripheral	Unprotected left main
Debulking before brachytherapy	Severe lesion angulation
Debulking for in-stent restenosis	Heavily calcified lesions
Debulking before stenting	Coronary perforation
Saphenous vein grafts: Ostial, focal, anostamosis, and thrombotic lesions	Coronary dissection
Total occlusions: coronary and peripheral	
Bifurcation lesions	
Lesions that cannot be crossed or dilated with a balloon	

The excimer laser can be used with femoral, brachial, or radial approach. If needed, it can be delivered with "double wire" technique because it does not interact with the material of the guidewire. Depressed left ventricular function is not a contraindication; in fact, the device gains considerable success in these compromised patients. Because severe bradycardia and heart block are exceedingly rare, prophylactic temporary pacemakers are not required.

12. What are the benefits of laser angioplasty in ACS?

Laser application carries several benefits, including rapid removal of the thrombus, vaporization of procoagulant reactants, absence of a systemic lytic state, facilitation of adjunct balloon angioplasty, stenting, augmentation of t-PA activity, and suppression of platelet aggregation.

13. Which laser catheters are available for coronary revascularization?

There are two types of approved excimer laser catheters. Concentric catheters vary in size from 0.9, 1.4, 1.7, and 2.0 mm. The 1.4-, 1.7-, and 2.0-mm lasers are manufactured with the optimally spaced fibers technology, and the 0.9-mm lasers, which is the smallest debulking device available, is produced with the traditional fiber-packing technology. Eccentric catheters for "quadrant debulking" that are similar to DCA are available in sizes of 1.7 and 2.0 mm.

14. What are the components of safe laser technique?

The most severe complications of laser intervention include perforation, dissection, and acute vessel closure. The most important aspect of safe laser angioplasty is the use of heparinized saline flush for removal of contrast and dilution of blood at the ablation site. This technique is crucial because dye has a significant potentiating effect on peak pressure wave generation. We recommend delivery of 2 to 3 trains of laser emission followed by retraction of the laser catheter into the guide catheter and injection of intracoronary nitroglycerin. The laser catheter can be then readvanced or a larger laser catheter can be used for further debulking.This "pulse and retreat" laser technique minimizes acoustic injury. Lasing during retraction of the catheter along the lesion is currently recommended. Energy fluence is usually set at 45 mJ/mm^2, 25 Hz; however, higher energy 60 mJ/mm^2, 40 Hz is considered beneficial for thrombotic or resistant lesions. A "wireless" lasing technique for selected patients with total SFA occlusions or total aorto-ostial saphenous graft occlusions has recently been introduced.

15. Does the composition of the target lesion affect the laser energy levels required for debulking?

In a multicenter study involving the investigational mid-infrared, solid-state, pulsed-wave holmium:YAG laser (2.1 μ wavelength), 1862 symptomatic patients with significant CAD were treated. Analyzing the effect of lesion composition on laser energy levels required for debulking, investigators discovered that restenosis lesions, known to be composed of smooth muscle proliferation, needed more laser pulses for ablation than *de novo* lesions, which usually contain thrombus, cholesterol plaque, and fibrosis. A similar observation had recently been made regarding angiographic thrombotic lesions in acute MI and unstable angina. The thrombotic lesions appear to require a higher level of excimer laser energy compared with nonthrombotic lesions.

16. Can lasers be used for peripheral revascularization?

Perpheral atherosclerotic arterial disease is a major cause of lower extremity ischemia and limb loss. Limitations of percutaneous balloon angioplasty for peripheral revascularization are noted in long lesions and total occlusions. Laser energy has been shown to effectively treat these lesions, and cases of major complications are infrequent. Professor Biamino from Germany pioneered laser for peripheral revascularization applications, especially in total, long SFA occlusions. In experience with 318 consecutive patients who received excimer laser angioplasty of 411 SFA, total occlusions averaging 19±6 cm in length, Biamino's group recorded a 91% procedural success. The excimer laser has recently also been tested in inferopopliteal arterial disease and appears to provide efficient and safe means of revascularization for patients with non-healing ulcers. An interesting development has recently emerged regarding potential application of laser energy for treatment of acute thrombotic stroke and acute ischemic-thrombotic syndromes. The catheters available for peripheral lasing vary in size from 2.0 to 2.5 mm.

BIBLIOGRAPHY

1. Anderson JL: Why does thrombolysis fail? Breaking through the reperfusion ceiling. Am J Cardiol 80: 1588–1990, 1999.
2. Cannon CP: Overcoming thrombolytic resistance. J Am Coll Cardiol 34:1395–1402, 1999.
3. Dahm JB, Topaz O, Weonckhaus C, et al: Laser-facilitated thrombectomy: A new therapeutic option for treatment of thrombus-laden coronary lesions. Cath Cardiovasc Intervent 56:365–372, 2002.
4. Das TS: Percutaneous peripherial revascularization with excimer laser: equipment, technique and results. Laser Med Sci 16:101–107, 2001.
5. Grelich PE, Carr ME, Zekert SL, Dent RM: Quantitative assessment of platelet function and clot structure in patients with severe coronary artery disease. Am J Med Sci 307:15–20, 1994.
6. Grundfest WS, Litvack F, Forrester J, et al: Laser ablation of human atherosclerotic plaque without adjunct tissue injury. J Am Coll Cardiol 5:929–933, 1985.
7. Kwok OH, Prpic R, Gaspar J, et al: Angiographic outcome after intracoronary X-Sizer helical atherectomy and thrombectomy: first use in humans. Cath Cardiovasc Intervent 55:133–139, 2002.
8. Nishida T, Nakamura M, Tsunda T, et al: A case of acute myocardial infarction treated with a new thrombectomy system. Cath Cardiovasc Intervent 55:239–243, 2002.
9. Rosenschein U, Faul G, Erbel R, et al: Percutaneous transluminal ultrasonic therapy of occluded saphenous vein grafts. Circulation 99:26–29, 1999.
10. Scheinert D, Laird JR, Schroeder M, et al: Excimer laser-assisted recanalization of long, chronic superficial femoral artery occlusions. J Endovasc Therapy 8:156–166, 2001.
11. Singh M, Reeder GS, Ohman EM, et al: Does the presence of thrombus seen on a coronary angiogram affect the outcome after percutaneous coronary angioplasty? An angiographic trials pool data experience. J Am Coll Cardiol 38:624–630, 2001.
12. Singh M, Tiede DJ, Mathew V, et al: Rheolytic thrombectomy with AngioJet in thrombus-containing lesions. Cath Cardiovasc Intervent 56:1–7, 2002.
13. Sullenbarger JT, Dalton RD, Nasser A, Matar FA: Adjunct abcixiab improves outcomes during revascularization of totally occluded saphenous vein grafts using TEC. Cath Cardiovasc Intervent 46:107–110, 1999.
14. Topaz O, Bernardo N, Desai P, Janin Y: Acute thrombotic-ischemic coronary syndromes: the usefulness of TEC. Cath Cardiovasc Intervent 48:406–420, 1999.
15. Topaz O, Perin EC, Jesse RL, et al: Power thrombectomy in acute coronary syndromes. J Invas Cardiol 2003, in press.
16. Topaz O, Rosenbaum EA, Luxenberg MG, Schumacher A: Laser assisted coronary angioplasty in patients with severely depressed left ventricular function: quantitative coronary arteriography and clinical results. J Intervent Cardiol 8:661–669, 1995.
17. Topaz O, McIvor M, Stone GW, et al: Acute results, complications and effect of lesion characteristics on outcome with solid-state, pulsed-wave mid-infrared laser angioplasty system: final multicenter report. Laser Surg Med 22:228–239, 1998.
18. Topaz O, Bernardo NL, McQueen RA, et al: Effectiveness of excimer laser coronary angioplasty in acute myocardial infarction or in unstable angina pectoris. Am J Cardiol 87:849–855, 2001.
19. Topaz O: Lasers. In Topol EJ (ed): Textbook of Interventional Cardiology, 4th ed. Philadelphia, W.B. Saunders, 2003, pp 675–703.
20. Topaz O, Minisi AJ, Bernardo NL: Comparison of effectiveness of excimer laser angioplasty in patients with acute coronary syndromes versus those without normal left ventricular ejection fraction. Am J Cardiol [in press].

21. EMBOLIC PROTECTION DEVICES

Fernando A. Cura, M.D.

1. How frequently does distal embolization occur?

Since the introduction of percutaneous coronary intervention (PCI), we have been under the impression that embolization is a rare event, confined chiefly to revascularization of degenerated saphenous vein grafts (SVGs). Angiographic evidence of distal embolization has been described from 0.1% during elective angioplasty to 15.0% among SVG or acute myocardial infarction (MI) interventions. However, almost every patient undergoing percutaneous revascularization has particulate matter retrieved when an embolic filter device is used.

With more systematic assessments of cardiac enzymes—specifically, creatine kinase (CK), its MB isoform, and troponin—evidence has begun to clarify the incidence of periprocedural MI. The reported incidence of CK-MB elevation after PCI is between 25 and 37%. One third of those are elevations above three times the upper limit of normal. Factors that may cause elevated CK-MB levels include not only distal embolization but also side branch occlusion, thrombus formation, and coronary spasm. This suggests that although embolization is extraordinarily common, approximately one third of patients actually suffer some extent of measurable myocyte damage. Perhaps most patients still experience some embolization but do not go on to myonecrosis either because the burden of particulate matter is much less or because there are adaptive responses to accommodate the process.

With the availability of imaging technology that includes magnetic resonance imaging (MRI) and transcerebral and transcranial Doppler, microvascular obstruction has been documented in a far greater proportion of patients than ever conceived during carotid interventions. Although the occurrence of ischemic stroke after carotid stenting is relatively low ($< 2\%$), cerebral microembolization detected by transcranial Doppler is reported in virtually every patient undergoing the procedure. In a transcanial Doppler study, an average of 74 distal emboli per procedure has been observed during balloon angioplasty and stenting.

2. What is the clinical importance of coronary distal embolization?

The linkage between microvascular obstruction and an unfavorable long-term clinical prognosis has been established in many series. Furthermore, therapeutics shown to reduce microvascular obstruction have improved clinical outcomes. The degree of risk is proportional to the magnitude of the increase in cardiac enzymes. The cause and long-term consequences of relatively low-grade subclinical CK-MB elevations (or troponin) remains somewhat conjectural. It appears that CK-MB elevations more than three times the normal level definitely increase the risk of late infarction or cardiac death. Lesser elevations above the range of normal may also portend a modest increase in risk.

3. When does embolization occur during angioplasty?

The incidence of microemboli occurring during carotid angioplasty and stenting was studied by transcranial Doppler monitoring in the different phases of the procedure. Microembolization was detected in the middle cerebral artery during guidewire crossing, balloon dilatation, stent implantation, and after postdilatation. However, the mean number of microemboli is highest during balloon predilation than subsequent stenting. Direct stenting without balloon predilation was associated with less embolization than seen with the combination of balloon predilation and subsequent stenting.

4. How frequent is distal embolization with different interventional strategies?

The lowest incidence of myonecrosis is during balloon angioplasty. Although directional and rotational atherectomy improve angiographic results compared with balloon angioplasty, postprocedural infarction occurs at least twice as often with these technologies. The incidence associated with stent placement is comparable to and possibly higher than that of balloon angioplasty; however, it was recently reported that direct stenting without predilatation reduces this complication.

However, the use of antiplatelet agents, particularly the glycoprotein (GP) IIb/IIIa inhibitors, as well as clopidogrel in patients acute coronary syndromes (ACS) has been shown to reduce the incidence of postprocedural MI. Moreover, the use of embolic protection devices during SVG intervention has also demonstrated a reduction in acute ischemic events.

5. What subgroup of patients is at increased risk of embolization?

It is important to recognize a certain profile of individuals who are most apt to shower emboli at the time of a revascularization procedure. The diffuseness of disease, plaque burden, friability of the atheromatous lesion, and presence of thrombus seem to be the most likely predisposing features. In particular, patients with aged and diffusely diseased SVGs are at the highest risk of postprocedural MI. The risk of developing CK-MB elevation is about 50% during SVG intervention, mainly because of the more friable atherosclerotic or thrombotic components of plaques.

The incidence and magnitude of observed elevations are twice higher for patients with unstable rather than stable angina, in particular among patients with acute MI. Myocardial contrast echocardiography has shown that 25% or more of patients with what appeared to be brisk epicardial flow after reperfusion therapy (Thrombolysis in Myocardial Infarction [TIMI] 3 grade using conventional contrast dye angiographic assessment) did not have tissue level reperfusion corresponding to microvascular obstruction. The use of percutaneous thrombectomy and embolic protection devices may result in significant improvement of clinical outcomes. Patients with unstable coronary syndromes may experience similar benefit because of the increased risk of distal embolization of thrombotic lesions. Diabetics have an increased mortality rate after PCI that could be attributed to the diffuseness of atherosclerotic involvement and extent of preexisting microvascular disease that reduces the adaptive capacity to embolization.

6. Who should be considered for embolic protection devices?

Distal embolization after angioplasty in degenerated SVGs results in high rates of postprocedural myonecrosis and subsequent mortality. However, this risk does not appear to be significantly reduced with GP IIb/IIIa inhibition. Macroscopically visible red or yellow debris is extracted in more than 90% of patients. The recently published Saphenous vein graft Angioplasty Free of Emboli Randomized (SAFER) trial has demonstrated a significant reduction in major adverse cardiac events among patients treated with embolic protection devices, the PercuSurge GuardWire Temporary Occlusion and Aspiration System (Medtronic AVE, Santa Rosa, CA). There was a profound reduction (42% relative) in the 30-day primary endpoint of death, MI, or revascularization (9.6% for GuardWire patients versus 16.5% for control patients; $P = 0.004$). This predominantly reflects a reduction in MI of all magnitudes (see table below). In addition, final TIMI grade 3 flow was higher for the GuardWire group compared with the control arm, and distal protection offered similar benefit against ischemic events, whether or not the operator had decided to pretreat with a platelet GP IIb/IIIa receptor blocker.

CLINICAL ENDPOINT (30 DAY)	GUARDWIRE ($N = 406$)	CONTROL ($N = 395$)	P
MI	8.6	14.7	0.008
Q-wave MI	1.2	1.3	NS
Non–Q-wave MI (> three times normal CK-MB)	7.4	13.7	0.006
Death	1.0	2.3	0.170

On the other hand, most of the neurologic complications after carotid stenting are caused by intracerebral embolism of fragmented plaques or clots. The risk of embolization appears to be highest in elderly patients; those with ulcerated, thrombotic, long, and multiple lesions, and echolucent plaques; and among symptomatic patients. However, every plaque generates some amount of embolic material. Thus, for the individual patient, a neurologic event during the stent procedure cannot be predicted with certainty and a cerebral protection system is therefore desirable for every patient. Different embolic protection devices are currently used to prevent post-procedural stroke.

Embolic protection devices have been also tested in patients undergoing percutaneous native coronary, renal, and vascular intervention, with retrieval of atherosclerotic material in almost every patient. However, the clinical benefits of these devices is under investigation.

7. What are the histologic findings of the embolized material?

The composition, quantity, and size of embolic particulate debris depend on the characteristics of the lesion treated. Between 50% and 90% of patients have grossly visible particulate material aspirated. The aspirated particles ranged from 22 to 667 per patient, and their size ranged from 3.6 to 5262.0 μm in maximum diameter (mean, 203 $\pm$ 256 μm). However, the majority of particles are less than 96 μ. Light microscopy revealed that the particles consisted predominantly of necrotic core with cholesterol clefts, lipid-rich macrophages, fibrin material, old and fresh thrombi, and calcific plaque fragments (Figs. 1 and 2). Fibrous caps and smooth muscle cells were identified, but these appeared relatively sparse.

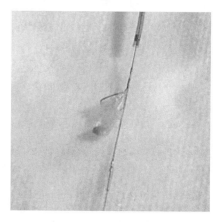

FIGURE 1. FilterWire (Boston Scientific, Natick, MA) with captured emboli.

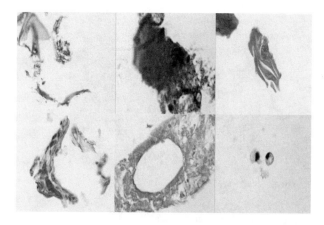

FIGURE 2. Example of collected debris.

8. What types of embolic protection systems are available for SVG intervention?

Recently, a few devices have been designed to trap embolic material in the coronary circulation, in particular during SVG intervention. These devices fall into two general types: 1) distal balloons that occlude the artery during intervention with aspiration of debris with a small catheter and 2) filters that trap debris during intervention and are then collapsed and retrieved.

9. Name the embolic protection devices available for SVG intervention.

The PercuSurge GuardWire system (Medtronic AVE, Santa Rosa, CA) consists of a 190-mm long hollow 0.014-inch guidewire with a central lumen connected to a compliant balloon with a maximum diameter of 5.0 mm reached at an inflation pressure less than 2 atm (Fig. 3).

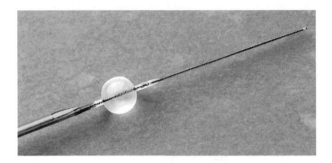

FIGURE 3. GuardWire Temporary Occlusion and Aspiration System (Medtronic AVE, Santa Rosa, CA).

The GuardWire catheter is advanced distal to the lesion and inflated to maintain complete lumen occlusion. During occlusion of the distal graft, the interventional procedure is performed through the dedicated hollow 0.014-inch guidewire. At the end, a monorail aspiration catheter (connected to a 20-cc vacuum syringe) is used to evacuate atherosclerotic or thrombotic debris.

The AngioGuard Filter System (Cordis, Johnson & Johnson, New Brunswick, NJ) consists of a 0.014-inch angioplasty guidewire with an expandable umbrella-type filter at the distal tip that uses a 100-μ, laser-drilled holes in a polymeric shelve that, when opened, trap debris. The filter is expanded by eight nitinol struts and have four radiopaque markers. The manufactured filter sizes are 4.0, 5.0, and 6.0 mm. The porous membrane permits normal distal blood flow while trapping potential emboli by filtration. By collapsing the umbrella, the filtered debris can be captured and removed (Fig. 4). These devices are currently undergoing multicenter evaluation (SAFE study) with promising preliminary results.

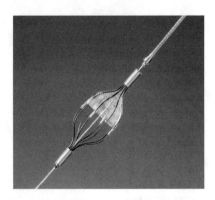

FIGURE 4. AngioGuard XP Filter Configuration (Cordis, Johnson & Johnson).

The EPI FilterWire (Boston Scientific, Natick, MA) is a filter protection system that is currently under clinical investigation. It consists of a polyurethane filter that has distal pores 80 μm in diameter. The filter is delivered by a 3.8-Fr delivery catheter (Fig. 5). The filter is expanded by a nitinol loop at the proximal end of the filter that adapts to the vessel size.

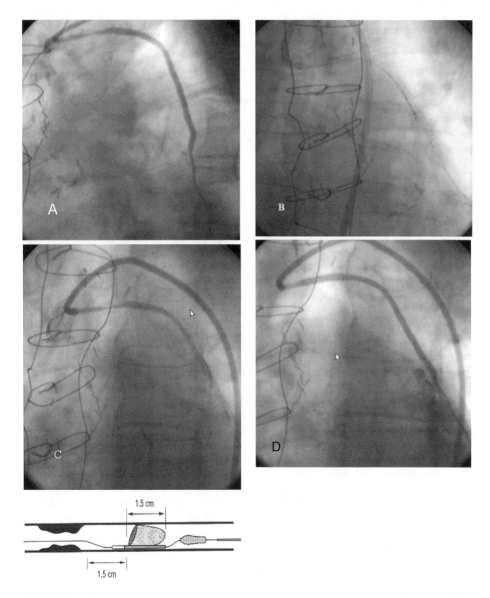

FIGURE 5. *A*, Severe proximal complex lesion in saphenous vein graft to left anterior descending (LAD) coronary artery. *B*, EPI FilterWire crossing the lesion. *C*, Expanded filter in vessel. *D*, Successful angiographic result.

10. What types of embolic protection systems are available for carotid intervention?

The common goal of these devices is the distal capture of any material that may be set free during stenting of the target lesion. This is achieved by distal temporary occlusion of the target artery with subsequent aspiration of blood and debris through the placement of a filtration device distal to the lesion or by proximal catheter occlusion of the common and external carotid arteries; this establishes protection by reversing blood flow in the target vessel.

11. Name the type of emboli protection devices available for carotid intervention.

The PercuSurge GuardWire system (Medtronic AVE, Santa Rosa, CA), which is similar to the coronary system, comprises three components: the GuardWire temporary occlusion catheter, the MicroSeal adapter, and the aspiration catheter. The GuardWire is manufactured in 0.014- and 0.018-inch diameters, with lengths of 190 and 300 cm. The guidewire carries at its distal end an elastomeric balloon that can be inflated at low pressure. The size of the elastomeric balloon varies to accommodate vessel diameters from 4.0 to 6.0 mm.

Recently, a variety of temporary arterial filter systems designed to capture and remove particulate matter released during carotid stenting has become available. The NeuroShield Cerebral Protection System (MedNova Ltd., Galway, Ireland), AngioGuard system (Cordis Corp., Johnson & Johnson, New Brunswick, NJ), EPI FilterWire (Boston Scientific, Natick, MA), and TRAP vascular filtration system (Microvena Corporation, White Bear Lake, MN) share similar characteristics.

There are two flow-reversal systems, the MO.MA system (INVATEC, Concesio, Italy) and the Parodi Anti-Emboli System (ArteriA, San Francisco, CA), by which the external and the common carotid artery are occluded by soft balloons that are located at the tip of the catheter and the sheath, respectively, in order to establish a flow reversal from the involved internal carotid artery to the sheath. The Parodi Anti-Emboli System establishes backflow by connecting the arterial sheath with a venous sheath that is placed into the femoral vein. A filter, which is located between the arteriovenous shunt, prevents the embolic particles from entering the venous system.

12. What risks are associated with using embolic protection devices?

The majority of the systems are first-generation devices; therefore, some of the filters still have a large crossing profile with the subsequent risk of distal embolization while crossing high-grade stenoses. Other technical complications of the filters include spasm and vessel dissection at the site of the system placement. Distal embolization associated with transient occlusion with large amount of embolized debris while using filter protection systems or incomplete material retrieved with aspirate devices has been described. Moreover, the balloon occlusion–type devices cause distal ischemia that may not be tolerated by some patients.

13. What are the limitations of embolic protection devices?

Specific anatomical considerations may contraindicate the use of a protection device. These considerations include the presence of an abnormal vessel segment distal to the target lesion and not enough distal length to place the device ($\geq \sim 30$ mm is needed). In the case of balloon occlusion system during carotid intervention, the tolerance may be jeopardized in the presence of total occlusion of the contralateral carotid artery with ipsilateral vertebral or intracranial disease.

Some limitations of the devices are important to highlight. The aspiration catheter of the balloon occlusion system may not remove all particles trapped in the arteries. In addition, angiography cannot be performed while the distal balloon is inflated, making assessment of lesion morphology and stent placement more difficult. The filter-type devices have a finite lower limit in the size of particles that can be captured; the practical lower limit for pore size appears to be 50 μm. Smaller microparticulate matter can still get through the filter, although particles that small may have no clinical significance. It is still early in the development of these catheter- and guidewire-based systems; making them as atraumatic as possible, with the lowest profile and highest torque-ability, will require further iterative engineering. Without question, several emboli protection devices will evolve and ultimately be incorporated into the daily practice of PCI and peripheral revascularization.

BIBLIOGRAPHY

1. Baim DS, Wahr D, George B, et al: Randomized trial of a distal embolic protection device during percutaneous intervention of saphenous vein aorto-coronary bypass grafts. Circulation 105:1285–1290, 2002.

2. Califf RM, Abdelmeguid AE, Kuntz RE, et al: Myonecrosis after revascularization procedures. J Am Coll Cardiol 31:241–251, 1998.

3. Grube E, Gerckens U, Yeung AC, et al: Prevention of distal embolization during coronary angioplasty in saphenous vein grafts and native vessels using porous filter protection. Circulation 104:2436–2441, 2001.

4. Macdonald S, Venables GS, Cleveland TJ, Gaines PA: Protected carotid stenting: safety and efficacy of the MedNova NeuroShield filter. J Vasc Surg 35:966–972, 2002.

5. Markus HS, Clifton A, Buckenham T, Brown MM: Carotid angioplasty: detection of embolic signals during and after the procedure. Stroke 25:2403–2406, 1994.

6. Ohki T, Parodi J, Veith FJ, et al: Efficacy of a proximal occlusion catheter with reversal of flow in the prevention of embolic events during carotid artery stenting: an experimental analysis. J Vasc Surg 33:504–509, 2001.

7. Piana RN, Paik GY, Moscucci M, et al: Incidence and treatment of "no-reflow" after percutaneous coronary intervention. Circulation 89:2514–2518, 1994.

8. Qureshi AI, Luft AR, Janardhan V, et al: Identification of patients at risk for periprocedural neurological deficits associated with carotid angioplasty and stenting. Stroke 31:376–382, 2000.

9. Reimers B, Corvaja N, Moshiri S, et al: Cerebral protection with filter devices during carotid artery stenting. Circulation 104:12–15, 2001.

10. Tardiff BE, Califf RM, Tcheng JE, et al: Clinical outcomes after detection of elevated cardiac enzymes in patients undergoing percutaneous intervention: IMPACT-II Investigators: Integrilin (eptifibatide) to Minimize Platelet Aggregation and Coronary Thrombosis-II. J Am Coll Cardiol 33:88–96, 1999.

11. Topol EJ, Yadav JS: Recognition of the importance of embolization in atherosclerotic vascular disease. Circulation 101:570–580, 2000.

12. Webb JG, Carere RG, Virmani R, et al: Retrieval and analysis of particulate debris after saphenous vein graft intervention. J Am Coll Cardiol 34:468–475, 1999.

22. INTRAVASCULAR ULTRASOUND

Samir R. Kapadia, M.D.

1. What is an intravascular ultrasound (IVUS) examination?

IVUS examination involves introduction of a small (~ 1 mm in diameter) catheter with an ultrasound probe in coronary arteries to examine the vessel lumen and vessel wall. It is an invasive procedure that is most commonly performed by an interventional cardiologist in the cardiac catheterization laboratory. This technique is now commonly available and fairly frequently used in clinical practice to answer specific questions related to vessel wall and lumen morphology. It is the only clinically available technique that currently provides *in vivo*, high-resolution images of the coronary artery wall.

2. What is the typical resolution of IVUS imaging?

High ultrasound frequencies (20–50 MHz) are used for intravascular imaging, which allows high-resolution imaging. High frequency can be effectively used because the transducer is placed in close proximity to the vessel wall, compensating for less penetration of the high-frequency ultrasound. This is in contrast to surface echocardiography in which 5.0 to 7.5 MHz frequencies are used to allow for appropriate penetration of ultrasound. The use of high frequency provides excellent resolution because the ultrasound wavelength, which determines the maximum resolution, is inversely proportional to the frequency. At 30 MHz, the wavelength is approximately 50 μm, which permits axial resolution of approximately 100 to 150 μm. Determinants of lateral resolution are more complicated and depend on the imaging depth and beam shape. Typically, lateral resolution for a 30-MHz device averages approximately 250 to 300 μm at distances most prevalent in coronary imaging. The thickness of the slice of coronary artery imaged (beam width) is approximately 300 μm. (Fig. 1)

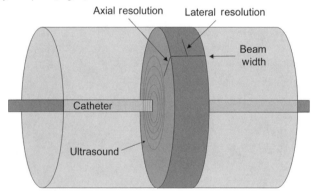

FIGURE 1. Typical resolution of an IVUS image.

3. What are the different types of ultrasound catheters?

Two different types of transducer designs have emerged: mechanically rotated devices and multi-element electronic arrays. These two approaches exhibit significantly different characteristics, which can influence both image quality and handling properties.

Mechanical probes use a drive cable that runs the length of the catheter that rotates a single piezoelectric transducer element mounted near the distal catheter tip. For most mechanical ultrasound systems, a rotation rate of 1800 rpm is used, yielding 30 images per second. Image quality is better than that of electronic arrays, but the rotating shaft can introduce artifacts if uniform rotation of shaft cannot be achieved because of vessel tortuosity or other mechanical reasons.

In the electronic systems, an annular array of multiple piezoelectric transducer elements is activated sequentially to generate an image. The electronic signals are processed by several ultra-miniaturized integrated circuits near the catheter tip. Accordingly, only two flexible conductive wires are required within the catheter shaft, which yields a flexible catheter. Currently available annular array catheters yield somewhat inferior images compared with mechanical catheters, particularly in the areas close to catheter (i.e., near field).

4. How do a normal and diseased arteries look when they are examined with IVUS?

In a normal coronary artery, the discrete echodense layer at the lumen–wall interface represents the tunica intima. The tunica media is visualized as a distinct subintimal echolucent layer, which is limited by an outer echodense external elastic membrane (EEM). The outer edge of the adventitia is indistinct because it merges into the surrounding perivascular connective tissue. The vessel size is conventionally determined as EEM area. The echodense intima and adventitia with the echolucent medial layer in between give the arterial wall a trilaminar appearance. However, this characteristic pattern is not a universal finding during *in vivo* examinations. In 30% to 50% of normal coronary segments, the very thin intimal layer poorly reflects ultrasound and leads to dropout of signals, which results in a monolayer appearance of the arterial wall.

The blood within the vessel lumen exhibits a characteristic pattern of echogenicity. The lumen is characterized by blood flow seen as subtle, finely textured echoes moving in a characteristic swirling pattern. Plaque is seen as an echodense layer between the lumen and external elastic membrane (Fig. 2). Calcification, fibrous capsule, and echolucent areas (presumably lipid pools) can be visualized in some plaques. Diameter stenosis and area stenosis of the vessel can be measured directly at the lesion site.

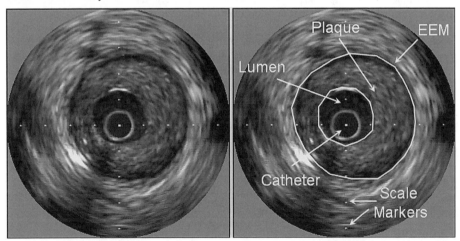

FIGURE 2. IVUS image of a diseased coronary artery with a circumferential plaque. The catheter is seen in the center of the lumen. The lumen is seen as a dark area circumscribed by the intimal layer. Plaque is seen between the intima and EEM. The echolucent area just beneath the EEM represents media. The distance between the markers is 1 mm.

5. What are the different methods available to visualize a coronary artery, and how does IVUS compare with them?

Angiography, magnetic resonance imaging (MRI), computed tomography (CT) scan and IVUS are the currently available techniques used to visualize coronary arteries.

Angiography allows rapid visualization of the entire coronary tree. However, it only allows visualization of the lumens of the vessels. It has many limitations (Table 1). MRI and CT scan currently do not have resolution comparable to angiography or IVUS for coronary imaging. Image acquisition time and motion of the heart are the major challenges in improving resolution for these very promising noninvasive technologies to visualize coronary arteries.

IVUS allows precise visualization of the plaque and coronary artery lumen with high resolution. Currently, it is the only technique to allow *in vivo* visualization of the coronary artery wall with high resolution. However, it is invasive, and longitudinal reconstruction of the entire coronary artery can be time consuming and difficult. Accordingly, it is best used as a complementary technique to angiography when angiography cannot provide definite answers.

Table 1. Limitations of Angiography

Limitations related to two-dimensional imaging
1. Eccentric plaques
2. Bifurcation lesions
3. Complex lumen shapes (e.g., after angioplasty, ruptured plaque)
4. Coronary artery motion and overlap
Limitations related to the inability to visualize the vessel wall
1. Vessel remodeling
2. Diffuse disease
3. Characterization of haziness (e.g., calcification, dissection, eccentric plaque)
4. Characterization of plaque structure

6. What is arterial remodeling, and what is its significance in imaging coronary arteries?

Remodeling refers to the changes in arterial dimensions associated with the development of atherosclerosis lesion. Initial development of a plaque affects the vessel size (i.e., EEM area) more than the lumen of the artery. The plaque grows outward in the arterial wall for some time and then starts encroaching upon the lumen. This focal arterial enlargement at atherosclerotic lesion sites was initially described by Glagov et al in a necropsy study of left main coronary arteries. In lesions with area stenosis less than 30% to 40%, the increase in arterial size "overcompensated" for the plaque deposition, leading to an increase in lumen area. With more advanced lesions (area stenosis > 40%), the degree of arterial enlargement or remodeling was less evident and worse disease resulted in a smaller lumen area. IVUS has allowed the *in vivo* study of remodeling and has confirmed these necropsy observations.

Compensatory remodeling has several clinical implications. It represents one possible explanation for the frequent underestimation of the severity of atherosclerotic disease by contrast angiography. Similarly, it may influence the angiographic estimation of the true size of the coronary artery, which is crucial for the success of coronary interventions. Negative remodeling (i.e., constriction of the vessel) has been implicated in restenosis after balloon angioplasty. Recent IVUS studies have found a relationship between the extent of remodeling and the clinical presentation in patients with coronary artery disease (CAD). It appears that whereas patients with unstable angina frequently have positively remodeled large plaques, patients with stable angina frequently have negatively remodeled relatively small plaques.

7. What is the role of IVUS in assessing indeterminate lesions by coronary angiography?

Occasionally, despite multiple projections, the severity of certain lesions is difficult to ascertain by angiography. For these ambiguous lesions, IVUS provides a method for accurate quantification of plaque and lumen. In intermediate lesions, IVUS area stenosis greater than 70%, minimal lumen diameter 1.8 to 2.0 mm or less, and minimal lumen area 4.0 mm^2 or less reliably identify functionally significant coronary stenoses. For left main coronary artery, these thresholds are less clear, but minimal lumen diameter 3 to 4 mm or less and minimal lumen area 7.0 to 9.0 mm^2 or less are considered to be significant.

8. What are the applications of IVUS in stenting?

IVUS can provide useful information regarding the vessel size, amount of calcification, eccentricity of plaque, and involvement of the ostium. In certain patients, this information can be very useful in planning the interventional strategy and selecting devices. After deployment of a stent, IVUS examination can help to determine proper apposition of the stent struts, peristent dissections, or significant plaque prolapse. Multiple studies have attempted to determine whether routine use of IVUS to guide stenting makes a clinically significant difference in outcome after stenting. Although some evidence suggests that routine use of IVUS can improve outcomes, the reduction in restenosis is relatively small. Furthermore, it adds to the time and cost of the procedure. Accordingly, routine use of IVUS to guide stenting is not practical. However, when there is doubt regarding the reference diameter or the adequacy of the stent result, low threshold should be exercised in using IVUS guidance.

9. What is the role of IVUS in atherectomy?

The presence of significant superficial calcification can be identified by IVUS when directional atherectomy (DCA) is not typically successful. Adequacy of debulking can be investigated with IVUS because many IVUS studies have demonstrated substantial residual plaque burden after atherectomy despite good angiographic results. However, the role of DCA in the era of stenting remains questionable.

IVUS imaging has confirmed the principle of differential cutting with high-speed rotational atherectomy. As in the case of DCA, IVUS demonstrates a large residual plaque burden after rotational atherectomy. However, IVUS imaging before rotational atherectomy may not be feasible in most patients because rotational atherectomy is mostly used in severely calcified vessels where IVUS catheter can be difficult to deliver.

10. What are the major areas where IVUS has helped in understanding transplant CAD?

Transplant CAD includes atherosclerosis lesions present in donor hearts before transplantation and lesions of transplant vasculopathy that develop after transplantation. IVUS studies have helped to understand many aspects of these disease processes.

IVUS studies have shown that transmission of donor atherosclerosis is very common ($\sim$ 50%) despite normal angiograms. However, the donor atherosclerosis lesions do not predispose to transplant vasculopathy or worse outcome. The progression of donor lesion is most pronounced in first 2 years after transplantation and seems to be related to high cholesterol (mainly triglycerides) in recipients.

Early lesions of transplant vasculopathy (TV) are present in 50% of patients at 1 year, and these lesions are morphologically difficult to distinguish from atherosclerosis lesions, although they are more frequently concentric and diffuse. At 5 years, almost 80% of the patients have TV lesions. TV lesions are more severe in patients with significant change in their cholesterol from baseline. It has also been shown that cholesterol lowering decreases the rate of progression of TV lesions. Furthermore, the detection of severe TV lesions by IVUS 1 year after transplantation predicts worse long-term outcome in recipients. In summary, IVUS information is very useful in clinical and research investigations of TV.

11. What is an optimally deployed stent by IVUS?

Optimal stent deployment is variably defined in different trials. Suggested relative stent expansion criteria, which compare the minimal stent area with that of the reference segments, include 90% or more or 100% of the distal and 80% or 90% or more of the average reference lumen areas. A target minimal stent area greater than 7 or 8 mm^2 can be used as a rapid criterion for identifying an optimal stent result; however, obviously this number is dependent on the normal reference diameter of the vessel. Some laboratories aim at reaching a lumen symmetry index greater than 0.7, determined as the minor in-stent diameter divided by the major diameter. Minor dissections detected by IVUS do not seem to affect outcome.

12. What are IVUS-derived endpoints for atherosclerosis regression trials?

In atherosclerosis regression-progression trials, IVUS-derived measurements are now used as endpoints. The best method to quantify atherosclerosis burden is to measure as many possible frames from a slow motorized pullback. Motorized pullback is necessary to calculate the longitudinal extent of atherosclerosis plaque because it allows steady, constant speed of pullback. Typically, motorized pullback is performed at 0.5 mm/sec. The cross-sectional slices at each 1 mm are measured and the plaque volume is calculated by multiplying the plaque area with the longitudinal distance. The change in plaque volume at baseline is compared with that on follow-up examination, usually 1 to 2 years apart. Lumen and vessel volume can also be followed for better understanding of the pathophysiology of atherosclerosis.

13. How safe is IVUS examination?

IVUS is safe with very low complication rate, commonly reported to be 1% to 3%; the most frequent complication being transient arterial spasm, which responds rapidly to intracoronary nitroglycerin. The major complication rate (i.e., dissection or vessel closure) occurs in fewer than 0.5% of patients. Almost all major complications occur in patients undergoing IVUS examination to aid interventional procedure in severely atherosclerotic arteries rather than in patients undergoing diagnostic imaging for moderately diseased arteries. Moreover, IVUS examination does not seem to accelerate the progression of atherosclerosis.

14. What are the most common artifacts in an IVUS image?

The most common and important artifact, NURD (non-uniform rotational distortion), arises from uneven drag on the drive cable of the mechanical catheters, resulting in visible distortion of the image (Fig. 3). It can sometimes be minimized by using coaxial guiding catheters or lubricants or not overtightening the hemostatic valve. The "ring-down" artifact is produced by acoustic oscillations in the piezoelectric transducer that obscure the near field, resulting in an acoustic catheter size larger than its physical size. Geometric distortion can result from imaging in an oblique plane (i.e., a plane not perpendicular to the long axis of the vessel). This is particularly a problem in tortuous vessels. IVUS catheters that are not properly flushed give a starry appearance from microbubbles.

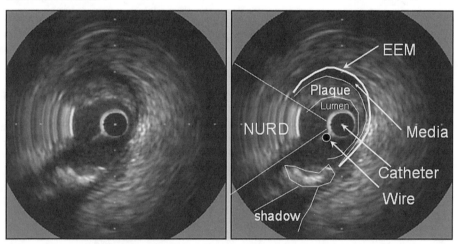

FIGURE 3. An example of NURD artifact. It is seen as smearing of the pixels caused by uneven drag on the drive cable. In this image, coronary calcification is seen, which casts acoustic shadow. The catheter, guidewire (with its shadow), and plaque are well visualized.

15. Are there other applications of IVUS beyond coronary imaging?

IVUS can be used to investigate any intravascular structure. This is particularly useful in measurement of aortic size and the relationship of renal artery origin to aortic aneurysm in endovascular treatment of abdominal aortic aneurysms. A 12.5-MHz probe is usually used for visualizing larger arteries. Mechanical catheters have been used for intracardiac echocardiography to identify precise morphology, but this method does not allow Doppler interrogation of flow. Because of this reason, it has fallen out of favor, especially with advent of better phase array intracardiac echocardiography probes (e.g., Acunav).

16. What is the role of IVUS in radiation therapy?

The success and safety of brachytherapy depends on delivering the precise dose to the artery wall. Because the vessel wall is not seen on angiography, the accurate dose delivery is possible only with IVUS measurement of treatment segment. Furthermore, IVUS has proven useful in clarifying the mechanisms of benefit and refining the techniques in brachytherapy. Radiation effects are strongly influenced by the dose delivered to the media or adventitia, which is dependent on the thickness and composition of the plaque and the position of the catheter in the lumen. Shielding of normal vessel in eccentric plaque and routine guidance of IVUS for radiation treatment are some of the rapidly evolving research areas.

BIBLIOGRAPHY

1. Kapadia SR, Nissen SE, Ziada KM, et al: Development of transplantation vasculopathy and progression of donor-transmitted atherosclerosis: comparison by serial intravascular ultrasound imaging. Circulation 98:2672–2678, 1998.
2. Kapadia SR, Nissen SE, Tuzcu EM: Impact of intravascular ultrasound in understanding transplant coronary artery disease. Curr Opin Cardiol 14:140–150, 1999.
3. Kapadia SR, Nissen SE, Ziada KM, et al: Impact of lipid abnormalities in development and progression of transplant coronary disease: a serial intravascular ultrasound study. J Am Coll Cardiol 38:206–213, 2001.
4. Mintz GS, Nissen SE, Anderson WD, et al: American College of Cardiology Clinical Expert Consensus Document on Standards for Acquisition, Measurement and Reporting of Intravascular Ultrasound Studies (IVUS): a report of the American College of Cardiology Task Force on Clinical Expert Consensus Documents. J Am Coll Cardiol 37:1478–1492, 2001.
5. Nissen SE: Application of intravascular ultrasound to characterize coronary artery disease and assess the progression or regression of atherosclerosis. Am J Cardiol 89(suppl B):24–31, 2002.
6. Nissen SE, Yock P: Intravascular ultrasound: novel pathophysiological insights and current clinical applications. Circulation 103:604–616, 2001.
7. Schoenhagen P, Nissen S: Understanding coronary artery disease: tomographic imaging with intravascular ultrasound. Heart 88:91–96, 2002.
8. Tuzcu EM, Kapadia SR, Tutar E, et al: High prevalence of coronary atherosclerosis in asymptomatic teenagers and young adults: evidence from intravascular ultrasound. Circulation 103:2705–2710, 2001.
9. Ziada KM, Kapadia SR, Tuzcu EM, Nissen SE: The current status of intravascular ultrasound imaging. Curr Probl Cardiol 24:541–566, 1999.

23. PRESSURE AND DOPPLER SENSOR GUIDEWIRES*

Morton J. Kern, M.D.

1. How does the Doppler signal measure flow?

Intracoronary flow velocity is measured by a steerable, flexible angioplasty guidewire with a piezoelectric ultrasound transducer mounted at the tip (FloWire; JOMED Inc., Uppsala, Sweden). The speed (velocity) of red blood cells flowing past an ultrasound-emitting and -receiving crystal can be measured by the Doppler phase shift in frequency:

$$Velocity\ (cm/sec) = (F1*F2)*C/2*F2*Cos\ (\Phi)$$

Where:
Velocity = velocity of coronary blood flow
Freq 1 = transmitting frequency of the Doppler crystal
Freq 2 = returning frequency to the Doppler crystal
Constant = speed of sound in blood
Cos Φ = angle of incidence at the crystal

Volumetric flow in the epicardial artery can be obtained by multiplying the flow velocity above by the vessel cross-sectional area (cm^2) measured by online quantitative imaging techniques, yielding a value in cm^3/sec. Definitions of coronary vasodilatory reserve (CVR), relative CVR, and fractional flow reserve (FFR) have been previously discussed. The total cross-sectional area of the 0.014-inch guidewire is $0.164\ mm^2$ or less than 21% cross-sectional area of a 1-mm diameter catheter. Velocity measurements obtained with the Doppler guidewire techniques have been validated both *in vitro* and *in vivo* by Doucette et al. and Labovitz et al.

2. What is the reproducibility of Doppler measurements?

The reproducibility of intracoronary Doppler measurements was examined by Gaster et al. Intra- and inter-observer variability of online and offline measurements was compared in 108 patients referred for coronary angioplasty. For two measured coronary flow reserve (CFR) values, the limit of agreement between the two measurements was 27% to 39% of the first measured value. At a CFR value of 2.5, for a 95% confidence interval (CI), the next measurement would be within 1.8 to 3.5. An initial CFR value of 3 or more indicated that all subsequent CFR values would be 2.5 or more. All patients with initial CFR values of 2.0 or less had reproducible CFR values within the 95% CI of 2.5 or less. The authors indicated that CFR measurements were most reproducible for values around 2.5, allowing lesion triage according to hemodynamic significance.

3. How does a stenosis influence arterial flow?

A significant epicardial stenosis produces characteristic alterations in phasic flow patterns, hyperemic capacity, and distal flow relative to a normal proximal flow value. In vessels greater than 2 mm in diameter, a nominal ($< 15\%$) decrease in flow velocity can be expected from proximal to distal, secondary to diffuse disease and arterial branches. However, because blood flow velocity and vessel cross-sectional area decrease concordantly from proximal to distal, the respective flow proximal to distal flow velocity ratio should be close to unity.

Critical stenosis also impairs maximal hyperemia and reduces coronary vasodilatory reserve.

4. What is adenosine, and what does it do?

Adenosine is a naturally occurring nucleoside that is formed within the myocytes from either dephosphorylation of adenosine triphosphate (ATP) or cyclic adenosine monophosphate (cAMP)

---

*Some sections reproduced from Kern MJ: Curriculum in coronary physiology. Cath Cardiovas Diag 54: 376–400, 2001.

or from S-adenosyl homocysteine. It is rapidly removed from the blood by both a high-affinity red blood cell uptake mechanism and a direct deamination, with a half-life in human blood of less than 20 seconds. Adenosine interacts with purinergic subclass A_2 receptors to increases cytosolic cAMP as the second messenger for vasomotion. Because of its unique position in ATP metabolism, adenosine appears to be an important endogenous regulator of coronary blood flow during both stress and ischemia. Adenosine produces maximal coronary hyperemia and effects atrioventricular nodal conduction.

5. How does intravenous compare with intracoronary adenosine for use with FFR?

The vasodilatory effects of adenosine are primarily on the microcirculation, with little effect on the epicardial conduit arteries. Both intracoronary and intravenous adenosine infusions produce maximal hyperemia in humans. Heart transplant patients appear to be especially sensitive to intracoronary adenosine injections. The standard dose of intracoronary adenosine is 18 to 40 μg (i.e., with smaller doses used for right coronary artery injections.)

Jeremias et al. examined differences in FFR between intracoronary (IC) (15–20 μg in the right and 18–24 μg in the left coronary artery) and intravenous (IV) adenosine (140 μg/kg/min) in 52 patients with 60 lesions. Mean percent stenosis was 56% ± 24% (range, 0% to 95%). The mean FFR was 0.78 ± 0.15 with a range of 0.41 to 0.98. There was a strong, significant, linear relationship between IC and IV adenosine ($r = 0.978$; $P < 0.001$). The differences in measured FFR between IC and IV methods was −0.004 ± 0.03. A small random scatter in both directions of FFR was 8.3%, where intracoronary adenosine FFR was ≥ 0.05 compared with IV FFR, suggesting a suboptimal IC hyperemic response in some patients. Changes from basal heart rate and blood pressure were greater with IV adenosine. Two patients taking IV — but none taking IC adenosine — had side effects of bronchospasm and nausea. These data indicate that IC adenosine is equivalent to IV infusion for determination of FFR in large majority of patients. However, in a small percentage of people in whom coronary hyperemia may be suspected to be suboptimal with IC adenosine, a repeated higher IC adenosine dose may be helpful.

6. How much IC adenosine should be used for CVR?

The use of incremental dosing of IC adenosine for the measurement of CVR has been recommended by Segni et al. who divided 457 patients into two groups, those with normal coronary arteries and those with intermediate (40%–70%) coronary artery disease. CVR was measured after incremental doses of adenosine, (12–54 ug i.c. for the left coronary arteries [LCA] 6 to 42 ug i.c. for the right coronary artery [RCA]). Only 40% of the patients showed maximal CVR values after the first administered dose; 39% of patients with normal arteries and 27% of patients with intermediate disease required incremental dosing to achieve a CVR greater than 2.5. The author suggested repeating IC adenosine until a plateau of CVR is achieved. Therefore, it is recommended to use IC bolus adenosine 18 to 30 μg for the RCA and 24 to 40 μg for the LCA.

7. Can ATP or dobutamine be used to induce maximal coronary hyperemia?

Although unavailable in the United States, ATP (adenosine 5′-triphosphate) may also be used to stimulate maximal hyperemia. IC ATP of 0.5, 5, 15, 30, and 50 μg, respectively, compared favorably with papaverine responses without significant hemodynamic or electrocardiographic changes. Maximal coronary vasodilation could be safely obtained with IC ATP doses of 15 μg or more.

Dobutamine (10–40 μg/kg/min IV) was compared with IC adenosine in 22 patients with single-vessel CAD. Peak dobutamine infusion produced similar distal coronary pressure and pressure ratios (P_d/P_a 60 ± 18 vs. 59 ± 18 mm Hg; FFR 0.68 ± 0.18 and 0.68 ± 0.17, respectively; all $P = NS$). An additional bolus of IC adenosine given at peak dobutamine in nine patients failed to change the FFR. IV dobutamine acted like adenosine and fully exhausted myocardial resistance. Coronary reserve and left ventricular ischemic responses can thus be obtained in the catheterization laboratory lab if needed.

8. What is provisional stenting, and when is it used?

Provisional stenting has been proposed whereby balloon angioplasty guided by angiographic anatomy and a physiologic endpoint is performed, and stenting is only done when endpoint criteria are not met. Five multicenter trials proved the concept of provisional stenting. However, provisional stenting using coronary flow, pressure, or intravascular ultrasound (IVUS) has not become common practice for several reasons. The results of routine stenting without adjunctive technology are excellent. A large percentage of provisional stenting procedures still require stenting because of suboptimal anatomic physiologic results. Provisional stenting is more time consuming than routine stenting. In some analyses, routine stenting appears less costly than provisional stenting, and any cost differential is offset by the increased procedure time to use adjunctive technology (IVUS and coronary flow or pressure). Because significant reductions in major adverse clinical events after stenting are evident, provisional stenting seems unlikely to supplant routine stenting in clinical practice.

9. Do physiologic endpoints provide prognostic data?

Major predictors of adverse cardiac events after stent implantation can be determined by intracoronary Doppler and quantitative coronary angiography. Haude et al. examined both absolute and relative coronary reserve and angiographic results in 150 patients 6 months after stenting. Thirty-three of the 150 patients developed adverse cardiac events with relative CVR less than 0.88, an incidence of 6.8%. A combination of relative CVR greater than 0.88 and percent diameter stenosis less than 11% predicted an adverse cardiac event rate of 1.5%. The measurement of relative CVR and percent diameter stenosis after stenting were highly significant for identifying patients at risk for major adverse cardiac events 6 months after stenting (Fig. 1). Serruys et al. also note that even in stented patients, a high CVR was associated with lower 6-month target lesion revascularization (TLR) rates.

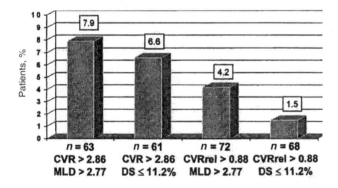

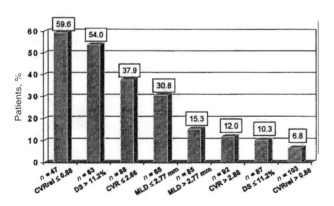

FIGURE 1. Incidence of MACE at follow-up in patient subgroups with coronary stent implantation selected by cutoff values for morphometric and functional parameters (*top*) or their combination (*bottom*). Reproduced with permission from Haude et al: Circulation 103:1212–1217, 2001.

10. What is the relationship between FFR and restenosis?

Fujita et al. examined the relationship between FFR and angiographic restenosis in 32 patients after PCI. After intervention, coronary stenosis diameter was improved from 68% ± 13% to 23% ± 15%. There was no correlation between pressure gradients at rest or during hyperemia or FFR with the percent diameter of stenosis after intervention. On follow-up angiography at 6 months in all patients, angiographic restenosis (percent diameter stenosis > 50%) occurred in four patients (12.5%). There was no correlation between resting pressure gradient and percent diameter stenosis at follow-up, but the hyperemic pressure gradient and FFR correlated with percent diameter stenosis ($r = 0.559$, $P < 0.01$; $r = 0.703$; $P < 0.0001$, respectively), indicating that hyperemic pressure gradients and FFR may be useful in predicting of restenosis. Further examination in large patient numbers shows a direct relationship between low restenosis rates and high FFR.

11. How are coronary physiologic and IVUS measurements related?

In 73 patients, Abizaid et al. reported that a minimum lumen cross-sectional area of less than 4.0 mm^2 or mean lumen diameter (MLD_{IVUS}) of less than 2.0 mm has a diagnostic accuracy of 92% for identification of diseased vessels with a CVR of less than 2.0. quantitative coronary arteriography (QCA) lesion length, but not lumen diameter, was an independent predictor of CVR. A similar study comparing IVUS, QCA, and FFR in 42 patients with 51 stenoses also demonstrated that QCA alone was not accurate in determining physiologic lesion significance assessed by either IVUS or FFR. There was, however, a strong correlation between minimal lumen area by IVUS less than 3.0 mm^2 and CSA_{IVUS} stenosis greater than 60% with a measured FFR less than 0.75 (IVUS sensitivity, 83%; specificity, 92% respectively).

Briguori et al. also found that the percent area stenosis and lesional length had a significant inverse correlation to FFR ($r = -0.58$, $P < 0.001$; $r = -0.41$, $P < 0.004$, respectively). Hanekamp et al. found that a normal FFR after stent deployment indicates good stent implantation. In 31 patients with 81 paired IVUS and FFR measurements, an FFR greater than 0.94 indicated a 91% concordance in the ability to predict suboptimum stent deployment ($P < 0.00001$). QCA alone showed a low concordance rate with either IVUS or FFR (48% and 46%, respectively).

A similar U.S. multicenter trial of 84 patients compared IVUS results and FFR for determining optimal stent placement. Isolated coronary artery lesions had stent placement with increasing inflation pressures and serial IVUS measurements. Starting at 10 atmospheres and increasing serially by two atmospheres, FFR was checked until it was greater than 0.94 or 16 atmospheres was achieved. IVUS measurements were then performed. Over the range of IVUS criteria, the highest sensitivity, specificity, and predictive accuracy of FFR were 80%, 30%, and 42%, respectively. Receiver operator characteristics (ROC) curves defined an optimal FFR at 0.96 or more. At this threshold, sensitivity, specificity, and predicted accuracy of FFR were 75%, 58%, and 62%, respectively. With a high concordance to FFR and IVUS, the negative predicted value was 88%. Significantly better diagnostic information was achieved in patients receiving the highest IC adenosine doses (≥ 30 μg) during FFR measurements. The study concluded that an FFR of 0.96 or less after stent deployment predicted suboptimal IVUS criteria of deployment. However, an FFR of more than 0.96 did not reliably predict an optimal stent result.

Van Liebergen et al. demonstrated improved hyperemic coronary flow after optimized stent implantation guided by IVUS in 20 patients. When maximal hyperemia after optimal balloon angioplasty (guided by IVUS imaging) is achieved, further flow increases after stenting are not expected. The absence of functional residual luminal obstruction after IVUS-guided balloon angioplasty may explain similar clinical outcomes reported for percutaneous transluminal coronary angioplasty results in the provisional stent studies.

Criteria for optimal FFR, QCA, and IVUS values in the assessment of optimal stent deployment in an *in vitro* model were examined by Matthys et al. FFR and QCA, as well as IVUS measurements, were obtained in 4-mm diameter tubes with varying stenoses from 40% to 60%. When flow rates varied from 50 to 150 mL/min, FFR increased by 2% to 7%. At 100 mL/min, FFR increased by only 0.8% from suboptimal to optimal deployment. The gain in FFR between suboptimal and optimal deployment was less than 5% for flows at 100 mL/min, but FFR may increase 15% to 20% for changes in blood flow from 50 to 150 mL/min. The authors concluded that IVUS and QCA were more appropriate for the assessment of optimal stent deployment. This data appear to be supported by that of Fearon et al. in a multicenter trial.

12. Do Doppler parameters after stenting have prognostic value?

Intracoronary Doppler parameters predicted major adverse cardiac events after stent implantation. Haude et al. measured distal and relative CVR in 150 patients after PTCA stenting with 6-month follow-up. The results revealed that major adverse cardiac events in 33 patients at 6 months were associated with reduced CVR (2.96 ± 0.87 vs. 2.40 ± 0.7, $P = 0.001$), relative CVR (1.02 ± 0.24 vs. 0.81 ± 0.24, $P = 0.001$), and minimal luminal diameter (2.98 ± 0.56 mm vs. 2.11 ± 0.74 mm, $P = 0.001$). A postintervention relative CVR of more than 0.88 was the best single predictor, with an incidence of 6.8% major adverse cardiac events. A combination of relative CVR greater than 0.88 and a percent diameter stenosis less than 11.2% was associated with incidence of major adverse cardiac events of only 1.5%.

13. Do patients with chronic total occlusions have microvascular disease?

In patients with chronic total occlusion, microvascular dysfunction may be more commonly encountered than previously expected. Werner et al. found reduced coronary flow reserve after successful recanalization and stenting of chronic total occlusions of more than 4 weeks' duration in 42 patients. Coronary flow reserve was less than 2.0 in 55% of all patients. In a subgroup of patients with simultaneous pressure and flow velocity recordings, 52% of patients showed CFR less than 2 and FFR greater than 0.75, confirming significant microvascular dysfunction. Both CFR and FFR were reduced in only two patients (8%). A low CFR was associated with higher average peak velocity (36 ± 17 vs. 22 vs. 12 cm/sec, $P = 0.006$). Doppler parameters did not change in the first 24 hours after recanalization. The authors concluded that patients with diabetes or hypertension had a lower CFR than those without this comorbidity, but that microvascular dysfunction was still observed in 55% of chronic total occlusions independent of impairment of regional microvascular dysfunction. Neither CFR nor FFR alone is appropriate for assessing angioplasty results in patients with chronic total occlusion, and combined measurements help differentiate microvascular from residual coronary stenosis.

14. How does left bundle branch block (LBBB) affect coronary flow?

Phasic coronary flow velocity patterns and CVR may be abnormal in patients with LBBB. Thirteen patients with LBBB and normal arteries underwent stress thallium scintigraphy after cardiac catheterization. Eleven control subjects without LBBB were also examined. Whereas the time to maximum peak diastolic flow velocity was longer for patients with LBBB (134 ± 19 ms vs. 105 ± 12 ms, $P < 0.05$), acceleration was slower (170 ± 54 vs. 279 ± 96 cm/s^2, respectively, $P < 0.05$). CVR in patients with exercise perfusion defects was lower in patients without perfusion defects and in the control group (2.7 ± 0.3, 3.7 ± 0.5, and 3.4 ± 0.5; all $P < 0.05$). The investigators indicated that LBBB causes early diastolic blood flow impairment in the left anterior descending artery (LAD) because of diastolic compressive resistance from delayed ventricular relaxation and that scintigraphic perfusion defects in these patients were associated with lower coronary flow reserve, also supporting abnormalities of the microvascular function.

15. How is coronary physiology used for patients with acute myocardial infarction (MI)?

An impaired CVR appears related to the degree of residual stenoses and the amount of viable myocardium and microcirculatory injury in the region adjacent to the infarct. Mazur et al. measured CVR in 32 patients who underwent PTCA 6.9 ± 3.4 days after acute MI. Patients were classified into two groups according to the presence (20 patients) or absence (nine patients) of improvement in LV wall motion (LVWM) on echocardiographic study performed after 7 weeks after baseline study. Coronary flow reserve in the infarct related artery was significantly higher in the LVWM recovery group (1.43 ± 0.57 vs. 0.98 ± 0.70, $P = 0.0001$) compared with the no LVWM recovery group.

Because microvascular stunning partially recovers over time, a highly variable acute condition limits the use of physiologic measurements in the first days of the index event. Some investigators reported postinfarction CVR greater than 1.3 may be associated with preservation of the microcirculation, but others found no relationship between CVR and myocardial viability by scintigraphy. CVR did not differentiate between patients with extensive versus small infarctions, suggesting that CVR cannot resolve the regional microcirculation nor be directly related it to the extent of myonecrosis.

The capacitance of viable myocardium should be reflected in phasic flow characteristics. Kawamoto et al. measured systolic average peak flow velocity and diastolic flow velocity deceleration time (DDT) in 23 patients with acute anterior MI and found that if the systolic APV was greater than 6.5 cm/sec or the DDT greater than 600 ms, there was greater LVWM recovery within the infarcted region and improved regional LVWM on follow-up echocardiography (Fig. 2). Similarly, Tsunoda et al. evaluated continuous flow velocity measurements for 18 ± 4 hours after successful angioplasty in 19 patients with acute anterior MI. Two divergent flow response groups were identified. In patients in whom average peak velocity (APV) increased after only a transient decline, regional wall motion and overall LV systolic function improved (ejection fraction [EF] increased $17 \pm 9\%$). However, if the APV progressively decreased throughout the next day, LV systolic function did not improve (EF increased only $4 \pm 9\%$; $P = 0.007$).

Viable myocardium   Nonviable myocardium

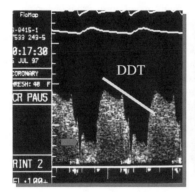 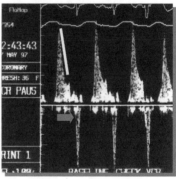

FIGURE 2. Phasic coronary blood flow patterns immediately after recanalization in infarct patients. In viable myocardium, antegrade flow is dominant during systole (*left*). Diastolic peak velocity showed normal deceleration. In this case, LV function was well preserved by effective reperfusion.

In patients from the nonviable group, early systolic retrograde flow is dominant and antegrade flow is decreased (*right*). Diastolic peak velocity showed rapid deceleration. In this case, little functional recovery was seen despite successful recanalization. Reproduced with permission from Kawamoto et al: Circulation 100: 339–345, 1999.

16. What is the use of early systolic flow reversal and diastolic deceleration time?

To further examine coronary flow velocity immediately after primary coronary stenting for acute MI, Wakatsuki et al. examined LAD flow velocity after primary stenting in 31 patients with their first MI. The patients were divided into groups by the presence or absence of early systolic flow reversal (ESFR), regional wall motion abnormalities, and EFs and were then compared at follow-up. The change in regional wall motion was significantly greater in the non-ESFR group than in the ESFR group. There was a significant improvement in LVEF when there was no early systolic flow reversal compared with the presence of systolic flow reversal, and the diastolic to systolic flow ratio correlated positively with change in regional wall motion. These data indicate that the coronary flow velocity pattern measured immediately after successful primary stenting is predictive of LV functional recovery in patients with acute MI.

The differentiation between two types of thrombolysis in myocardial infarction (TIMI) grade 2 flow can also predict improvement in LVWM recovery after stenting. Akasaka et al. studied TIMI flow in 35 patients having successful recanalization for acute anterior MI after stenting. LVWM recovery was present in patients who had TIMI 2 flow with reduced APV and prolonged deceleration time (type 1) compared with patients who had systolic flow reversal and rapid deceleration time (type 2). Stenting increased TIMI 2 flow to TIMI 3 flow in more patients with type 1 than type 2 (67% vs. 0% patients). TIMI 2, type 2 flow pattern, was associated with persistent and poor LVWM recovery.

17. How does CVR relate to the reperfusion injury syndrome?

Coronary blood flow reserve is related to LV function and infarct size, depending on the extent of reperfusion injury after acute MI. Feldman et al. examined 21 patients with an anterior MI treated less than 12 hours after the onset of angioplasty and reperfusion. Coronary flow reserve, LVEF, infarct size, and LV end-systolic volume were evaluated before and immediately afterward. Ten of 21 patients with "reperfusion syndrome" (i.e., increased ischemia after thrombolysis) had ST segment elevation despite recanalization and post-PTCA CVRs of 1.2 compared with patients without reperfusion syndrome with CVRs of 1.6, ($P < 0.005$). Infarct size at 6 weeks and predischarge LV end-systolic volume index were larger, and LVEF was lower in patients with reperfusion syndrome and low coronary flow reserve compared with those without the similar electrocardiographic reperfusion syndrome (Fig. 3). The authors concluded that these individuals have a transiently lower CVR with sustained LV dysfunction, larger infarct size, and greater microcirculatory perfusion injury

These findings suggest that maneuvers that might maintain or produce flow augmentation (e.g., an intraaortic balloon pumping or adenosine) might result in improved myocardial salvage. Improved microcirculatory responses after new antiplatelet pharmacology appear to promote recovery of LV function. Neumann et al. measured CVR and regional LV function immediately after stenting and again 14 days later in two groups of acute MI patients, a control group treated with standard heparin, and another group treated with heparin and glycoprotein IIb/IIIa inhibition with abciximab. Improved coronary vascular function demonstrated by increased hyperemia was coupled with improved regional systolic LVWM in the abciximab group compared with the standard therapy group.

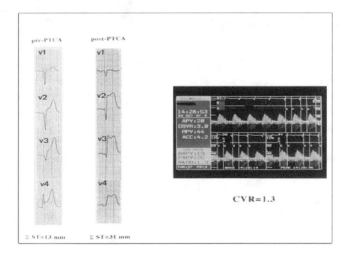

FIGURE 3. *A,* Electrocardiographic and coronary flow patterns in a patient with reperfusion syndrome. Primary PTCA of the mid-LAD was performed 245 minutes after the onset of chest pain. *Left,* Electrocardiogram (ECG) pattern. Thirty seconds after reperfusion, the patient complained of increased chest pain. The ECG shows additional elevation of ST segment. *Right,* Flow velocity pattern in the distal LAD 10 minutes after successful PTCA. *Bottom left* and *right screens* indicate base (BAPV = 19 cm/sec) and adenosine-induced hyperemic (PAPV = 26 cm/sec) APVs, respectively. Residual coronary velocity reserve (RATIO) is 1.3. Reproduced with permission from Feldman et al: J Am Coll Cardiol 35:1162–1169, 2000. *(continued)*

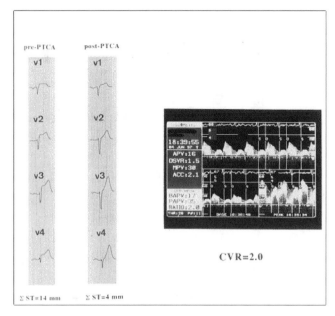

B

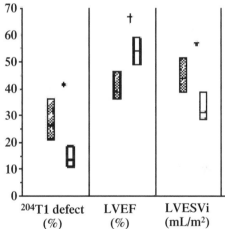

C

FIGURE 3. (*continued*) *B*, Electrocardiogram and coronary flow patterns in a patient without reperfusion syndrome. Primary PTCA of the mid-LAD was performed 255 minutes after the onset of chest pain. *Left,* Electrocardiogram (ECG) pattern. The patient experienced a gradual decline of chest pain. The ECG obtained 1 minute after reperfusion shows a partial resolution of ST segment elevation. *Right,* Flow velocity pattern in the distal LAD 10 minutes after successful PTCA. *Bottom left* and *right screens* indicate base (BAPV = 17 cm/sec) and adenosine-induced hyperemic (PAPV = 35 cm/sec) APVs, respectively. Residual coronary velocity reserve (RATIO) is 2.0. Reproduced with permission from Feldman et al. J Am Coll Cardiol 35:1162–1169, 2000.

C, Infarct size and LV function. Six weeks after acute MI, patients with reperfusion syndrome (*hatched boxes*) had a larger infarct size (% ^{201}Tl defect) and a lower radionuclide LVEF than patients without RS (*open boxes*). Patients with RS had also a larger pre-discharge LV end-systolic volume index (LVESVi). Each box displays median and 95% confidence interval (*P=0.001; †P=0.004). Reproduced with permission from Feldman et al. J Am Coll Cardiol 35:1162–1169, 2000.

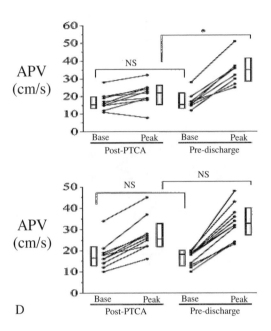

FIGURE 3. (*continued*) D, Individual time-averaged peak velocities (APVs) under basal conditions (base) and adenosine-induced hyperemia (peak), after PTCA and at pre-discharge follow-up. *Top,* In patients with reperfusion syndrome (RS), basal APV is stable over time, but hyperemic APV improves significantly. *Bottom,* whereas basal APV is stable over time, peak APV does not increase significantly in patients without RS. Each box displays median and 95% confidence interval (*$P <$ 0.005). Reproduced with permission from Feldman et al. J Am Coll Cardiol 35:1162–1169, 2000.

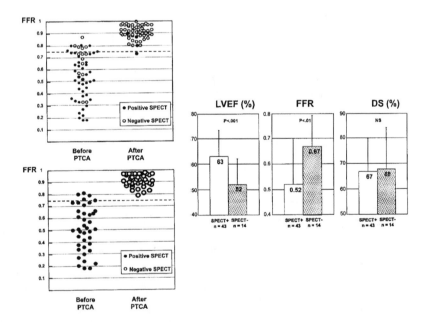

FIGURE 4. *Left panel,* Values of FFR before and after angioplasty according to results of sestamibi SPECT myocardial perfusion imaging in patient population as a whole (*top*) and in patients with truly positive and truly negative SPECT imaging (*bottom*). *Right panel,* Values of LVEF, FFR, and diameter stenosis (DS) according to results of SPECT imaging. At a similar degree of stenosis, patients with positive SPECT imaging results have better preserved LVEF and lower FFR than patients with negative SPECT imaging results, suggesting a larger amount of viable tissue. This corroborates that for same anatomic obstruction, the value of FFR depends on mass of myocardium at risk. Reproduced with permission from De Bruyne et al. Circulation 104:157–162, 2001.

18. When can FFR be used with acute MI?

FFR can be useful in patients with recent but not acute MI, as described by De Bruyne et al. Although an FFR value of 0.75 can distinguish normal and abnormal noninvasive stress testing in stable patients with normal LV function, the responses in patients with prior MI, DeBryne et al. examined FFR in 57 patients more than 6 days after MI. Single-photon emission computed tomography (SPECT), imaging and FFR were compared before and after coronary intervention. The sensitivity and specificity of FFR 0.75 or more was for normal SPECT imaging; 82% and 87%, respectively. The concordance between FFR and SPECT was 85% ($P < 0.001$). When only true positive and true negative SPECT imaging results were considered, corresponding values of 87%, 100%, and 94% were observed (Fig. 4). Patients with positive SPECT results before angioplasty had significant lower FFR than patients with negative SPECT results before the procedure. There was a higher LVEF and similar degree of diameter stenosis with the higher FFR. A significant inverse correlation was found between LVEF and FFR. These data indicate that the FFR value of 0.75 distinguished patients with positive from negative SPECT imaging results at least 6 days after acute MI, and that for a similar degree of stenosis, FFR was related to the mass of viable myocardium. Because of the dynamic responses of an acutely infracted myocardial bed, FFR responses in the first 48 hours may not reflect the true significance of the target lesion.

BIBLIOGRAPHY

1. Abizaid A, Mintz GS, Pichard AD, et al: Clinical, intravascular ultrasound, and quantitative angiographic determinants of the coronary flow reserve before and after percutaneous transluminal coronary angioplasty. Am J Cardiol 82:423–428, 1998.
2. Akasaka T, Yoshida k, Kawamoto T, et al: Relation of phasic coronary flow velocity characteristics with TIMI perfusion grade and myocardial recovery after primary percutaneous transluminal coronary angioplasty and rescue stenting. Circulation 101:2361–2367, 2000.
3. Anderson HV, Carabello BA: Provisional versus routine stenting—routine stenting is here to stay. Circulation 102:2910–2914, 2000.
4. Bartunek J, Winjs W, Heyndrickx GR, de Bruyne B: Effects of dobutamine on coronary stenosis: physiology and morphology comparison with intracoronary adenosine. Circulation 100:243–249, 1999.
5. Berne RM: Cardiac nucleotides in hypoxia: possible role in regulation of coronary blood flow. Am J Physiol 204:317–322, 1963.
6. Briguori C, Anzuini A, Airoldi F, et al: Intravascular ultrasound criteria for the assessment of the functional significance of intermediate coronary artery stenoses and comparison with fractional flow reserve. Am J Cardiol 87:136–141, 2001.
7. Caracciolo EA, Wolford TL, Underwood RD, et al: Influence of intimal thickness on coronary blood flow responses in orthotopic heart transplant recipients: a combined intravascular Doppler and ultrasound imaging study. Circulation 92:II182–II190, 1995.
8. De Bruyne, B, Pijls N, Barunek J, et al: Fractional flow reserve in patients with prior myocardial infarction. Circulation 104:157–162, 2001.
9. DiMario C, Moses JW, Anderson TJ, et al. on behalf of the DESTINI Study Group (Doppler Endpoint STenting INternational Investigation): Randomized comparison of elective stent implantation and coronary balloon angioplasty guided by online quantitative angiography and intracoronary Doppler. Circulation 102:2938–2944, 2000.
10. Doucette JW, Corl PD, Payne HM, et al: Validation of a Doppler guide wire for intravascular measurement of coronary artery flow velocity. Circulation 85:1899–1911, 1992.
11. Dupouy P, Pelle G, Garot P, et al: Physiologically guided angioplasty in support to a provisional stenting strategy: immediate and six-month outcome. Cathet Cardiovasc Intervent 49:369–375, 2000.
12. Fearon W, Luna J, Samady H, et al: Fractional flow reserve compared with intravascular ultrasound guidance for optimizing stent depoyment. Circulation 104:1917–1922, 2001.
13. Feldman l, Himbert D, Juliard J, et al: Reperfusion syndrome: relationship of coronary blood flow reserve to left ventricular function and infarct size. J Am Coll Cardiol 35:1162–1169, 2000.
14. Fujita H, Inoue N, Matsuo Y, et al: Fractional myocardial flow reserve (FFRmyo) after coronary intervention as a predictor of chronic restenosis. J Invas Cardiol 11:527–532, 1999.
15. Gaster A, Korsholm L, Phayssen P, et al: Reproducibility of intravascular ultrasound and intracoronary Doppler measurements. Cathet Cardiovasc Intervent 53:449–458, 2001.
16. Hanekamp CEE, Koolen JJ, Pijls NHJ, et al: Comparison of quantitative coronary angiography, intravascular ultrasound, and coronary pressure measurement to assess optimum stent deployment. Circulation 99:1015–1021, 1999.

17. Haude M, Baumgart D, Verna E, et al: Intracoronary Doppler and quantitative coronary angiography-derived predictors of major adverse cardiac events after stent implantation. Circulation 103:1212–1217, 2001.

18. Jeremias A, Whitbourn RJ, Filardo SD, et al: Adequacy of intracoronary versus intravenous adenosine-induced maximal coronary hyperemia for fractional flow reserve measurements. Am Heart J 140: 651–657, 2000.

19. Joye JD, Cates CU, Farah T, et al: Cost analysis of intracoronary Doppler determination of lesion significance: preliminary results of the PEACH study. J Invas Cardiol 1:27, 1995.

20. Kawamoto T, Yoshida K, Akasaka T, et al: Can coronary blood flow velocity patters after percutaneous transluminal coronary angiography predict recovery of regional left ventricular function in patients with acute myocardial infarction. Circulation 100:339–345, 1999.

21. Kern MJ, Aguirre FV, Bach RG, et al: Interventional physiology rounds: fundamentals of translesional pressure-flow velocity measurements. Cathet Cardiovasc Diagn 31:137–143, 1994.

22. Kern MJ, Deligonul U, Tatineni S, et al: Intravenous adenosine: continuous infusion and low dose bolus administration for determination of coronary vasodilatory reserve in patients with and without coronary artery disease. J Am Coll Cardiol 18:718–729, 1991.

23. Labovitz AJ, Anthonis DM, Cravens TL, Kern MJ: Validation of volumetric flow measurements by means of a Doppler-tipped coronary angioplasty guide wire. Am Heart J 126:1456–1461, 1993.

24. Lafont A, Dubois-Rande JL, Steg PG, et al. for the F.R.O.S.T. Study Group: The French Randomized Optimal Stenting Trial: a prospective evaluation of provisional stenting guided by coronary velocity reserve and quantitative coronary angiography. J Am Coll Cardiol 36:404–409, 2000.

25. Matthys K, Carlier S, Segers P, et al: In vitro study of FFR, QCA, and IVUS for the assessment of optimal stent deployment. Cathet Cardiovasc Intervent 54:363–375, 2001.

26. Mazur W, Bitar JN, Lechin M, et al: Coronary flow reserve may predict myocardial recovery after myocardial infarction in patients with TIMI grade 3 flow. Am Heart J 136:335–344, 1998.

27. Neumann FJ, Blasini R, Schmitt C, et al: Effect of glycoprotein Iib/Iia receptor blockade on recovery of coronary flow and left ventricular function after the placement of coronary artery stents in acute myocardial infarction. Circulation 98:2695–2701, 1998.

28. Pijls NHJ, Klauss V, Siebert U, et al: Coronary pressure measurement after stenting predicts adverse events at follow-up: a multicenter registry. Circulation 105:2950–2954, 2002.

29. Segni ED, Higano ST, Rihal CS, et al: Incremental doses of intracoronary adenosine for the assessment of coronary velocity reserve for clinical decision making. Cathet Cardiovasc Intervent 54:34–40, 2001.

30. Serruys PW, Di Mario C, Piek J, et al. for the DEBATE Study Group: Prognostic value of intracoronary flow velocity and diameter stenosis in assessing the short- and long-term outcomes of coronary balloon angioplasty: the DEBATE study (Doppler Endpoints Balloon Angioplasty Trial Europe). Circulation 96:3369–3377, 1997.

31. Serruys PW, de Bruyne B, Carlier S, et al. on behalf of the Doppler Endpoints Balloon Angioplasty Trial Europe (DEBATE) II Study Group: Randomized comparison of primary stenting and provisional balloon angioplasty guided by flow velocity measurement. Circulation 102:2930–2937, 2000.

32. Skalidis EI, Kochiadakis GE, Koukouraki SI, et al: Phasic coronary flow pattern and flow reserve in patients with left bundle branch block and normal coronary arteries. J Am Coll Cardiol 33:1138–1142, 1999.

33. Sonoda S, Takeuchi M, Nakashima Y, Kuroiwa A: Safety and optimal dose of intracoronary adenosine 5′-triphosphate for the measurement of coronary flow reserve. Am Heart J 135:621–627, 1998.

34. Tsunoda T, Nakamura M, Wakatsuki T, et al: The pattern of alteration in flow velocity in the recanalized artery is related to left ventricular recovery in patients with acute infarction and successful direct balloon angioplasty. J Am Coll Cardiol 32:338–344, 1998.

35. Van Liebergen RAM, Piek JJ, Koch KT, et al: Hyperemic coronary flow after optimized intravascular ultrasound-guided balloon angioplasty and stent implantation. J Am Coll Cardiol 34:1899–1890, 1999.

36. Wakatsuki T, Nakamura M, Tsunoda T, et al: Coronary flow velocity immediately after primary coronary stenting as a predictor of ventricular wall motion recovery n acute myocardial infarction. J Am Coll Cardiol 35:1835–1841, 2000.

37. Werner G, Ferrari M, Richartz B, et al: Microvascular dysfunction in chronic total cornary occlusions. Circulation 104:1129–1134, 2001.

38. Wilson RF, Wyche K, Christensen BV, et al: Effects of adenosine on human arterial circulation. Circulation 82:1595–1606, 1990.

24. VASCULAR CLOSURE DEVICES

Oscar C. Muñoz, M.D., and Javier Jimenez, M.D.

1. Why were vascular closure devices introduced in the catheterization laboratory armamentarium?

Advances in coronary and peripheral intervention had led to the use of larger profile devices as well as aggressive anticoagulation strategies; both needed more reliable closure of vascular puncture sites. Moreover, the tendency to optimal resource utilization, increase patient comfort, and increase outpatient intervention had prompted the rapid development in vascular sealing techniques to achieve fast and effective hemostasis. A decrease in the incidence of access-related complications, although desirable, has not been the reason for these innovations.

2. What closure devices are currently available?

Several vascular closure devices are available to achieve hemostasis after percutaneous coronary intervention (PCI). VasoSeal (Datascope Corp., Mahwah, NJ) is a plug made of biodegradable bovine collagen; Duett (Vascular Solutions, Inc., Minneapolis, MN) and BioSeal are thrombin-containing biosealant gels that are delivered to the tissue surrounding the arteriotomy; Angio-Seal (St. Jude Medical, St. Paul, MN) is a vascular "sandwich" with polymer, anchor, and collagen plug; Perclose (Abbott Laboratories, Abbott Park, IL) is a percutaneous suture; and Femostop (Bard, Inc., Billerica, MA) is a pneumatic compression girdle (not closure).

3. What are the indications for the use of vascular closure devices?

Vascular closure devices significantly reduce the time to hemostasis and time to movilization. Also, they offer a predictable closure of the arteriotomy site. Therefore, they are indicated in patients who require a continuous antiplatelet or anticoagulant therapy postcatheterization, patients who require early mobilization (e.g., those with low back pain syndrome), or when a reduction in the burden of medical staff is advised.

4. How does VasoSeal work?

VasoSeal is a purified bovine (biodegradable) collagen sponge that is inserted in the soft tissue tract over the arterial puncture site. This device is deployed through a sheath, but it remains extravascular. It induces platelet activation and aggregation with release of clotting factors, resulting in thrombus formation. No manipulations of the puncture hole are required, but occlusive compression of the artery proximal to the puncture site is necessary during deployment (requires two operators) and nonocclusive compression for 5 to 10 minutes after deployment.

5. How do Duett and Bioseal work?

Duett was first used clinically in July 1997. It is a thrombin-containing gel that is applied to the tissue surrounding the arteriotomy. It requires a balloon to be inflated within the artery to prevent leakage of thrombogenic material into the vessel.

6. How does Angio-Seal work?

Angio-Seal is delivered through a sheath at the puncture site; the three components that make up the device (i.e., collagen plug, flat rectangular polymer anchor, and connecting suture) are all bioabsorbable. The plug has a lactide and glycolide anchor attached to a 24- to 28-mg collagen sponge by an absorbable suture. The device is contained in a carrier tube. The carrier tube containing the plug is inserted through the sheath, deploying the anchor within the arterial lumen. This results in plugging of the anterior arterial wall puncture site by the anchor and collagen plug.

7. How does Perclose work?

The Perclose device consists of a sheathlike device that contains two or four lancelike needles that are connected at their tips to one or two suture loops. The introducer sheath is exchanged for the device and advanced until a pulsatile backbleeding indicates that the lancelike needles can retrogradely be deployed. Finally, by pulling back the ring-shaped handle, the arterial wall is captured by the sutures. Then needles are removed, the device is partially withdrawn, the sutures are cut, and a square knot is tied.

8. What are the advantages and disadvantages of vascular closure devices?

DEVICE	ADVANTAGES	DISADVANTAGES
VasoSeal	Improves patient comfort Allows early sheath removal Extravascular Easy to learn Does not enlarge puncture hole Simple conversion to standard external compression Can be used in diseased arteries Early repuncture	No difference in bleeding or hematoma compared with manual compression Relies only on thrombus plug Requires two operators High failure rate in obese patients (weight > 90 kg) Ambulation delay (1–3 hours)
Duet and BioSeal	Do not enlarge puncture hole One operator needed Simple conversion to standard extternal compression Inmediate repuncture	Rely solely on thrombus plug Potential intravascular administration of procoagulant Used in diseased vessels? Ambulation delay (1–3 hours)
Angio-Seal	Significant decrease in bleeding and hematoma compared with manual compression Easy to learn One operator needed No need for external compression Early ambulation possible	Intraluminal anchor Enlarged puncture hole Repuncture delay (weeks) Contraindicated in diseased arteries
Perclose	Excellent hemostasis Secure suture closure Almost immediate ambulation Immediate repuncture Closes larger punctures	Significant learning curve Enlarges puncture hole Contraindicated in diseased arteries.

9. What variables influence the outcome of vascular closure?

The success of vascular closure is influenced by the level of anticoagulation of the patient at the moment of closure, sheath size, physician learning curves (mainly for the Perclose device), location of puncture site, patient's body habitus, vessel site, and presence of local atherosclerotic disease.

10. What are the contraindications to the use of vascular closure devices?

The contraindications depend partially on the type of device used. In general, it is preferred not to use vascular closure devices if an artery other than the common femoral artery was punctured; if more than a single wall puncture was required; in patients punctured through a vascular graft, clinically significant vascular disease, or uncontrolled hypertension (> 180 mmHg systolic blood pressure), or preexisting autoimmune disease; in patients who have known allergies to beef products, collagen or collagen products, or polyglycolic or polylactic acid polymers for the Vaso-Seal, Duett, and Angio-Seal devices; patients with a bleeding disorder, including thrombocytopenia (< 100.000 platelet count), thromboasthenia, von Willebrand's disease, or anemia (hemoglobin < 10 mg/dL; hematocrit < 30); patients who are pregnant or lactating; pediatric patients or others with small femoral artery size (< 4 mm in diameter); and if early repuncture of the same arteriotomy site is expected (for Angio-Seal or VasoSeal).

11. What are the potential complications associated with the use of vascular closure devices?

The potential complications of the use of vascular closure devices in general are not different from those in manual closure techniques. The complications include bleeding, hematoma, arteriovenous fistula, pseudoaneurysm, retroperitoaneal hemorrhage, access site–related blood transfusion, vascular occlusion, access site infection, vascular surgery, and complete vascular occlusion. Rare complications such as granulomatous reactions have been reported with bovine collagen injection.

12. Are vascular complications more frequent when arteriotomy closure devices are used than whith manual compression?

This issue remains controversial; several former studies found no significantly greater incidence of major complications with the use of closure devices. A recent trial by Dangas et al. concluded that the use of vascular closure devices after PCI was associated with higher vascular complication rates than hemostasis with manual compression. Specifically, ACD use was associated with a more frequent occurrence of hematoma, desease in hematocrit level, and vascular surgical repair.

13. Are vascular closure devices safe in patients treated with intravenous (IV) glycoprotein GP IIb/IIIa inhibitors?

A large study in which 2009 patients had manual compression, the Angio-Seal device was used in 411 patients and the Perclose device was used in 408 patients demonstrated that Angio-Seal and Perclose devices have a similar overall risk as manual compression, even in patients treated with IV GP IIb/IIIa platelet inhibitors. However, the incidence of retroperitoneal hemorrhage among patients treated with both closure devices was significantly higher compared with manual compression (1.0% for Angio-Seal, 0.8 % for Perclose vs. 0.1% for manual compression; $P = 0.01$). This risk might be caused by accidental puncture of the posterior artery wall or periarteriotomy artery wall not prevented with compressive methods in patients treated with potent platelet inhibitors and anticoagulation regimens.

14. What is the SyvekPatch?

The SyvekPatch (Marine Polymer Technologies, Danvers, MA), an external device used to control bleeding from vascular access sites and percutaneous catheters, consists of a poly-N-acetyl glucosamine polymer, which is isolated from a microalga. Mechanism studies suggest that the SyvekPatch involves both clot formation and local vascoonstriction as part of its hemostatic effect. The patch is applied locally and manually compressed for 10 minutes in diagnostic procedures and 20 minutes after interventional procedures after activated clotting times (ACTs) are below 300 seconds. A recently published study by Nader et al. reported rapid control of bleeding on a total of 1000 patients with only one major complication (0.1%; pesudoaneurym) and few minor complications (1.3%).

BIBLIOGRAPHY

1. Balzer JO, Scheinert D, Diebold T, et al: Postinterventional transcutaneous suture of femoral artery access sites in patients with peripheral arterial occlusive disease. Cathet Cardiovasc Intervent 53:174–181, 2001.
2. Criado FJ, Abul-Khoudoud O, Martin JA, et al: Current developments in percutaneous arterial closure devices. An Vasc Surg 14:683–687, 2000.
3. Cura FA, Kapadia SR, L'Allier PL, et al: Safety of femoral closure devices after percutaneous coronary interventions in the era of glycoprotein IIb/IIIa platelet blockade. Am J Cardiol 86:780–782, 2000.
4. Dangas G, Mehran R, Kokolis S, et al; Vascular complications after percutaneous coronary interventions following hemostasis with manual compression versus arteriotomy closure devices. J Am Coll Cardiol 38:638–641, 2001.
5. Ernst SM, Tjonjocgin RM, Schrader R, et al: Immediate sealing of arterial puncture sites after cardiac catheterization and coronary angioplasty using a biodegradable collagen plug: results of an international registry. J Am Coll Cardiol 21:851–855, 1993.

6. Nader RG, Garcia JC, Drushal K, et al: Clinical evaluation of the SyvekPatch in consecutive patients undergoing interventional, EPS and diagnostic cardiac catheterization procedures. J Invas Cardiol
   14:305–307, 2002.

7. Rosenfield K, Goldstein JA, Safian RD: Medical and peripheral vascular complications. In Safian RD,
   Freed MS (eds): The Manual of Interventional Cardiology, 3rd ed. Royal Oak, MI, Physicians Press,
   2001, pp 489–492.

8. Shrake KL, Mayer SA: A cost analysis of complications associated with arterial closure following diagnostic and therapeutic cardiac catheterization. J Cardiovas Manage 26:33, 1998.

9. Tavris D, Gross T, Gallauresi B, et al: Arteriotomy closure devices: the FDA perspective. J Am Coll Cardiol 38:642–644, 2001.

10. Ward SR, Casale P, Raymond R, et al: Efficacy and safety of a hemostatic puncture closure device with
   early ambulation after coronary angiography. Am J Cardiol 81:569–572, 1998.

V. Percutaneous Coronary Artery Interventions: Indications and Applications

25. CORONARY INTERVENTIONS FOR STABLE ANGINA

Neil Sawhney, M.D., and Barry Sharaf, M.D.

1. What is the evidence supporting PCI over medical therapy in patients with stable angina?

One would think that with over 1 million angioplasties performed per year that there would be strong evidence in favor of angioplasty. Unfortunately, this is not the case. There have been very few trials comparing PCI with medical therapy, and the results have been less than conclusive. The ACME trial in 1992 studied 212 patients with positive stress tests, angina, and single-vessel disease randomized to initial therapy with balloon angioplasty versus medical therapy. The PTCA patients had significantly less angina and were able to go significantly longer on the treadmill than the medically treated group. However, there was no difference in death or MI between the groups and the PTCA patients had more repeat PTCA and CABG. The MASS trial looked at patients with only proximal LAD disease and randomized to PTCA versus surgery versus medicine in 214 patients. The results were identical to the ACME trial, in which patients in the PTCA versus medicine arms had no difference in mortality or infarction rates, but PTCA (or surgery) resulted in greater symptomatic relief.

Relevant Trials in Percutaneous Revascularization

TRIAL	YEAR	N=	DESIGN	FINDING
VA Cooperative	1972	686	CABG vs Med tx	Survival benefit in high-risk patients with CABG. Benefit lost by 11 yrs
European Coronary Surgery Study	1973	768	CABG vs Med tx	Survival benefit with CABG by 5 years primarily due to 3-v dz and 2-v dz with significant prox LAD stenosis
CASS	1975	780	CABG vs Med tx	No difference in mortality at 5 years except in subgroup with 3-v dz and EF<50%
ACME	1992	212	Med tx vs PTCA in 1-vessel disease	No difference in MI or death. PTCA arm with less angina with average increase in ETT by 1.6 minutes
RITA-2	1997	1018	Med tx vs multivessel PTCA	Less angina and longer ETT times with PTCA, but more death and NQMI in PTCA arm
ACIP	1995	558	Med tx vs revascularization (PTCA or CABG) for pts with ischemia but minimal angina	Less ischemia and less 1-year mortality in revascularization group than in the group treated medically to relieve angina

(continued)

Relevant Trials in Percutaneous Revascularization (Continued)

TRIAL	YEAR	N=	DESIGN	FINDING
AVERT	1999	341	Low-risk patients with mild angina and normal LV function randomized to max dose statin vs PTCA	At 18 months, patients receiving PTCA had higher LDL cholesterol and more ischemic events
MASS	1995	214	Pts with 1V high-grade proximal LAD stenosis tx med vs PTCA vs CABG	No difference in death or MI in any arm. Less angina in both recascularization arms with least in CABG arm
CABRI	1995	1154	Multivessel PTCA vs CABG	At 6.5 years, no difference in MI or mortality. Greater need for repeat intervention with PCI
BARI	1996	1809	Multivessel PTCA vs CABG	At 5 years, no difference in survival except in diabetic subgroup. Greater need for repeat revascariztion in PTCA group
ERACI-II	2001	450	Multivessel PCI with stenting vs CABG	Only trial to show a mortality benefit in the PCI group but mainly driven by very high surgical mortality (>12% vs 0.9% for PCI)
ARTS	2001	1205	Mulitvessel PCI with stenting vs CABG	At 1 year, no difference in MI or mortality. Greater need for repeat intervention with PCI
SOS	2002	988	Mulitvessel PCI with stenting vs CABG	At 2 years, no difference in MI or mortality. Greater need for repeat intervention with PCI
RAVEL	2002	238	Drug eluting stent vs standard stent	At 6 months, 0% restenosis in DES arm vs 26.6% in standard stent arm. 1 yr MACE in 5.8 vs 28.8%, respectively

2. Are there any data supporting medical therapy over PCI?

The RITA-2 trial published in 1997 is the largest trial to study PTCA versus medical therapy. This trial enrolled over 1000 patients and had 2.7 years of follow up. While it confirmed the benefits of PTCA with increased exercise times and decreased angina as seen in ACME and MASS, RITA-2 also suggested possible harm from PTCA with an excess of death and nonfatal MI occuring 6.3% versus 3.3% of patients treated medically (p = 0.02). The AVERT trial studied a more contemporary concept of aggressive lipid lowering versus PCI in 341 patients with mild stable angina and normal LV function. In this group of patients, there were 36% fewer ischemic events in the medically treated group. As compared with the patients who were treated with PCI, the patients who received atorvastatin had a significantly longer time to the first ischemic event (p = 0.03). Most of the events in the PCI group were likely due to restenosis.

The ongoing Clinical Outcome Utilizing Revascularization and Aggressive Drug Evaluation (COURAGE) trial will be the largest study to compare optimal medical therapy and percutaneous revascularization. This study will apply intensive medical management in all patients, and study the incremental benefit of revascularization. It is hoped that COURAGE will better define the role of modern PCI in the age of aggressive lipid lowering therapy.

3. When should one perform PCI over medical therapy?

PCI should never be done "over" medical therapy. It should be regarded as a complementary therapy rather than an alternate one. This has been the major criticism of the AVERT trial, that aggressive medical therapy *with* PCI was not evaluated. Taken as an aggregate, the data suggest that PCI should be done if the patient has severe angina especially if "failing" medical management, or is intolerant of medications, AND if PCI can be done with reasonable chance of success and with limited risk.

4. Is PCI ever indicated in asymptomatic or minimally symptomatic patients?

The majority of patients with asymptomatic ischemia or with minimal angina should be treated medically, as most trials have only shown that PCI reduces anginal symptoms more than medications. One trial, the ACIP trial, enrolled patients who had ischemia both on treadmill and on ambulatory monitoring. Most of these patients had early positive stress tests and multivessel disease. In these high-risk patients, patients did better when revascularized by either surgery or PCI rather than when medically treated. At 12 weeks, this was demonstarted by less ischemia on ambulatory monitoring and an increase in total treadmill time. At 1 year follow-up, mortality was 4.4% in the angina-guided therapy group, 1.6% in an ischemia-guided therapy group, and 0% in the revasculariztion group. At 2 years, this benefit over angina-guided therapy persisted. Thus there may be a subgroup of patients with severe ischemia but minimal symptoms who may benefit from PCI.

5. Should women be referred for revascularization less often than men?

In the past, female gender was a strong predictor of worse outcomes from both PTCA and surgery, leading some to refer women for revascularization less often than men. Women are under-represented in most PCI trials, and so most of the data supporting this approach came from registries and subgroup analysis. For example, in the 1985 NHLBI PTCA registry, women were less likely to have angiographic or clinical success, were more likely to suffer coronary artery dissection post-PTCA, and had six times higher in-hospital mortality following PTCA and a five times higher mortality from emergent CABG. In the 1995 NHLBI PTCA registry, the procedural success, in-hospital death or myocardial infarction rates, and need for coronary artery bypass graft surgery were similar in women and men. While it is true that the 1-year mortality (6.5% vs 4.3%, p = 0.02) and the combined end point of death/MI/CABG (18.3% vs. 14.4%, p = 0.03) were higher in women than in men, the women tended to be older and have more co-morbid conditions than the men. After controlling for these factors, gender was no longer a significant predictor of death or MI at 1 year. Thus current management strategies should not take gender into account when deciding on PCI versus medical management.

6. When performing PCI in a patient with multivessel disease, should complete revascularization be the goal?

For the majority of patients, coronary angioplasty and CABG achieve similar mortality endpoints, with the major difference between the two strategies being patients in the PCI groups require a greater number of subsequent revascularizations. While the primary cause for this is assumed to be restenosis, some have argued that the trials are weighted against PCI because equivalence of complete revascularization was neither required nor evaluated by the majority of these trials. For example, in only 64% of BARI patients was complete revascularization even attempted in the PCI arm. In the CABRI trial, only 29% of patients received complete revascularization by PCI. Provocatively, this completely revascularized CABRI subgroup had a higher event-free survival when compared with the incompletely revascularized patients (69% vs 57%; p = 0.01). Similarly, a combined subgroup analysis from the BARI and CABRI trials showed patients with complete revascularization had a significantly higher event-free survival than patients with incomplete revascularization. This difference was primarily due to a higher incidence of subsequent bypass procedures in the incomplete revasculariztion group (10.0% vs 2.0%; p < 0.05). Despite these data, three other PCI versus CABG trials did require an attempt to achieve equivalence in revascularization: RITA, GABI, and ERACI. The repeat intervention rate was not lower in these trials than in those that accepted non-equivalence of revascularization. The most recent data, reflecting more current therapies, come from the ARTS trial. The ARTS trial also compared multivessel angioplasty versus CABG. In this trial, there was an intention for comparable revascularization and 89% of patients received intracoronary stents. Despite the requirement for comparable revascularization, completeness was achieved in 84.1% of bypass patients and only 70.5% of Angioplasty patients. Again in the ARTS trial, there was a significant difference in event-free survival in complete versus incomplete revascularization groups with a trend towards higher mortality in the incomplete revascularization group. In summary, the strive for complete revascularization has not shown a clear mortality benefit over more traditional approaches but seems to decrease or at least delay the number of patients who require subsequent CABG.

7. What are limitations of PCI and CABG trials?

While PCI and CABG have evolved substantially over the years, perhaps the greatest advances in the care of patients with CAD have been the advances in medical therapy. For example, when the original CABG versus medical therapy trials were done, even aspirin was not standard therapy for CAD. The recognition of the benefits from aspirin, beta blockers, ACE-inhibitors and statins has made most trials of the 1980s obsolete. Advances in CABG surgery have included increasing use of arterial conduits and technical improvements leading to cosmetic improvements and better neurologic outcomes. In the same time period, PCI has advanced by quantum leaps. The advent of stents along with the adjuvant use of glycoprotein IIb/IIIa inhibitors and thienopyridines has significantly improved PCI outcomes. For example, most of the trials comparing PCI with CABG for patients with multi-vessel CAD were in the "pre-stent" era. The majority of the late events in the PCI subgroups were due to restenosis and would be expected to be impacted significantly by the availability of stents. This has further rendered much of the 1990s trials obsolete. The ongoing revolution in PCI technology, for example, with drug eluting stents, will likely continue to make even our most contemporary trials such as the ARTS trial obsolete.

8. What should be done with patients with medically refractory ischemia but at particularly high risk for surgery?

There are surprisingly little data in this arena, as no major PCI trial required medically refractory ischemia for entry, and most trials excluded patients who were high risk for surgery or PCI. One trial, the VA AWSOME trial, suggests that these unstable high-risk patients had similar outcomes whether managed with PCI or with CABG.

9. Should surgery ever be recommended for single-vessel disease?

Many would never consider patients with single-vessel CAD for surgical revascularization. Indeed, the CASS trial in the early 1980s was unable to demonstrate a survival benefit in patients with single-vessel coronary artery disease treated with CABG versus medical therapy. Several recent trials have studied PCI verses single-vessel CABG for proximal LAD stenosis. The most recent and perhaps most provocative trial studied 220 symptomatic patients with very proximal LAD stenosis and randomized to minimally invasive bypass with a LIMA versus PCI with stenting and followed for 6 months. In this very select population of patients (bifurcation lesions, ostial lesions, total chronic occlusions, and multivessel disease all being excluded), the percentage of patients free from angina at 6 months was 79% in the surgical group and 62% in the stenting group (p = 0.03). The difference was primarily related to a 29% incidence of restenosis. Interestingly, of the 110 surgical patients, 18 percent had anastomotic lesions of 50% or greater with 5 patients requiring PCI, 5 required conversion to open thoracotomy, 3 required reoperation for anastomosis occlusion, and 2 patients had the anastomosis erroneously placed on the 1st diagonal. Furthermore, while there was no statistical difference in mortality, 3 patients in the surgical group died and none in the stenting group. The results are similar to previous trials such as the MASS trial which also suggest better anginal relief and less repeat procedures with conventional single-vessel bypass over PCI but at a cost of greater invasiveness. As previously mentioned, while restenosis was 29%, subgroup analysis showed type A, B, and C lesions to have resenosis rates of 18, 26, and 56%, respectively. This suggests that while PCI is certainly safe, some patients with proximal LAD anatomy may be better suited for PCI than others. At the current time, surgical revascularization should be considered in proximal LAD coronary artery disease when anatomy is unfavorable for PCI or when more sustained freedom from angina is desired. Whether further advances in PCI with intracoronary radiation and drug eluting stents further improves these results remains to be seen.

10. Should PCI ever be performed in diabetics with multivessel disease?

Yes. While in the majority of patients, multivessel angioplasty and surgery have equivalent outcomes, the BARI trial showed diabetics to have a significant long-term survival benefit from surgical revascularization over angioplasty. CABG has thus become the standard for diabetics with multivessel disease. However, there are other important considerations when choosing a revascularization strategy for a diabetic. The obvious limitation of BARI was the lack of stent and IIb/IIIa inhibitor use, leading to substandard results compared to current practice. More interesting is that of the patients screened with multi-vessel CAD amenable to PTCA and CABG, less than 1/3 were enrolled and randomized in BARI. The majority of patients in fact had therapy directed by physician preference, and in these patients (BARI Registry), diabetics did not have a survival benefit from surgery. While it is not clear which factors account for the difference, one can speculate that perhaps cardiologists were less likely to refer their patients for the trial if their patients were more likely to have a high surgical risk or were less likely to receive a LIMA. Perhaps they were more likely to refer to surgery for those with more diffuse CAD and when completeness of revascularization by angioplasty was unlikely. So while it is true that the diabetics in BARI with multivessel PCI had worse survival than the surgical group, the advances in PCI, the patients' overall surgical risk, their likelihood of receiving a LIMA, and their overall noncardiac survival must all be considered in deciding on an initial revascularization strategy. It is hoped that the ongoing BARI-2 trial will further define the role of multivessel PCI in diabetics.

11. What role should decreased decreased left ventricular function play in one's decision to perform PCI for stable angina?

In all major registries, PCI mortality is higher in patients with depressed ejection fractions. Thus left ventricular function must be a major consideration before deciding to undertake PCI. Furthermore, the older CABG versus medicine trials from the late 1970s and early 1980s have also suggested that surgical revascularization provides a mortality benefit in patients with left ventricular dysfunction. While this may or may not still be true, surgery does offer more complete revascularization to the majority of patients. In patients with severe LV dysfunction in whom PCI is performed, careful consideration must be made as to how the patient will tolerate PCI-induced ischemia. In some cases, prophylactic right heart catheterizations and IABP or cardiopulmonary support systems may be warranted.

12. How will drug eluting stents change the management of PCI?

Based on the results of the First in Man, RAVEL, and most recently SIRIUS trials, sirolimus eluting stents are on the verge of FDA approval and release. The results of the three trials are consistent with decreased rates of restenosis and target vessel revascularization in all lesion types irregardless of vessel size and lesion or stent length, without major adverse cardiac events. The magnitude of reduction in restenosis is greater than that seen in trials of stenting versus balloon angioplasty. The in-stent inhibition of neo-intimal hyperplasia and subsequent restenosis is virtually complete. Restenosis at the stent margins still occurs likely as a result of incomplete stent coverage of balloon-injured segments. Potential changes in management of PCI patients will depend on the cost of the devices but may include stenting of longer lengths of artery surrounding severe stenoses to ensure complete stent coverage of injured segments (from "normal to normal") and perhaps stenting of non-"culprit" and stenoses of borderline severity as well as stenoses not yet identified as either symptom or ischemia producing.

BIBLIOGRAPHY

1. American College of Cardiology/AHA Task Force on Assessment of Diagnostic and Therapeutic Cardiovascular Procedures: Guidelines for percutaneous transluminal coronary angioplasty. J Am Coll Cardiol 37(8):2215–2239, 2001.

2. Bypass Angioplasty Revascularization Investigation (BARI) Investigators: Comparison of coronary bypass surgery with angioplasty in patients with multivessel disease. N Engl J Med 335:217, 1996.
3. CABRI Trial Participants: First-year results of CABRI (Coronary Angioplasty verses Bypass Revasularization Investigation). Lancet 346:1179, 1995.
4. Folland ED, Hartigan PM, Parisi AF, et al: Percutaneous transluminal coronary angioplasty versus medical therapy for stable angina pectoris. J Am Coll Cardiol 29:1505, 1997.
5. Hueb WA, Belloti G, de Oliveria SA, et al: The Medicine, Angioplasty, or Surgery Study (MASS): A prospective, randomized trial of medical therapy, balloon angioplasty, or bypass surgery for single proximal left anterior descending artery stenosis. J Am Coll Cardiol 26:1600, 1995.
6. Parisi AF, Folland ED, Hartigan P: A comparison of angioplasty with medical therapy in the treatment of single-vessel coronary artery disease. N Engl J Med 326:10–16, 1997.
7. Pitt B, Waters D, Brown WV, et al: Aggressive lipid-lowering therapy compared with angioplasty in stable coronary artery disease. N Engl J Med 341:70–76, 1999.
8. Pocock SJ, Henderson RA, Rickards AF, et al: Meta-analysis of randomized trials comparing coronary angioplasty with bypass surgery. Lancet 346:1184, 1995.
9. RITA-2 Trial Participants: Coronary angioplasty versus medical therapy for angina: The Second Randomized Intervention Treatment of Angina (RITA-2) trial. Lancet 350:461, 1997.
10. Rogers WJ, Bourassa MG, Andrews TC, et al: Asymptomatic cardiac ischemia pilot (ACIP) study: Outcome at one year for patients with asymptomatic cardiac ischemia randomized to medical therapy or revascularization. J Am Coll Cardiol 26:594–605, 1995.
11. van den Brand MJ, Rensing BJ, Serruys PW, et al: The effect of revascularization on event-free survival at one year in the ARTS trial. J Am Coll Cardiol 39:559–564, 2002.
12. Yusuf S, Zucker D, Peduzzi P, et al: Effect of coronary artery bypass graft surgery on survival: Overview of 10-year results from randomized trials by the Coronary Artery Bypass Surgery Trialists Collaboration. Lancet 344:563, 1994.

26. CORONARY INTERVENTION FOR UNSTABLE ANGINA

Cesar Jara, M.D., and Eduardo de Marchena, M.D.

1. What is unstable angina?

The classical definition involves any increase in the usual pattern of angina (i.e., frequency, duration, or elicited by a lower level of activity), rest angina, or new-onset angina at least Canadian Cardiovascular Society (CCS) class III (walking one to two blocks on the level, climbing one flight of stairs). However, a better definition is as part of the acute coronary syndrome (ACS), which involves any clinical symptoms compatible with acute myocardial ischemia. ACS includes acute myocardial infarction (MI), either ST segment elevation or non–ST segment elevation (NSTEMI), and unstable angina (UA). Therefore, at presentation, overlap exists between NSTEMI and UA (Fig. 1).

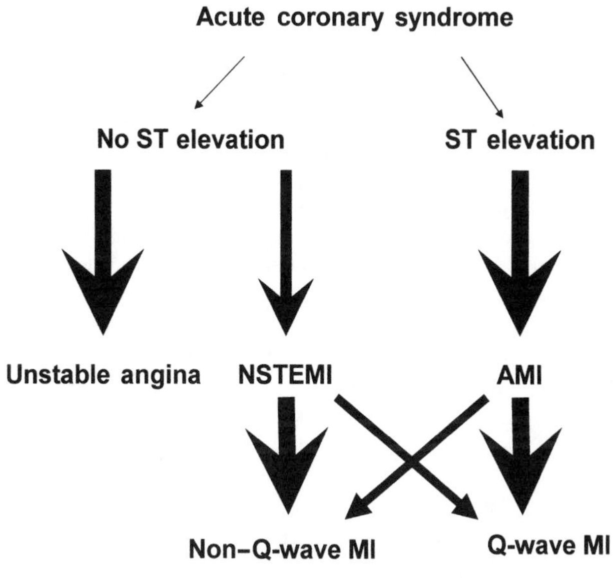

Acute coronary syndrome

No ST elevation   **ST elevation**

Unstable angina   NSTEMI   **AMI**

Non–Q-wave MI   **Q-wave MI**

FIGURE 1. Acute coronary syndrome: unstable angina, non–ST elevation MI and ST elevation MI. Clinical approach with initial ECG for rapid triage and adequate treatment. Adapted from Braunwald E. Circulation 98:2219–2222, 1998.

2. What causes UA/NSTEMI?

It is an imbalance between myocardial oxygen supply and demand, with five nonexclusive causes: non-occlusive thrombus in a ruptured preexisting plaque (the most common cause), dynamic obstruction (vasoconstriction), progressive mechanical obstruction, inflammation or infection, and secondary UA/NSTEMI (e.g., fever, anemia, hypoxemia and hypotension).

Microembolization of plaque debris (platelet aggregates, thrombus, or components of the disrupted plaque) accounts for several cases of ischemia and infarction.

3. Who should be considered for percutaneous coronary intervention (PCI)?

Patients with markers of *high risk* certainly benefit from an invasive strategy with PCI: recurrent ischemia or angina despite adequate medical therapy; recurrent ischemia or angina with clinical heart failure or new or worsening mitral insufficiency; hemodynamic instability; sustained ventricular tachycardia; new ST segment depression of at least 0.05 mV; transient (< 20 min) ST segment elevation of at least 0.1 mV in two or more contiguous leads; T-wave inversion of at least 0.3 mV in two or more contiguous leads; elevated troponin; depressed left ventricular (LV) systolic function (ejection fraction < 40%); PCI within past 6 months; history of coronary bypass graft surgery (CABG) and high risk findings on stress testing.

Patients with no markers of high risk could also be considered for an invasive approach if they are suitable candidates for revascularization.

4. Why should an early invasive strategy be favored?

Recent large randomized trials have proven beyond doubt that coronary intervention is superior to an initial conservative strategy in *high-risk patients* with the appropriate *adjunctive device or medical therapy*. In the FRISC II trial, the combined endpoint of death and MI at 1 year occurred in 10.4% of the patients assigned to the invasive strategy versus 14.1% assigned to the more conservative strategy ($P = 0.005$). In the TACTICS-TIMI 18 trial at 6 months, the rate of the combined endpoint of death, nonfatal MI, and rehospitalization for an ACS was 15.9% with use of the early invasive strategy and 19.4% with use of the conservative strategy ($P = 0.025$). Prior randomized trials (TIMI IIIB, MATE, VANQWISH) failed to show a clear advantage because of an initial increased risk of cardiac events associated with PCI. The answer lies in the pathophysiology of UA (Fig. 2).

Stenting, the use of glycoprotein (GP) IIb/IIIa receptor antagonists, and clopidogrel account for most of the improved outcomes in an early invasive strategy by:

- Treating the unstable ruptured plaque and preventing dissection and vasoconstriction
- Eliminating thrombus and distal microembolization

Therefore, an early invasive approach, by defining the coronary anatomy, provides adequate risk stratification for rapid disposition of the patient and early identification of the subgroup at high risk for adverse outcome and highly likely to benefit from prompt revascularization by PCI or CABG.

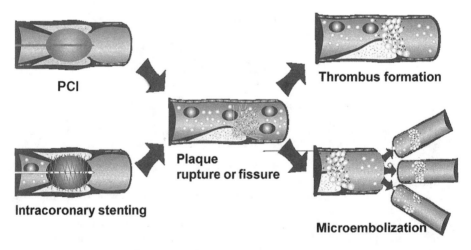

FIGURE 2. Pathophysiology of UA/NSTEMI. Therapy is aimed to control thrombus formation with microembolization (e.g., GP IIb/IIIa antagonists) and plaque rupture (e.g., PCI with stenting). Adapted from White HD: Unmet therapeutic needs in the management of acute ischemia. Am J Cardiol 80:2–10, 1997.

5. List the indications for revascularization with PCI or CABG in UA/NSTEMI.

CORONARY ARTERY DISEASE	TREATMENT OPTIONS
• Left main disease	CABG
• Left main disease and not candidate for CABG	Consider PCI
• Three-vessel disease with EF $<$ 0.50	CABG
• Multivessel disease, including proximal left anterior descending coronary artery (LAD)	CABG or PCI (most favor CABG)
• Multivessel disease, including proximal LAD with EF $>$ 0.50 and no diabetes	PCI
• One or two-vessel disease without proximal LAD and large area of ischemia	PCI or CABG
• One-vessel proximal LAD	PCI or CABG
• Multiple SVG stenosis, including LAD graft	CABG
• Focal SVG stenosis	PCI (high risk of embolization)

Adapted from ACC/AHA 2002 guideline update for the management of patients with UA/NSTEMI. ACC 51st annual scientific session. March 2002, Atlanta, GA.

6. How "early" is an early invasive approach?

In most of the studies, procedures were performed usually within 12 to 48 hours after adjunctive medical therapy was started (e.g., median of 22 hours in TACTICS-TIMI 18 trial). Although not mandatory, immediate angiography is an option, especially in unstable patients.

7. What is the proper adjunctive medical therapy for PCI in UA or NSTEMI?

Besides the usual anti-ischemic therapy (e.g., beta-blockers and nitrates), antithrombotic and antiplatelet therapy are imperative for the success of an early invasive approach.

Aspirin (ASA), clopidogrel, unfractionated heparin (UFH), or low-molecular-weight heparin (LMWH) and GP IIb/IIIa antagonists should be used in combination during PCI in high-risk patients.

8. Should we always try to use a GP IIb/IIIa antagonist during PCI in high-risk patients with UA/ NSTEMI? Which one?

The answer is a definite yes. A clear reason for the success of an early invasive approach is the adjunctive use of a GP IIb/IIIa antagonist. However, the choice of GP IIb/IIIa antagonist is not as clear.

Abciximab (ReoPro) is the most studied of this group of drugs, with clearcut benefit during PCI (EPIC, EPILOG, EPISTENT, and TARGET trials). However, the GUSTO-IV trial did not show any benefit with worse outcome if an early invasive approach is not planned during the first 48 hours. Therefore, abciximab should be used only with an early invasive strategy and planned PCI. The dose is 0.25 mg/kg intravenous (IV) bolus followed by infusion of 0.125 µg/kg/min (maximum 10 µg/min) for 12 to 24 hours.

Eptifibatide (Integrilin) is more flexible and can be used for either early invasive or conservative therapy. Even though initial data was not as strong as for abciximab, most likely because of underdosing and the heterogeneity of the population, recent trials (ESPRIT and INTERACT) have shown adequate safety and benefit for PCI in UA/NSTEMI. The dose is 180 µg/kg IV bolus followed by infusion of 2 µg/kg/min for up to 72 hours or 24 hours after PCI. If immediate PCI is planned, a second 180 µg/kg IV bolus should be given 10 minutes after the first bolus.

Tirofiban (Aggrastat), in spite of being the GP IIb/IIIa antagonist used in the TACTICS-TIMI 18 trial, is the least effective. Direct comparison with abciximab in the TARGET trail showed less protection during PCI for UA/NSTEMI, although a lower dose was used in this trial. The safety profile is very good. The dose is 0.4 µg/kg/min IV bolus for 30 minutes followed by an infusion of 0.1 µg/kg/min for up to 96 hours or at least 12 hours post-PCI.

9. Should UFH or LMWH be used during PCI in patients with UA/NSTEMI?

A large body of data derived from several clinical trials (ESSENCE, TIMI 11B, and INTERACT) favors the use of LMWH in *high-risk patients,* specifically enoxaparin, despite contentions of subtherapeutic dosing in the UFH patients. The wide variation in the therapeutic range (PTT) observed with UFH is the most likely explanation for this finding.

The only caveats for the widespread use of LMWH are increased cost, the lack of adequate monitoring (there is no activated clotting time or ACT), and vascular sheath removal (usually 8 hours after last dose). This can change after a rapid point-of-care technology recently developed that determines a LMWH "clotting time" (ACT equivalent) is tested and validated.

UFH is still a reasonable option if it is the operator preference for accurate ACT surveillance during PCI and in patients with higher risk of bleeding with LMWH, such as elderly patients older than age 75 years and patients with renal failure. The target ACT is 250 to 300, and if a GP IIb/IIIa antagonist is used, the target ACT should be 200 to 250.

10. Are all LMWHs comparable during PCI?

Definitely not. In the FRISC 2 trial, the use of dalteparin did not decrease the risk of procedure-related myocardial damage in the invasive group. Furthermore, the long-term benefit seen in the invasive group was not related to its use. There is also insufficient data in the combined use with GP IIb/IIIa antagonists.

Currently available information shows that enoxaparin is the LMWH of choice for PCI in UA/NSTEMI.

11. Can LMWH be combined with GP IIb/IIIa antagonists during PCI for UA/NSTEMI?

The answer is yes, with improved cardiovascular endpoints in *high-risk patients* and no significant increase in major bleeding. Trials of enoxaparin with GP IIa/IIIa antagonists have shown added benefit and adequate safety profile (NICE-4, INTERACT trials).

The dose of enoxaparin is 1 mg/kg subcutaneously (SQ) every 12 hours. No additional dose is needed if PCI performed within 8 hours of the last dose. If PCI occurs between 8 and 12 hours of the last SQ dose, an additional 0.3 mg/kg IV bolus should be administered.

The dose of enoxaparin should be reduced to 0.75 mg/kg if it is combined with abciximab. No change in dose is needed with eptifibatide (Integrilin).

12. How is clopidogrel used for PCI during UA/NSTEMI?

The data from the PCI-CURE and CREDO trials advocate the early use of clopidogrel with an initial oral bolus of 300 mg (preferably more than 6 hours before a planned PCI procedure) and daily use of 75 mg for at least 12 months. There is some increased risk of major bleeding in the group undergoing CABG during the first 5 days after stopping clopidogrel.

13. Are there any other medical therapies for PCI in UA or NSTEMI?

Early use of statins in ACS (e.g., atorvastatin) may promote plaque stabilization by decreasing inflammation, lowering macrophage content of plaques, and reducing the expression of proinflammatory cytokines. However, there is not yet any data for patients undergoing early PCI.

Bivalirudin, a direct thrombin inhibitor, is an alternative to UFH with apparently improved outcome and lower risk of major hemorrhage. However, its role in contemporary PCI remains to be defined. It is clearly indicated in patients with heparin-induced thrombocytopenia (HIT).

Thrombolysis is contraindicated in UA/NSTEMI and even intracoronary use because a large thrombus load has not shown consistent benefit.

14. Should ionic or non-ionic contrast agents be used?

Ionic contrast agents such as ioxaglate (hexabrix) should be preferred for PCI in UA/NSTEMI because of inhibitory effects in thrombosis and platelet aggregation producing a lower incidence of thrombosis, no-reflow phenomenon, and abrupt closure. However non-ionic contrast agents may be used if a meticulous technique (e.g., avoiding prolonged blood and contrast mixtures in syringes; wiping guidewires) and adequate systemic anticoagulation are ensured.

15. What is the success rate of PCI in patients with UA/NSTEMI?

The technical success rate of PCI is above 90% (e.g., 96% in the TIMI IIIB trial), similar to stable angina. However, the incidence of periprocedure complications is higher.

16. What complications are possible during PCI for UA/NSTEMI?

The average rate of complications has declined over the past decade: death, 0.5 to 1.0%; emergency CABG, 0.8 to 1.4%, and MI, 1% to 5%. The wide range of variation in the reported incidence of MI is related to the definition used (e.g., Q-wave MI vs. elevated troponin), changing the sensitivity of the diagnosis.

In any case, periprocedure MI or "micro-infarction" (i.e., mild elevated troponin) identifies patients with a higher risk of long-term cardiovascular complications.

17. What are the contraindications for an early invasive approach?

The presence of extensive comorbidity precludes an invasive strategy and makes a patient unsuitable for revascularization. It should be a case-by-case decision with extensive discussion of the risk-to-benefit ratio. Examples of such a clinical conditions are metastatic malignancy with poor life expectancy, intracranial disease with high risk of bleeding, dementia, and severe liver disease. There are other conditions that are less clear, such as very advanced aged with renal failure, in which the risk-to-benefit ratio is difficult to determine.

Other contraindications are the patient's personal preference and coronary artery disease (CAD) known to be unsuitable for revascularization.

18. Besides stenting, is there any role for other devices for PCI in patients with UA/ NSTEMI?

The role of the intraaortic balloon pump (IABP) in high-risk patients is controversial, with decreased ischemia and heart failure but overall not better long-term outcome. It is certainly recommended in patients with low EF or cardiogenic shock.

Distal embolic protection systems, particularly for PCI of saphenous vein grafts (SVGs), are a very attractive alternative to prevent downstream embolization of debris. Examples of such a devices are the AngioGuard Emboli Capture Guidewire (Cordis Corp., Miami Lakes, FL), a filter that permits normal distal blood flow while capturing emboli, and the GuardWire Plus (Medtronic AVE, Santa Rosa, CA), which has a distal ballon for temporary occlusion and a catheter for an aspiration system.

Drug-eluting stents (e.g., sirolimus and paclitaxel) are a promising tool, especially for diabetic patients and restenosis cases. The initial data show that these stents are superior to any other device, with 0% restenosis. They should be available in 2003. Future trials should include patients with UA/NSTEMI.

19. What is the outcome of PCI in women, diabetic patients, and elderly patients with UA/ NSTEMI?

Contrary to prior notion, the outcome of PCI in UA/NSTEMI for women is similar to men. Women tend to present with atypical symptoms at an older age and with more comorbidities.

Diabetic patients comprise about 20% of cases with UA/NSTEMI. They have a worse outcome after PCI because more extensive CAD and higher incidence of restenosis. Use of stenting with abciximab may improve these patients' long-term prognosis. CABG is favored, especially with an arterial conduit, although diabetic patients still fare worse than nondiabetic patients.

Elderly patients have a worse outcome after revascularization because of the presence of more comorbidities. However, they do benefit from an early invasive approach when compared with a conservative strategy. They also present with more atypical symptoms.

20. Does operator experience influence the outcome of PCI in patients with UA/NSTEMI?

Patients treated by high-volume physicians in high-volume hospitals have a lower risk of complications and better outcome. This raises concerns of performing PCI in hospitals without surgical backup and supports the current trends of training and board certification.

21. Could we review a clinical case?

Certainly. This is a 76 year-old woman with diabetes, hypertension, and hyperlipidemia with angina at rest, NSTEMI by cardiac enzymes, and abnormal ECG (deep T-wave inversions and ST segment depression in the precordial and inferior leads; Fig. 3A). Pre-PCI coronary angiography reveals complex subtotal occlusion of the proximal LAD (Fig. 3B). Post-PCI angiography with stenting and abciximab shows adequate results with TIMI 3 flow (Fig. 3C).

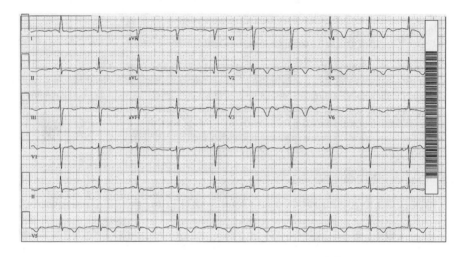

FIGURE 3A.

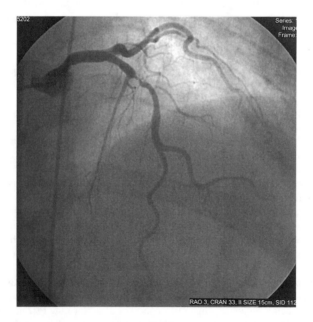

FIGURE 3B.

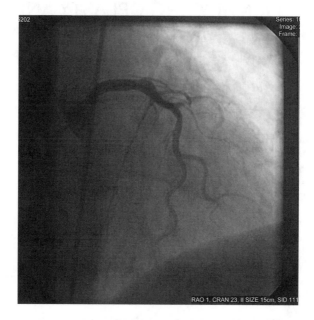

FIGURE 3C.

BIBLIOGRAPHY

1. ACC/AHA 2002 guideline update for the management of patients with Unstable Angina/ Non-ST-Elevation Myocardial Infarction: ACC 51st annual scientific session. March 2002, Atlanta, GA.
2. Antman EM, Cohen M, Radley D, et al. For the TIMI 11B and ESSENCE investigators: Assessment of the treatment effect of enoxaparin for unstable angina/non-Q wave myocardial infarction. TIMI 11B/ESSENCE Meta-analysis. Circulation 100:1602–1608, 1999.
3. Boden WE, O'Rourke RA, Crawford MH, et al: Outcomes in patients with acute non-Q wave myocardial infarction randomly assigned to an invasive as compared with a conservative management strategy. N Eng J Med 338:1785–1792, 1998.
4. Braunwald E: Unstable angina: an etiologic approach to management [editorial]. Circulation 98:2219–2222, 1998.
5. Cannon CP, Weintraub WS, Demopoulos LA, et al: Comparison of early invasive and conservative strategies in patients with unstable coronary syndromes treated with the glycoprotein IIb/IIIa inhibitor tirofiban: TACTICS-TIMI 18 investigators. N Eng J Med 344:1879–1887, 2001.
6. Effects of tissue plasminogen activator and a comparison of early invasive and conservative strategies in unstable angina and non-Q wave myocardial infarction: results of the TIMI IIIB trial. Circulation 89:1545–1556, 1994.
7. Freed M, Grines C, Safian R: The New Manual of Interventional Cardiology, 4th ed. Birmingham, MI, Physicians' Press, 1998.
8. Goodman SG: The integrilin and enoxaparin randomized assessment of acute coronary syndrome treatment (INTERACT) trail. J Am Coll Cardiol 40:8–9, 2002.
9. Mehta SR, Yusuf S, Peters RJ, et al: Effects of pretreatment with clopidrogel and aspirin followed by long-term therapy in patients undergoing percutaneous coronary intervention: the PCI-CURE study. Lancet 358: 527–533, 2001.
10. Simoons ML: Effect of glycoprotein IIb/IIIa receptor blocker abciximab on outcome in patients with acute coronary syndromes without early coronary revascularization: the GUSTO-IV ACS randomized trial. Lancet 357:1915–1924, 2001.
11. Topol EJ, Moliterno DJ, Herrmann HC, et al: Comparison of two platelet glycoprotein IIb/IIIa inhibitors, tirofiban and abciximab, for the prevention of ischemic events with percutaneous coronary revascularization. TARGET investigators. N Eng J Med 344:1888–1894, 2001.
12. Wallentin L, Lagerqvist B, Husted S, et al: Outcome at 1 year after an invasive compared with a non-invasive strategy in unstable coronary artery disease: the FRISC II invasive randomized trial. Lancet 356:9–16, 2000.

27. PRIMARY ANGIOPLASTY AND THROMBOLYSIS FOR ST SEGMENT ELEVATION ACUTE MYOCARDIAL INFARCTION

Luis E. Rechani, M.D., and Rafael F. Sequeira, M.D.

1. How common is myocardial infarction (MI)?

Annually, approximately 1.1 million people have an MI or fatal coronary event in the United States. In 1999, coronary artery disease (CAD) accounted for 529,659 deaths, and almost one half of these were out-of-hospital deaths. Coronary heart disease remains the leading cause of death despite a 54% reduction in age-adjusted mortality between 1963 and 1990.

2. What causes an acute MI?

The development of an occlusive thrombus within a coronary artery is the most common cause of ST elevation MI (STEMI), accounting for at least 80% to 90% of all cases. Thrombus formation typically occurs when rupture or erosion of an atherosclerotic plaque exposes procoagulant substances beneath the plaque surface, resulting in the generation of thrombin and stimulating platelet aggregation at the site.

3. Why are reperfusion strategies important in the management of STEMI?

A significant part of the improved outcome in patients with acute MI is associated with better treatment and, in particular, the widespread use of reperfusion strategies.

Timely reperfusion of jeopardized myocardium represents the most effective way of restoring the balance between myocardial oxygen and demand. Rapid restoration of blood flow can limit the degree of myocardial injury that develops after the development of an occlusive thrombus. The extent of protection appears to be related directly to the rapidity with which reperfusion is implemented after the onset of coronary occlusion. Rapid reperfusion can reduce infarct size, salvage damaged myocardium, improve healing of the myocardium, and lower morbidity and mortality.

4. What factors influence the benefits of reperfusion therapy?

The benefit of any reperfusion therapy is dependent not only on the early, complete, and sustained restoration of infarct-related artery flow but also on effective reestablishment of perfusion to the myocardium. Epicardial vessel patency and microvascular perfusion are not always closely partnered. This failure of reperfusion is thought to be the consequence of distal embolization of platelets and inflammatory cells resulting from lysis or disruption of the occlusive epicardial thrombus, as well as ischemia and reperfusion injury associated with inflammatory cell infiltration and tissue edema. Patients achieving a higher grade of perfusion in the infarcted artery have better long-term survival because of better left ventricular function, improved healing of the myocardium, and a reduction in arrhythmia complications.

5. What reperfusion strategies are currently in use for the management of STEMI?

a. Pharmacologic thrombolytic therapy

b. Percutaneous coronary intervention (PCI)

c. Combination of the above strategies

6. What are the advantages of thrombolytic therapy?

a. Restores patency of the affected blood vessel in up to 80% of cases

b. Widespread availability and use

7. What are the disadvantages of thrombolytic therapy?

a. Only 50% to 60% of patients achieve Thrombolysis in Myocardial Infarction (TIMI) grade 3 flow within 90 minutes

b. 30-day mortality rates are 6% to 8% in clinical trials but may be higher in clinical practice

c. Reocclusion of the infarct-related artery leading to increased mortality remains a problem

d. Intracranial hemorrhage with rates from 0.5% to 1.1%

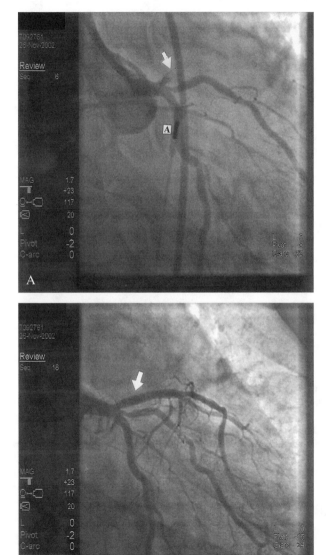

FIGURE 1. *A,* Anteroposterior caudal view of the left coronary artery demonstrating a total occlusion of the proximal left anterior descending (LAD) coronary artery during an acute MI (*Arrow*). The letter *A* denotes an intraaortic balloon pump catheter tip. *B,* An right anterior oblique caudal view reveals a patent LAD after successful PCI with stent (*arrow*). Slow flow is seen in the distal LAD.

8. What are the advantages of PCI?

a. Directly addresses the underlying coronary thrombus and atherosclerotic plaque

b. May provide more rapid and complete restoration of blood flow than fibrinolysis

c. Carries a low risk of precipitating intracranial bleeding events

Overall, primary angioplasty (i.e., percutaneous transluminal coronary angioplasty [PTCA] has been shown to restore blood flow to the affected artery in more than 90% of patients and is associated with a 1-year survival rate of 90% to 96% (Fig. 1).

9. What are the disadvantages of PCI?

a. Requires specific technical expertise and access to specialized facilities

b. Only 20% of U.S. hospitals have facilities for angiography, and only half of these have the capacity for performing emergency PTCA

10. Are there any contraindications to thrombolytic therapy?

Because of their generalized systemic effects there are several contraindications to their administration, as listed below.

Absolute contraindications to the administration of thrombolytic agents

   Prior intracranial hemorrhage

   Suspected aortic dissection

   History of intracranial neoplasm

   Active internal hemorrhage

Relative contraindications to the administration of thrombolytic agents

   Stroke within 1 year

   Markedly elevated blood pressure (BP) (> 180/110 mm Hg)

   Recent major surgery

   Recent internal hemorrhage

   Recent major surgery (< 3 weeks)

   Recent trauma (< 2–4 weeks)

   Prolonged cardiopulmonary resuscitation (> 10 minutes)

   Recent internal hemorrhage

   Active peptic ulcer disease

   Noncompressible vascular punctures

   Pregnancy

   Chronic severe hypertension

   Current use of anticoagulant therapy or known bleeding diathesis

Active menstruation is not a contraindication to the administration of thrombolytic therapy.

11. What are the complications of thrombolytic therapy?

Most complications from the administration of thrombolytic agents are related to hemorrhage. The most dreaded complication is an intracerebral hemorrhage because of the morbidity and mortality associated with this event. The incidence of intracerebral hemorrhage from the administration of a thrombolytic agent varies from 0.2% to 2.0% in the literature. Elderly patients and patients with markedly elevated BP are at the highest risk for developing an intracerebral hemorrhage. The incidence of total bleeding is approximately 20%, but major bleeding requiring transfusion of blood products or surgical intervention is much lower (~5%).

12. What complications are associated with PTCA?

Several types of complications may occur when patients undergo cardiac catheterization with coronary angiography and PTCA. These may be mechanical complications, including dissection or perforation of a coronary artery, acute thrombosis of a coronary artery or dissection of a peripheral artery at the site of access. Hemorrhage at the puncture site is one of the most common complications related to cardiac catheterization. However, major bleeding is relatively rare. Catheter manipulation may also lead to cholesterol embolization, stroke and arrhythmias. Complications can also occur associated with the administration of contrast agents. They include anaphalaxis in the most severe setting or contrast-induced nephropathy.

Complication Rates for Diagnostic Cardiac Catheterization

COMPLICATION	OCCURRENCES PER 10,000 PROCEDURES
MI	3
Stroke	6
Arrhythmia	33
Vascular complication	40
Death	8

13. What are the markers of successful reperfusion?
a. The detection and pattern of an increase in biochemical markers of myonecrosis, including myoglobin detected in the bloodstream (i.e., "early peaking")

b. Serial electrocardiograms; resolution of ST segment elevation by greater than 50% within 90 minutes of therapy is the most specific

14. What is the role of fibrinolytics combined with glycoprotein (GP) IIb/IIIa inhibitors?
Based on the recognition that platelets are a key component of arterial thrombosis and that antiplatelet therapy with aspirin provides major added benefit to fibrinolysis, the combination of fibrinolytic therapy and GP IIb/IIIa inhibitor therapy has been intensively studied. TIMI 14 (GUSTO V and ASSENT-3).

A greater extent of ST segment resolution with combination therapy has been observed together with a lower rate of reinfarction and a lesser need for urgent coronary intervention. However, no significant improvement in survival was seen and there was a trend for higher intracranial hemorrhage (ICH) rates with combination therapy in the patients older than age 75 years.

Other trials using combination therapy (INTEGRITI, FASTER) are currently ongoing.

15. Is there a benefit to combining fibrinolytics with low molecular weight heparins (LMWHs) or direct thrombin inhibitors?
In the past year, five randomized studies (HART, ENTIRE ASSENT-PLUS, AMI-SK, AS-SENT-3) consisting of 300 to 400 patients each have been performed evaluating LMWH and fibrinolytic therapy. LMWH was found to be at least as effective as unfractioned heparin as an adjunct to thrombolysis with a trend toward higher recanalization rates and less reocclusion at 5 to 7 days. Moreover, LMWH did not appear to increase major bleeding, including when given before routine acute angiography. Other larger trials (extract) are currently in progress.

An overview of 11 randomized trials evaluated direct thrombin inhibitors in more than 36,000 patients with acute coronary syndromes, including STEMI, showed no effect on mortality but a 25% reduction in reinfarction.

16. What is the role of rescue PCI?
Early PTCA (i.e., rescue angioplasty) after clinical failure of thrombolysis has been shown to improve patency of the infarct related artery in up to 90% of patients. Successful rescue PTCA may also salvage myocardium and reduce later ischemic events and mortality. However, despite these potential benefits, early PTCA was also associated with angiographic restenosis in up to 50% of vessels and the need for repeat target vessel revascularization in approximately 20% of patients.

17. Which adjunctive strategies in PCI have been shown to be of benefit?
Several large trials have shown that the use of stents reduces the likelihood of reocclusion after PTCA and improves some clinical outcomes, primarily the need for repeat procedures.

Recent trials have evaluated the interaction between stenting and antiplatelet treatment using abciximab in patients with STEMI who underwent primary PCI. This management strategy resulted in improved composite endpoints (i.e., death, recurrent MI, and target vessel revascularization).

18. What is facilitated PCI?

Facilitated early PCI refers to PCI after pharmacologic reperfusion therapy. It has the potential to fuse the best aspects of fibrinolysis and primary PTCA rapid reperfusion, improved patient stability, greater technical procedure success and TIMI 3 flow rates. In the SPEED trial, patients pretreated with pharmacologic reperfusion therapy had the highest TIMI 3 rates and a trend towards better outcomes. Larger trials are currently outgoing which should determine the use of this strategy in routine clinical practice.

19. Can reperfusion injury be controlled?

The concept that preventable damage occurs to the myocardium during the reperfusion process, either directly because of reperfusion or through ongoing ischemia, has led to attempts to treat with adjunctive therapy to reduce infarct size. Therapeutic approaches have included metabolic modulation; anti-inflammatory agents; alteration of cellular sodium, hydrogen, and calcium shifts; and physical cooling. Results to date have not shown a substantial clinical benefit; with better understanding of the process of cell damage in ischemia and reperfusion, methods to reduce infarct size and improve outcome should be possible.

BIBLIOGRAPHY

 1. Antman EM, Giugliano RP, Gibson CM, et al, for the TIMI 14 Investigators: Abciximab facilitates the rate and extent of thrombolysis: results of the Thrombolysis In Myocardial Infarction (TIMI) 14 trial. Circulation 99:2720–2732, 1999.
 2. Bashore TM, Bates ER, Berger PB, et al: Cardiac catheterization laboratory standards: Report of the American College of Cardiology Task Force on Clinical Expert Consensus Documents. J Am Coll Cardiol 37:2170–2214, 2001.
 3. Califf RM, Fortin DF, Tenaglia AN, Sane DC: Clinical risks of thrombolytic therapy. Am J Cardiol. 69(Suppl A):12–20, 1992.
 4. Dewood MA, Spores J, Notske R, et al: Prevalence of total coronary occlusion during the early hours of transmural myocardial infarction. N Engl J Med 303:897–901, 1980.
 5. Grines CL, Browne KF, Marco J, et al: A comparison of immediate angioplasty with thrombolytic therapy for acute myocardial infarction: the Primary Angioplasty in Myocardial Infarction Study Group. N Engl J Med. 328:673–679, 1993.
 6. The GUSTO Angiographic Investigators: The comparative effects of tissue plasminogen activator, streptokinase, or both on coronary artery patency, ventricular function and survival after acute myocardial infarction. N Engl J Med 329:1615–1622, 1993.
 7. ISIS-2 (Second International Study of Infarct Survival) Collaborative Group: Randomized trial of intravenous streptokinase, oral aspirin, both, or neither among 17,187 cases of suspected acute myocardial infarction: ISIS-2. Lancet 2:349–360, 1988.
 8. Montalescot G, Barragan P, Wittenberg O, et al: Platelet glycoprotein IIb/IIIa inhibition with coronary stenting for acute myocardial infarction. N Engl J Med 344:1895–903, 2001.
 9. Stone GW, Grines CL, Cox DA, et al: Comparison of angioplasty with stenting , with or without abciximab, in acute myocardial infarction. N Engl J Med 346:957–966, 2002.
10. Topol EJ, Califf RM, Van de Werf, et al: Reperfusion therapy for acute myocardial infarction with fibrinolytic therapy or combination reduced fibrinolytic therapy and platelet glycoprotein IIb/IIIa inhibition: the GUSTO V randomized trial. Lancet 357:1905–1914, 2001.

28. MULTIVESSEL CORONARY INTERVENTION

Ravish Sachar, M.D., and Deepak L. Bhatt, M.D.

1. What is the prognostic significance of multivessel coronary artery disease (CAD)?

The most commonly used classification system for CAD is based on the number of diseased vessels. However, cardiovascular risk cannot be accurately assessed solely by describing the coronary anatomy in terms of the number of vessels with stenoses 50% or greater. The inaccuracy of such a system stems from the fact that not all lesions carry the same significance. A subtotal occlusion of the proximal left anterior descending (LAD) carries a worse prognosis than a 60% midright coronary artery (RCA) lesion, but both are classified as single vessel disease. Furthermore, total atherosclerotic burden is likely a more sensitive marker for future cardiac events than the number of discrete stenoses. Areas of the coronary vasculature that appear to have mild or moderate disease, of which there are a large amount, are more likely to result in plaque rupture and myocardial infarction (MI) compared with the relatively smaller areas with discrete severe stenoses. Unfortunately, no accurate methods exist for quantifying the total extent of atherosclerosis that can be rapidly and safely used during angiography.

Nevertheless, several trials comparing coronary artery bypass grafting (CABG) with medical therapy have correlated prognosis with the number of diseased vessels. Almost all trials assessing the relative benefits of CABG versus medical therapy or percutaneous coronary intervention (PCI) have used the number of diseased epicardial vessels to risk stratify patients. Patients with the greatest risk profile have consistently been shown to derive the maximum benefit from CABG compared with medical therapy. Specifically, patients with three-vessel disease, proximal LAD disease, left main trunk (LMT) disease, left ventricular (LV) dysfunction, large ischemic burden, and Canadian Cardiovascular Society (CCS) class III or IV angina have been shown to have longer survival with CABG compared with medical therapy. Lower-risk patients with single- or double-vessel disease without LAD involvement and with normal LV function have had no survival advantage with CABG.

2. What is the role of stenting in patients with multivessel disease?

There has been an exponential growth in the use of coronary artery stents over the past decade, and the vast majority of PCIs performed currently use stents. Compared with percutaneous transluminal coronary angioplasty (PTCA), stenting reduces the incidence of abrupt vessel closure, the need for emergency bypass surgery, and the incidence of binary restenosis and target vessel revascularization (TVR). In the PTCA arm of the Bypass Angioplasty Revascularization Investigation (BARI) trial, stents were not used, and there was a 10% incidence of abrupt vessel closure, 7.1% of patients required emergency bypass surgery, and 54.5% required TVR over 5 years. Stenting in multivessel disease improves both short- and long-term outcomes after PCI and has been shown to be safe and effective with excellent angiographic success rates. In a nonrandomized study in Alberta, Canada, 11,661 patients with multivessel disease were treated with either CABG, stenting, or medical therapy and were subsequently followed up with for 5 years. Surgical revascularization or stenting resulted in better survival compared with medical therapy alone (91.4% vs. 91.9% vs. 82.9%, respectively). There was no difference in survival between CABG and stenting, except in patients with LMT lesions. Because this was not a randomized trial, these data cannot be used to directly compare multivessel stenting with CABG. One can, however, draw the conclusion that when the choice of revascularization therapy in multivessel disease is based on physician discretion, the results with the two strategies are equivalent.

3. For patients with multivessel CAD, which is better, PCI or CABG?

Several randomized trials have sought to answer this question (Table 1), and the answer depends on the endpoints used to define "better." Most trials have used a composite endpoint of death or nonfatal MI, with follow-up times ranging from 30 days to 6 years (Figs. 1 and 2).

Table 1. Randomized Trials of Multivessel Coronary Intervention versus Coronary Artery Bypass Grafting
(All data presented as CABG versus PCI)

TRIAL	YEAR	n	PCI	FOLLOW-UP	ENDPOINT	RESULTS	CONCLUSION
ERACI Single center	1993	127	PTCA	1 year	Death or MI	In-hospital mortality: 4.6% vs. 1.5%, P = NS In-hospital MI: 6.2% vs. 6.3%, P = NS 1-year mortality: 0% vs. 3.2%, P = NS 1-year MI: 1.8% vs. 3.2%, P = NS Repeat revascularization: 3.2% vs. 32%, P < 0.001	1. No difference in death or MI at 1 year 2. More repeat revascularization in patients with initial PTCA strategy
EAST Single center	1994	392	PTCA	3 years, 8 years	Composite of death, MI, defect on thallium	In-hospital mortality: 1% each group In-hospital MI: 10.3% vs. 3.0%, P = 0.004 3-year death, MI, thallium Defect: 27.3% vs. 28.8% 3-year mortality: 6.2% vs. 7.1%, P = 0.72 3-year MI: 19.6% vs. 14.6%, P = 0.21 Repeat revascularization: 14% vs. 63%, P < 0.001	1. No difference in composite endpoint 2. Lower rates of revascularization with CABG 3. 8-year follow-up: • Survival: 82.7% vs. 79.3%, P = 0.40 • Survival with 3 VD: 81.6% vs. 75.5%, P = 0.35 • Survival with 2 VD: 83.4% vs. 81.8%, P = NS
GABI Single center	1994	337	PTCA	1 year	1-year freedom from angina	Procedural MI: 8.1% vs. 2.3%, P = 0.022 Procedural mortality: 2.5% vs. 1.1%, P = 0.43 1-year death or MI: 13.6% vs. 6%, P = 0.017 Repeat revascularization: 6% vs. 44%, P < 0.001	1. Freedom from angina at 1 year equivalent for both groups 2. Not powered to detect differences in death or nonfatal MI
CABRI Multicenter	1995	1054	PTCA (stenting if needed)	1 year	One-year mortality	1-year mortality: 2.7% vs. 3.9%, P = 0.3 Repeat revascularization: 3.5% vs. 36.5%, P < 0.001	1. No difference in survival at 1 year 2. Fewer repeat revascularization procedures in CABG patients

Study	Year	N	Intervention	Follow-up	Endpoint	Results	Conclusions
BARI Multicenter	1996	1829	PTCA	Mean 5.4 years	Death or MI	In-hospital mortality: 1.3% vs. 1.1%, $P =$ NS In-hospital MI: 4.6% vs. 2.1%, $P < 0.01$ 5-year death or MI: 19.6% vs. 17.3%, $P = 0.84$ 5-year mortality: 10.7% vs. 13.7%, $P = 0.19$ 5-year MI: 11.7% vs. 10.9%, $P = 0.45$ Repeat revascularization: 8% vs. 54%	1. No significant difference in death or MI at 5 years 2. Patients randomized to PTCA had more repeat revascularization procedures
TOULOUSE Single center	1997	152	PTCA	5 years	Freedom from angina	5-year mortality: 10.6% vs. 13.2%, $P =$ NS 5-year MI: 1.3% vs. 5.3%, $P =$ NS Freedom from Angina: 94.7% vs. 78.9%, $P < 0.01$ Repeat revascularization: 3.9% vs. 25%, $P < 0.01$	1. More patients with freedom from angina in the CABG arm 2. Patients randomized to PTCA had more repeat revascularization procedures
RITA-1 Multicenter	1998	1011	PTCA	Median 6.5 years	Death or MI	In-hospital mortality: 3.6% vs. 3.1% In-hospital MI: 4.0% vs. 6.5% Death or MI: 16% vs. 17%, $P = 0.64$ Mortality: 9.2% vs. 7.9%, $P =$ NS MI: 7.1% vs. 9.7%, $P =$ NS Repeat revascularization: 10.8% vs. 44.3%	1. No difference in the primary endpoint of death or MI at median 6.5-year follow-up 2. More revascularization procedures among patients with an initial PTCA strategy
ARTS Multicenter	2001	1205	Stent	1 year	12-month death, MI, stroke, TIA, or TVR	1-year event-free survival: 87.8% vs. 73.8%, 1-year mortality: 2.8% vs. 2.5% 1-year MI: 4.0% vs. 5.3% Repeat revascularization: 3.5% vs. 16.8%	1. No difference in death or MI at 1 year 2. More repeat revascularization in the patients with an initial PCI strategy
ERACI II Multicenter	2001	450	Stent if vessel ≥ 3 mm	30 days, 1 year	1-year death, MI, TVR	30-day MACE: 12.3% vs. 3.6%, $P = 0.002$ 30-day MI: 5.7% vs. 0.9%, $P = 0.012$ 30-day death or MI: 11.4% vs. 1.8%, $P = 0.0001$ 1-year mortality: 8.5% vs. 3.1%, $P < 0.017$ 1-year MI: 6.3% vs. 2.3%, $P < 0.017$ Repeat revascularization: 4.8% vs. 16.8%, $P < 0.001$	1. Stenting associated with better survival and freedom from MI at 30 days and 1 year 2. Stenting associated with more repeat revascularization procedures

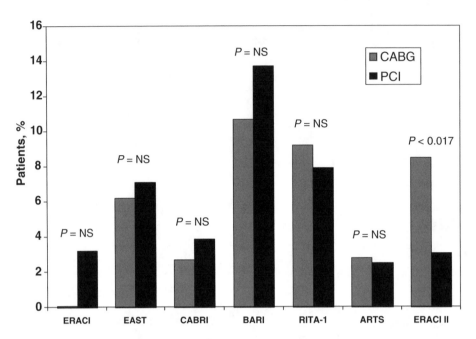

FIGURE 1. Randomized trials of CABG versus PCI trials: mortality rates. Almost all trials, with the exception of ERACI II, have found no significant difference in mortality between patients randomized to CABG or PCI.

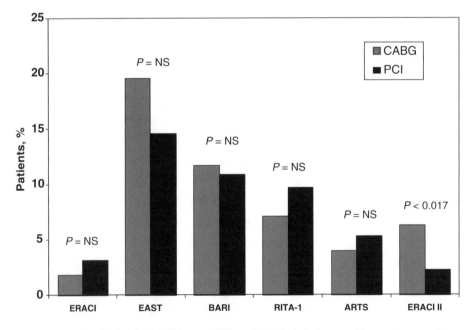

FIGURE 2. Randomized trials of CABG versus PCI: nonfatal MI. As is the case with mortality rates, almost all trials, with the exception of ERACI II, have found no significant difference in nonfatal MI between patients randomized to CABG or PCI.

Using this composite endpoint, most trials have found no difference between the two strategies among nondiabetics, with the exception of ERACI II, which found a significant difference in death and nonfatal MI favoring the percutaneous approach at 1-year follow-up. TVR, however, has consistently been higher in all trials among patients treated percutaneously, even with the use of stents (Fig. 3). Drug-eluting stents may tilt the tables in favor of PCI, but this remains to be seen. Diabetic patients treated percutaneously have consistently had higher rates of death, MI, and TVR, and this will be discussed further below.

In addition to these endpoints, other issues need to be considered. Newman et al. have shown a neurocognitive decline after 5 years in patients undergoing CABG. Others have found that although patients undergoing PCI return to work an average of 5 weeks sooner than those undergoing CABG, more patients undergoing CABG have freedom from angina at 1 year after surgery and higher functional status at 3 years. Finally, patients often present with strong opinions about which treatment they want. Thus, when deciding between CABG and PCI, in addition to the traditional endpoints, patient preference needs to be evaluated.

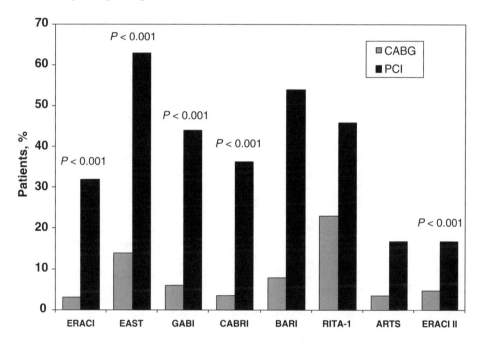

FIGURE 3. Randomized trials of CABG versus PCI: repeat revascularization. All trials have found that an initial strategy of PCI results in higher rates of revascularization compared with an initial strategy of CABG.

4. What clinical and anatomic factors must be considered when deciding on CABG or PCI?

After obtaining angiographic data, the following issues should be addressed before deciding on a treatment strategy:

1. The projected survival benefit of revascularization, if any
2. The nature and extent of the patient's symptoms and the likelihood of improvement with either treatment strategy
3. The anatomic and technical feasibility of CABG and PCI and the risks and benefits associated with either procedure
4. The presence of LMT disease and the extent of LV dysfunction, if any
5. The need for noncoronary cardiac surgery currently or in the near future

6. Comorbid conditions (e.g., diabetes, renal failure, congestive heart failure, chronic obstructive pulmonary disease, malignancy) and their effect on intraprocedural risk and postprocedural recovery

7. The risk of not revascularizing and instead treating the patient with medical therapy alone

8. Patient preference

5. What are the limitations of randomized trials comparing multivessel PCI with CABG?

Most of the randomized trials assessing PCI versus CABG have had stringent exclusion criteria, thereby excluding patients with prior CABG or PCI, LMT lesions, chronic total occlusions, or patients with recent MI. Patients in whom CABG has been shown to be superior to medical therapy (see previous discussion) were generally excluded. Each patient randomized had to have coronary anatomy suitable to either type of revascularization, and this was based on operator discretion. The resultant ratio of screened to enrolled patients has been very large ($\sim 5\%$ of patients screened were enrolled). For example, in the BARI trial, 25,200 patients were screened and 1829 were finally enrolled. Furthermore, approximately 60% of enrolled patients had two-vessel disease with a mean ejection fraction of 57%, and patients with diffuse disease without discrete lesions generally were not enrolled. Even in Arterial Revascularization Therapies Study (ARTS), the most recent trial in which stents were used, only 30% of patients had three-vessel disease. Although the reasoning behind these exclusions may be sound, the result has been a skewed patient population that is lower risk than the average population encountered in clinical practice. Therefore, the generalizability of these data is limited.

Furthermore, all published trials except two (ARTS and ERACI II) have used PTCA without stenting, and none of the trials has mandated the use of glycoprotein (GP) IIb/IIIa inhibitors. As a result, these trials do not represent the current standard of care in the United States. Over the past decade, the use of stents and GP IIb/IIIa inhibitors has drastically reduced the incidence of emergency CABG, periprocedural MI, and TVR in percutaneously treated patients. Additionally, advances in surgical technique, especially the rapidly growing use of off-pump CABG, limits the generalizability of surgical data from the randomized trials. Finally, none of the trials completed so far have been powered to detect a mortality difference between the two therapies.

6. What is the role of GP IIb/IIIa inhibitors in patients undergoing elective multivessel PCI?

Several trials have established a role for GP IIb/IIIa inhibitors during elective PCI, both with PTCA as well as with stenting. The EPISTENT trial randomized 2399 patients to stenting plus placebo, stenting plus abciximab, or PTCA plus abciximab and found a significant decrease in periprocedural events (30-day death and MI: 3.0% vs. 7.8%) and a significant decrease in 1-year mortality (1.0% vs. 2.4%) among stented patients who received abciximab compared with those who did not. In a long-term follow-up of patients enrolled in the EPIC, EPILOG, and EPISTENT trials, mortality was significantly higher among the placebo arms compared with the abciximab arms (12.6% vs. 10.2%). Abciximab and stenting have been shown to have a large benefit on the reduction of major adverse cardiac events (MACE) among patients with complex atherosclerotic lesions. However, the majority of patients in these trials had single-vessel interventions, and no trial has specifically evaluated the use of GP IIb/IIIa inhibitors for multivessel disease. One can, however, extrapolate the benefits seen in single-vessel disease to patients with multivessel disease. Additionally, pooled data from the EPIC, EPILOG, and EPISTENT trials demonstrated that abciximab significantly reduced the occurrence of death or MI in patients with multivessel disease.

7. Is there any benefit of CABG versus PCI in patients with multivessel disease and stable angina compared with patients with multivessel disease and unstable angina?

One randomized trial has examined this issue with the use of stents. de Feyter et al. randomized 755 patients with stable angina and 450 patients with unstable angina to CABG or coronary stenting. There was no difference between stenting and CABG in the composite endpoint of death, MI, or stroke at 1 year between patients with unstable angina (91.2% vs. 88.9%) and stable angina (90.4% vs.

92.6%). TVR was higher among stented patients (16.8% vs. 16.9%) compared with CABG (3.6% vs. 3.5%), but there was no difference in TVR between patients with unstable angina and stable angina.

8. Is there any benefit of CABG versus PCI in patients with acute MI?

Limited data address the issue to PCI versus CABG in the setting of acute MI. Logistically, it is difficult to answer this question because angiography will always be performed before bypass surgery. In most cases, only patients with coronary anatomy not amenable to PCI will be referred to surgery, thus selecting out a higher risk population being referred for surgical revascularization. It has been established, however, that emergent bypass surgery carries a higher mortality and morbidity rate compared with elective bypass surgery. Thus, in the setting of acute MI, it is preferable to treat the culprit lesion percutaneously. If there are other mitigating factors such as inability to treat the culprit lesion, cardiogenic shock with anatomy unsuitable for PCI, or mechanical complications such as papillary muscle rupture or a ventricular septal defect, the patient should be referred for emergent surgery, with the understanding that such patients have a high mortality risk. Patients with cardiogenic shock, in particular, benefit from revascularization of as much myocardium as possible.

9. In patients with acute MI and multivessel disease, should only the culprit lesion be treated, or should all stenoses be treated?

It has been estimated that 30% to 60% of patients presenting with acute MI have multivessel disease. In the era of decreased procedural complications because of stents and GP IIb/IIIa inhibitors, the ability to perform multivessel PCI for nonculprit lesions during primary angioplasty for acute MI has increased. However, no randomized trials have addressed this issue. The benefits of complete revascularization with multivessel PCI may be attenuated by increased procedural complications and the potential for nephrotoxicity caused by the contrast load. Retrospective studies suggest that event-free survival is higher for patients who only have the culprit vessel treated. One recent study reported a multicenter experience of 79 cases of multivessel PCI during acute MI and matched these with an equal number of control cases. Although there was a trend toward increased mortality in the patients who underwent multivessel intervention, there was no difference in the primary composite endpoint of death, reinfarction, repeat PCI, or bypass surgery. Consistent with these findings, a recent study has suggested that the severity of stenosis in nonculprit lesions may be exaggerated because of vasoconstriction caused by higher levels of circulating catecholamines during acute MI. Until a randomized trial is performed to address this issue, it is best to use a case-by-case approach. In cases in which the nonculprit lesion appears to have hemodynamic significance and is easily approachable, treatment can be justified. This is especially true in the setting of cardiogenic shock, in which improvement of flow to as much myocardium as possible is needed to improve ventricular function. Conversely, in cases in which the lesion is likely not responsible for symptoms, it may be best to treat only the culprit lesion at the time of the MI.

10. Should multivessel interventions be staged?

As multivessel interventions have become increasingly prevalent, the issue of staging procedures has become more relevant. In general, patients who are susceptible to the adverse effects of ionic contrast agents should be considered for staged procedures. This includes patients with renal insufficiency, LV dysfunction with elevated LV end-diastolic pressures, and patients who cannot lie flat for long periods of time. There has been only one study that has examined this issue. Nikolsky et al. followed 129 patients in whom PCI was conducted in a single session and 135 patients in whom the procedure was staged. There was an insignificant trend toward fewer events at 30 days and 1 year in the staged arm. However, this was a single-center study with a small sample size. There is currently no proven advantage of staging PCI in patients without comorbidities.

11. Do diabetics have worse outcomes after CABG than nondiabetics?

Diabetics who undergo CABG have worse short and long-term outcomes compared with nondiabetics. Carson et al. retrospectively reviewed the 1-month outcomes among diabetics ($n =$

41,663) and nondiabetics (n = 105,123) after CABG and found that all-cause mortality was significantly higher among diabetics (3.7% vs 2.7%). Diabetics also had higher in-hospital morbidity and infection rates than nondiabetics. Similarly, long-term survival after CABG among diabetics is worse than among nondiabetics. Barsness et al. published data from the Duke University database showing a higher 5-year mortality rate among diabetics with multivessel disease undergoing CABG compared with nondiabetics (26% vs. 14%). Insulin-dependent diabetics tended to have worse outcomes than those taking oral therapy.

12. Do diabetic patients with multivessel disease have similar outcomes with CABG and PCI?

Approximately 20% to 25% of patients enrolled in randomized trials are diabetic, and these patients have consistently been shown to have worse clinical and angiographic outcomes after PCI and CABG compared with nondiabetics. It is well established that diabetics have higher mortality, more periprocedural MIs and higher rates of restenosis and TVR compared with nondiabetics. Hypercoaguability, platelet hyperreactivity, and abnormal endothelial autoregulation have all been described and may be potential factors leading to the observed adverse outcomes. Insulin has been shown to increase levels of platelet-derived growth factor (PDGF), which stimulates vascular smooth muscle cells; this is consistent with clinical data showing that insulin treated diabetics have worse outcomes compared with diabetics who do not use insulin. Furthermore, diabetics tend to have more diffuse and distal disease, along with a higher prevalence of LV dysfunction.

Randomized trials comparing surgical and percutaneous revascularization strategies in diabetic patients have consistently shown a survival advantage for patients undergoing surgery. The largest randomized trial of CABG versus PCI, BARI, showed a significant 5-year survival advantage among diabetic patients treated with an initial strategy of CABG compared with PCI (80.6% vs. 65.5%). These findings have subsequently been reproduced in other trials comparing PTCA with CABG. The pathophysiologic reasons for better outcomes for diabetics after CABG are unclear. Diabetic arteries are more likely to have diffuse disease. Additionally, the presence of an alternative arterial conduit after CABG likely attenuates the effect of plaque rupture in the native vessels of a fragile population.

In the current era in which the majority of patients undergoing PCI receive stents, the applicability of earlier trials using PTCA only is questionable. Stenting has reduced the rates of restenosis and TVR among diabetics compared with PTCA alone and brought levels closer to those seen in nondiabetics. However, mortality and MI appear to remain higher in diabetics even with the use of stents. For example, in the ARTS trial, in which PCI was performed with stenting, 1-year TVR was slightly higher at 14.3% among diabetics compared with 11.7% among nondiabetics. These levels are much lower than the TVR levels seen in trials that used PTCA only. However, 1-year mortality among diabetics remained higher at 6.3% for the PCI arm and 3.1% for the CABG arm. It should be pointed out, however, that this difference did not reach statistical significance and that the study was not adequately powered to look at mortality in the diabetic subset. In fact, if one looks at the combined endpoint of death, MI, or stroke among diabetic patients at 1 year, there was no statistical difference between CABG and PCI (12.5% vs. 14.3%).

In general, the goal should be to achieve maximal revascularization. If both strategies appear to be equally feasible, current guidelines recommend that diabetics with multivessel disease be referred for CABG. As discussed later, however, the adjunctive use of GP IIb/IIIa inhibitors was not evaluated in any of these trials, and their effect on outcomes after multivessel PCI compared with CABG remains to be seen.

13. What is role of GP IIb/IIIa inhibitors during PCI in diabetic patients?

Although no randomized trials have specifically addressed the issue of multivessel stenting in diabetics, the beneficial effect of GP IIb/IIIa inhibition in terms of death, MI, and TVR after PCI in diabetics has been shown. In a pooled analysis of 1462 diabetic patients from the EPIC, EPILOG, and EPISTENT trials, abciximab was found to significantly decrease all-cause mortal-

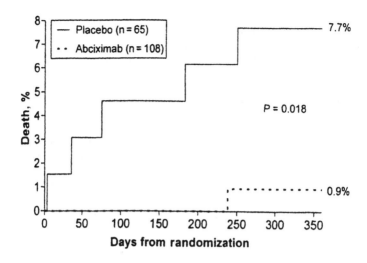

FIGURE 4. One-year mortality in diabetic patients undergoing multivessel intervention randomized to abciximab compared with placebo. (From Bhatt DL, et al: The importance of intravenous antiplatelet therapy with abciximab during percutaneous coronary intervention in diabetic patients. Cardiovasc Rev Rep 22:161–164, 2001, with permission.)

ity at 1 year follow-up from 4.5% to 2.5%, and non–Q-wave MI from 9.7% to 4.0%. Among diabetics undergoing multivessel PCI, the mortality rate with the use of abciximab was 0.9% compared with 7.7% with placebo (Fig. 4). In a subset analysis of 491 diabetic patients enrolled in EPISTENT, Marso et al. found that the 6-month combined endpoint of death, MI, and TVR occurred in 25.2% and 12.5% of patients in the stent–placebo and stent–abciximab arms, respectively. One-year mortality was decreased from 4.1% to 1.2% in patients treated with stent–abciximab. Angiographic outcomes were also improved among stented patients treated with abciximab, although other trials have not confirmed a role for abciximab in reducing restenosis.

The benefits of GP IIb/IIIa inhibition appear to be a class effect and are not limited to abciximab. The use of tirofiban in diabetic patients was validated in a subset analysis of the TARGET trial, in which there were similar rates of 1-year mortality and 6-month TVR among diabetic patients randomized to abciximab or tirofiban. Interestingly, in this trial, there were no significant differences in the 6-month composite endpoint of death, MI, and TVR (16.3% vs. 14.3%) and 1-year mortality (2.5% vs. 1.6%) among diabetics and nondiabetics.

The 1-year mortality rates in these trials that used GP IIb/IIIa inhibitors are about half the 6.1% mortality rate observed among patients randomized to stenting in the ARTS trial and are similar to the mortality rate among patients randomized to CABG. Because there have been no trials comparing the two modes of revascularization using stents and GP IIb/IIIa inhibitors, the mortality benefit of CABG compared with PCI when performed according to current standards of care needs to be reevaluated in a prospective randomized trial. Until then, the existing data overwhelmingly support the use of GP IIb/IIIa inhibition during PCI in diabetic patients. Unless there are contraindications, the routine use of GP IIb/IIIa inhibitors in all diabetic patients undergoing single- or multivessel stenting is highly recommended.

14. What is the cost differential between multivessel coronary intervention and CABG?

Although the initial cost of the surgical approach is higher than the percutaneous approach, the higher rate of TVR among percutaneously treated patients results in more delayed costs among such patients. The cost of multivessel intervention compared with CABG has been studied as part of several large randomized trials.

The BARI trial randomized 1829 patients with multivessel disease to PTCA or CABG and found that the initial cost of PTCA was considerably less than the cost of CABG ($21,113 vs. $32,347). However, because of the larger number of repeat revascularization procedures among patients randomized to PTCA, the cost differential between the two arms at 5 years was only $2664 ($56,225 vs. $58,889). The 5-year total cost of an initial PTCA strategy was significantly cheaper among patients with two-vessel disease ($52,930 vs. $58,498) but not in patients with three-vessel disease ($60,918 vs. $59,430).

More recently, the ARTS trial randomized 1205 patients to stenting ($n = 600$) or CABG ($n = 605$) and reported similar results. Although the initial cost per patient was $4212 lower for the percutaneous approach ($10,653 vs. $6441), this difference was reduced to $2973 by the end of the first year. If all patients in the trial had undergone CABG, the additional cost at 1 year would have been $21,329 per patient who survived event free. Two other randomized trials, Randomized Intervention Treatment of Angina (RITA)-1 (5 year mean cost £8842 vs. £9268) and ERACI (1-year mean cost, $12,320 vs. $11,160) found no difference in the total follow-up cost between the two procedures.

There are limitations to these data, and conclusions must be drawn while keeping these limitations in mind. The current widespread use of stents, thienopyridines, aggressive lipid-lowering therapy, and GP IIb/IIIa inhibitors has lowered rates of death, MI, and TVR and, thus, limits our ability to extrapolate data from the above trials to today's practice. With drug-eluting stents poised to revolutionize interventional cardiology, it remains to be seen if the higher initial cost of such stents will be justified by lower costs associated with TVR. Similarly, improvements in surgical techniques make it difficult to apply these data to current patients. As a general principle, however, the advantage of a lower up-front cost of the percutaneous approach is attenuated by higher subsequent costs of TVR in such patients.

15. What is the optimal treatment of patients with LMT disease or severe LV dysfunction?
Limited randomized data are available for patients with LMT disease or severe LV dysfunction because these patients were either excluded from CABG versus PCI trials or the studies were insufficiently powered to assess these subgroups. As a result, the majority of the data for such patients are from early trials that evaluated CABG versus medical therapy. Based on the higher mortality for such patients treated medically in these trials, current guidelines recommend that patients with LMT disease or severe three-vessel disease with LV dysfunction be referred for CABG. Whether these recommendations are modified by future trials that specifically include such patients remains to be seen.

BIBLIOGRAPHY

1. Abizaid A, Costa MA, Centemero M, et al. and the Arterial Revascularization Therapy Study Group: Clinical and economic impact of diabetes mellitus on percutaneous and surgical treatment of multivessel coronary disease patients: insights from the Arterial Revascularization Therapy Study (ARTS) trial. Circulation 104:533–538, 2001.
2. Barsness GW, Peterson ED, Ohman EM, et al: Relationship between diabetes mellitus and long-term survival after coronary bypass and angioplasty. Circulation 96:2551–2556, 1997.
3. Bhatt DL, Marso SP, Lincoff AM, et al: Abciximab reduces mortality in diabetics following percutaneous coronary intervention. J Am Coll Cardiol 35:922–928, 2000.
4. Bhatt DL, Chew DP, Topol EJ. The importance of intravenous antiplatelet therapy with abciximab during percutaneous coronary intervention in diabetic patients. Cardiovasc Rev Rep 21:161–164, 2001.
5. Carson JL, Scholz PM, Chen AY, et al: Diabetes mellitus increases short-term mortality and morbidity in patients undergoing coronary artery bypass graft surgery. J Am Coll Cardiol 40:418–423, 2002.
6. CASS Principal Investigators and Their Associates: Myocardial infarction and mortality in the Coronary Artery Surgery Study (CASS) randomized trial. N Engl J Med 310:750–758, 1984.
7. Cura FA, Bhatt DL, Lincoff AM, et al: Pronounced benefit of coronary stenting and adjunctive platelet glycoprotein IIb/IIIa inhibition in complex atherosclerotic lesions. Circulation 102:28–34, 2000.
8. de Feyter PJ, Serruys PW, Unger F, et al: Bypass surgery versus stenting for the treatment of multivessel disease in patients with unstable angina compared with stable angina. Circulation 105:2367–2372, 2000.
9. Dzavik V, Ghali WA, Norris C, et al. and the Alberta Provincial Project for Outcome Assessment in

Coronary Heart Disease (APPROACH) Investigators: Long-term survival in 11,661 patients with multivessel coronary artery disease in the era of stenting: a report from the Alberta Provincial Project for Outcome Assessment in Coronary Heart Disease (APPROACH) Investigators. Am Heart J 142:119– 126, 2001.

10. EPISTENT Investigators: Randomised placebo-controlled and balloon-angioplasty-controlled trial to assess safety of coronary stenting with use of platelet glycoprotein-IIb/IIIa blockade: evaluation of platelet IIb/IIIa inhibitor for stenting. Lancet 352:87–92, 1998.

11. Hanratty CG, Koyama Y, Rasmussen HH, et al: Exaggeration of nonculprit stenosis severity during acute myocardial infarction: implications for immediate multivessel revascularization. J Am Coll Card 40: 911–916, 2002.

12. Hlatky MA, Rogers WJ, Johnstone I, et al: Medical care costs and quality of life after randomization to coronary angioplasty or coronary bypass surgery: Bypass Angioplasty Revascularization Investigation (BARI) Investigators. N Engl J Med 336:92–99, 1997.

13. Marso SP, Lincoff AM, Ellis SG, et al: Optimizing the percutaneous interventional outcomes for patients with diabetes mellitus: results of the EPISTENT (Evaluation of platelet IIb/IIIa inhibitor for stenting trial) diabetic substudy. Circulation 100:2477–2484, 1999.

14. Nikolsky E, Halabi M, Roguin A, et al: Staged versus one-step approach for multivessel percutaneous coronary interventions. Am Heart J 143:1017–1026, 2002.

15. Roe MT, Cura FA, Joski PS, et al: Initial experience with multivessel percutaneous coronary intervention during mechanical reperfusion for acute myocardial infarction. Am J Cardiol 88:170–173, 2001.

16. Roffi M, Moliterno DJ, Meier B, et al. and the TARGET Investigators: Impact of different platelet glyco-protein IIb/IIIa receptor inhibitors among diabetic patients undergoing percutaneous coronary inter-vention: Do Tirofiban and ReoPro Give Similar Efficacy Outcomes Trial (TARGET) 1-year follow-up. Circulation 105:2730–2736, 2002.

29. PERCUTANEOUS INTERVENTION BEFORE NONCARDIAC SURGERY

Neerav Shah, M.D., and Eduardo de Marchena, M.D.

1. What is the basis for the principle of myocardial revascularization before noncardiac surgery?

Large observational studies involving coronary artery bypass grafting patients who required noncardiac surgery showed that patients who had bypasses before their noncardiac surgery had a lower perioperative mortality rate than their nonrevascularized counterparts. The incidence was similar to patients who had no significant coronary artery disease (CAD).

2. Have any randomized studies supported percutaneous coronary intervention (PCI) as reducing perioperative mortality from noncardiac surgery?

Although intuitively this strategy would appear to make sense, no evidence from randomized, placebo-controlled trials support the superiority of PCI over beta-blockers in lowering perioperative risk.

3. What questions should be addressed before deciding on PCI before noncardiac surgery?

- Is the patient at high risk for a clinical cardiac event (Canadian Class III or IV, unstable angina)?
- Does the patient have a large amount of myocardium at risk on noninvasive stress test?
- Is the surgical procedure considered high risk?
- Are the risks or mortality of PCI higher than the surgery itself?
- How urgent or emergent is the surgical procedure?
- Can the procedure be delayed for 4 to 6 weeks after PCI?
- Does the procedure require local or regional or general anesthesia?

4. Do any data support medical therapy alone in high-risk patients undergoing noncardiac surgery?

A study performed by Poldermans et al. showed that even in the setting of a positive dobutamine stress echocardiography, beta-blockade alone (bisoprolol) lowered the risk of death from 17% to 3.4% and nonfatal myocardial infarction (MI) from 17% to 0%. One caveat is that a head-to-head comparison between PCI and perioperative beta-blocker therapy has never been performed.

5. How much of a delay does an extended cardiac evaluation typically cause? Can this delay result in poor clinical outcomes?

A small study of 42 vascular surgery patients requiring extended cardiac evaluation showed that the median delay between initiation of cardiac evaluation and surgical procedure was 25 days. This resulted in amputation in two patients who might otherwise have been able to have revascularization procedures.

6. How long should a patient be off Plavix and aspirin (ASA) before surgery?

Both ASA and Plavix inhibit activity for the entire lifetime of the platelet, which is from 3 to 7 days. Therefore, antiplatelets should be stopped 7 days before surgery.

7. What conclusions can be drawn from studies involving PCI before noncardiac surgery?

Very few studies exist evaluating a PCI strategy before noncardiac surgery. In Posner et al.'s study listed below, although perioperative mortality was lower as was angina, there was an increased incidence of perioperative MIs. Kaluza et al. described a high mortality rate (20%) when

PCI and stent placement were done within 2 weeks of the noncardiac surgery. In summary, the benefit of elective intervention before noncardiac surgery appears limited. It is likely that the majority of CAD patients could safely undergo surgery with perioperative beta-blockade alone. In unstable coronary patients or high-risk patients, such as those who have a large amount of myocardium at risk based on noninvasive stress imaging, a PCI strategy should be entertained despite the limited data.

Posner et al.
142 patients with PCI within 90 days of noncardiac surgery vs. 142 nonrevascularized patients with CAD who underwent surgery with medical therapy alone.

	PTCA, %	**CAD (Medical Treatment), %**
Adverse cardiovascular events	26.1	28.2
Death	2.1	2.8
MI	7	3.5
Congestive heart failure	12	14.8
Angina	5.6	9.2

Kaluza et al.
40 patients who underwent PCI with stent placement < 6 wks before noncardiac surgery.
Death → Eight patients (all had surgery within 2 weeks of PCI)
MI → Seven patients (all had surgery within 2 weeks of PCI)
Bleeding → 11 patients (eight/11 within 2 weeks of PCI)

8. Who should have a preoperative cardiac catheterization?

The American Heart Association/American College of Cardiology guidelines state that class I indications for cardiac catheterization before noncardiac surgery are:
- Patients with high risk results on noninvasive study
- Patients with unstable angina symptoms
- Patients with significant angina (CC III or IV)
- Nondiagnostic or equivocal stress test results in a high-risk patient undergoing high-risk surgery

9. Do heparin-coated stents decrease the incidence of perioperative stent thrombosis?

In theory, this would probably appear to be true. However, no clinical trial data exist in this specific patient cohort.

BIBLIOGRAPHY

1. Eagle KA, et al: ACC/AHA guideline update for perioperative cardiac evaluation for non cardiac surgery: executive summary. J Am Coll Cardiol 39:542–553, 2002.
2. Gottlieb A, Banoub M, Sprung J et al: Perioperative cardiovascular morbidity in patients with coronary artery disease undergoing vascular surgery after percutaneous transluminal coronary angioplasty. Cardiothorac Vasc Anesth 12:501–506, 1998.
3. Huber KC, Evans MA, Breshnahan JF, et al: Outcome of noncardiac operations in patients with severe coronary artery disease treated successfully with coronary angioplasty. Mayo Clin Proc 67:15–21, 1992.
4. Kaluza GL, Lee JJ Jr, Raizner ME, et al: Catastrophic outcomes of noncardiac surgery soon after coronary stenting. J Am Coll Cardiol 35:1288–1294, 2000.
5. Khot UM, Ellis SG: The role of percutaneous intervention prior to noncardiac surgery. Am Coll Cardiol Curr J Rev (Mar–Apr):57–60, 2001.
6. Posner KL, Van Norman GA, Chan V: Adverse cardiac outcomes after non cardiac surgery in patients with prior percutaneous transluminal coronary angioplasty. Anasthes Analg 89:553–560, 1999.

VI. Complex Coronary Intervention

30. CALCIFIED LESIONS AND OSTIAL LESIONS

Glenn Barquet, M.D., and Alexandre C. Ferreira, M.D.

CALCIFIED LESIONS

1. How reliable is angiography for assessing coronary calcification?

The severity of coronary calcification seen angiographically has been correlated to increasing circumferential arcs and total length of calcium as measured using intravascular ultrasound (IVUS). However, the sensitivity of angiography in detecting coronary calcium ranges between 25% and 85% and provides only moderate sensitivity for detecting even severe coronary calcification. Along with only moderate sensitivity, the specificity is limited, with an angiographic false-positive rate of 11%.

2. What are the acute results with percutaneous transluminal coronary angioplasty (PTCA) alone for treatment of calcified lesions?

Acute success rates with PTCA alone have been reported to be as high as 92%. When compared with noncalcified lesions, the acute success rate is 3% to 20% lower. The reported relative risk of in-hospital major adverse cardiac events (MACE) with PTCA of calcified lesions verses noncalcified lesions varies between 1.0 and 5.6 depending on the group studied.

3. How does the morphology of a calcified lesion adversely affect outcome with PTCA alone?

Suboptimal lumen enlargement is directly related to a balloon's inability to expand ("crack") a lesion as well as elastic recoil. Calcified lesions generally require higher inflation pressures to overcome lesion rigidity, thereby increasing the risk of dissection. Dissections usually begin at the transition between calcified and noncalcified atheroma and are caused by unequal distribution of shear forces during balloon expansion. The need for increased inflation pressures to expand calcified lesions also increases the risk of balloon rupture. Interestingly, most studies fail to show an increased rate of restenosis with PTCA of calcified lesions versus noncalcified lesions.

4. What non-balloon device has become the treatment of choice for calcified lesions, and why?

Rotational atherectomy (RA) has found its greatest application in the treatment of calcified stenoses with published procedural success rates in excess of 90% and complication rates less than 5%. Rotablator (Boston Scientific, Natick, MA) preferentially ablates calcified atheroma, leaving a more concentric lumen. RA of calcified lesions has been shown to yield fewer dissections than PTCA alone. This is because of RA's ability to produce microfractures in the calcified atheroma, thereby making the plaque more compliant during subsequent PTCA or stenting. A comparative trial of Rotablator plus PTCA versus Rotablator plus stent (Rotastent) demonstrated a smaller final diameter stenosis with Rotastent (23% smaller final diameter stenosis [DS]). PTCA after RA is best suited for the treatment of smaller caliber vessels. During Rotastent procedures it is essential to confirm lesion expansion with PTCA before stent implantation because incomplete stent expansion increases the risk of stent thrombosis and restenosis.

5. Are other forms of atherectomy recommended for the treatment of calcified lesions?

No. Directional coronary angioplasty (DCA) is not recommended. The initial DCA trials incorporated technologies that demonstrated a limited ability to debulk moderate to heavily calcified lesions. This was partly because of design limitations (i.e., cutter strength and window size). Advances in DCA design may show greater promise with flexible housing, larger window sizes, and stronger titanium cutters.

Transluminal extraction atherectomy (TEC) is also not recommended because of its limited ability to treat hard-calcified plaques. TEC does have the advantage of being smaller profile and more trackable than DCA and can traverse beyond proximal calcified segments in order to treat more distal noncalcified lesions.

6. Does the depth of calcium affect device selection for treatment of a lesion?

Yes. Superficial calcium at the intima–lumen interface has greater potential to impede efforts at primary angioplasty and stenting than does deep calcium at the media–adventitia border. Rotablator debulking is more ideally suited for superficial ± deep coronary calcification.

7. How does the length of a calcified lesion affect the results with RA?

Longer calcified lesions treated with RA result in greater downstream embolization of incompletely pulverized calcium. This has been shown to increase the "no-reflow" phenomenon and non–Q-wave myocardial infarction (MI). To combat this dilemma, interventions on lengthy calcified lesions should include use of smaller initial burr sizes with slow passes and stepwise increases in burr size to improve pulverization and final angiographic results.

OSTIAL LESIONS

8. Define the two major types of ostial lesions encountered in invasive cardiology.
- **Aorto-ostial:** Stenosis located at the aortic junction with either the left main (LM) coronary artery, right coronary artery (RCA), or saphenous vein graft
- **Branch ostial** ("origin lesion"): Stenosis located at the bifurcation of a major epicardial coronary artery with a branch vessel (e.g., LM–left anterior descending coronary artery, RCA-posterior descending artery [PDA])

Both ostial lesion types occur at the immediate origin of a major epicardial coronary artery. More liberal definitions include lesions that originate in the first 3 to 5 mm of a major epicardial coronary artery.

9. What lesion characteristics make ostial stenoses challenging to treat via percutaneous means?

Ostial lesions have increased rigidity, which counteracts attempts to expand ("crack") a lesion. In addition, elastic recoil is more pronounced at ostial lesions, partly accounting for increased restenosis rates. Aorto-ostial lesions present a unique challenge to angioplasty alone because plaque tends to displace into the aorta only to later shift back (similar to renal angioplasty). Ostial intervention trials have also demonstrated a higher incidence of coronary dissection versus non-ostial stenoses. Procedural challenges include difficulty achieving guiding catheter support, ostial guiding catheter-induced trauma, and greater need for high-pressure inflations. Therefore, treatment of ostial lesions requires meticulous emphasis on technique as well as appropriate application of available technologies to address both elastic recoil (stents) and altering the physics of plaque morphology (debulking).

10. Describe the role of angioplasty in the treatment of ostial lesions and its inherent limitations.

Procedural success rates with angioplasty for the treatment of ostial stenosis have improved over the past 2 decades. Clinical trials throughout the late 1980s reported success rates between 80% and 85%. More recent trials have demonstrated procedural success rates approaching 100%

depending on lesion location. However, angiographic restenosis rates have remained remarkably constant (between 40% and 50%). Elastic recoil is largely responsible for the loss of acute gains in luminal diameter. This has produced a shift in clinical practice away from PTCA alone toward incorporating debulking techniques and stenting of ostial lesions. PTCA has found its greatest application in conjunction with these interventional devices. The two most frequent roles of PTCA are predilation of ostial lesions in vessels smaller than 2.5 mm and postdilation to optimize final lumen diameter and stent apposition. During predilation, longer balloons or cutting balloons are preferred to avoid antegrade or retrograde displacement during balloon inflation ("watermelon seed" effect). Particular vigilance must be observed during balloon inflation of branch ostial lesions to avoid obstructing flow in nondiseased branch vessels.

11. Describe the technical features common to most percutaneous interventions performed on ostial lesions.

Beginning with guiding catheter selection, attention to anatomic takeoff of the LM or RCA is crucial in order to achieve coaxial alignment whenever possible. If dampening pressures are encountered with a standard guiding catheter, exchange for a catheter with sideholes should be performed. Guidewire selection is more individualized, with operator preference predominating. While advancing the chosen device for intervention, the guiding catheter should be positioned just outside the ostium of the LM or RCA. After the chosen device is properly positioned, the guiding catheter may be retracted slightly into the aorta. With PTCA, careful balloon positioning is crucial in order to avoid inflation within the guiding catheter that may lead to balloon rupture. Frequent small contrast dye injections and referencing anatomic landmarks are often necessary to achieve proper device position. IVUS has demonstrated clinical efficacy in defining normal vessel diameter, as well as extent and composition of ostial lesions.

12. Which atherectomy devices are most commonly used for debulking ostial lesions?

DCA is an effective means of debulking ostial, noncalcified, eccentric, and ulcerated lesions. It is most often recommended for larger vessels (> 2.5 mm) and has been shown to achieve procedural success rates between 70% and 97%. As opposed to PTCA, the proximal housing of the DCA may reside within the guiding catheter during debulking. Compared with PTCA alone, DCA portends an increased risk of non–Q-wave MI. DCA has been shown to lessen plaque shift and poststent neointimal hyperplasia, which some experts present in support of its use in the treatment of ostial lesions.

Clinical trial experience with RA has yielded success rates ranging between 91% and 98%. RA is particularly useful in the treatment of calcified lesions. Initial conservative burr sizing is recommended with a final burr-to-vessel ratio of less than 0.8, thereby reducing the risk of dissection. Slack in the guidewire should be avoided because it may lead to complications attributable to proximal guidewire kinking.

13. Describe the pertinent features of stent design, placement, and expected outcome for the treatment of ostial stenosis.

Stent specifications for the treatment of ostial stenoses should include the following characteristics: flexible, low profile, radiopaque, slotted, and tubular design. Balloon predilation is recommended to assess plaque stiffness with final high-pressure balloon inflations to ensure stent–vessel contact. Primary stenting is not recommended with ostial lesions. The proximal 1 mm of the stent should extend into the aorta to ensure coverage of the entire lesion. Flaring of the 1 mm extending into the aorta with a larger balloon may be performed to optimize results. Results form various clinical trials with ostial lesions revealed procedural success rates between 93% and 100%. Angiographic restenosis rates varied between 25% and 35%.

14. Is there a role for debulking before to stent implantation?

Yes. The use of combined modalities has proven to be highly effective in achieving larger acute gains in lumen size when stenting is used as the final common modality. Using a combined approach, the entirety of the plaque's physical properties is more fully addressed. Initial debulking optimizes stent deployment, reduces plaque shift, and increases minimum luminal diameter. Subsequent stenting counteracts both elastic recoil and negative remodeling while more fully expanding the vessel. However, stenting alone versus a combined approach yields a similar 1-year event-free survival and target vessel revascularization with a significantly longer total procedure time.

BIBLIOGRAPHY

1. Boehrer JD, Ellis SG, Pieper K, et al: Directional atherectomy versus balloon angioplasty for coronary ostial and non-ostial left anterior descending coronary artery lesions: results from a randomized multicenter trial. J Am Coll Cardiol 25:1380–1386, 1995.
2. Colombo A, Itoh A, Maiello L, et al: Coronary stent implantation in aorto-ostial lesions: immediate and follow-up results. J Am Coll Cardiol 27(Suppl A)::253, 1996.
3. Fitzgerald P, Ports T, et al: Contribution of localized calcium deposits to dissection after angioplasty: an observational study using IVUS. Circulation 86:64–70, 1992.
4. Fitgerald PJ, Stertzer SH, et al: Plaque characteristics affect lesion and vessel response to coronary rotational atherectomy: an intravascular ultrasound study. J Am Coll Cardiol (March; Suppl A):353, 1994.
5. Hoffman R, Mintz GS, et al: Comparative early and nine-month results of rotational atherectomy, stents, and combination of both for calcified lesions in large coronary arteries. Am J Cardiol 8:552–557, 1998.
6. Kurbaan AS, Kelly PA, Sigwart U: Cutting balloon angioplasty and stenting for aorto-ostial lesions. Heart 77:350–352, 1997.
7. Mintz GS, Pichard AD, et al: Determinants and correlates of target lesion calcium in coronary artery disease: A clinical, angiographic and intravascular ultrasound study. J Am Coll Cardiol 29:268–274, 1997.
8. Motwani JG, Raymond RE, Franco I, et al: Effectiveness of rotational atherectomy of right coronary artery ostial stenosis. Am J Cardiol 85:563–567, 2000.
9. Safian RD, Freed MS: The Manual of Interventional Cardiology, 3rd ed. Royal Oak, MI, Physicians Press, 2001.
10. Tan K, Sulke N, Taub N, et al: Percutaneous transluminal coronary angioplasty of aorta ostial, non-aorta ostial, and branch ostial stenoses. J Am Coll Cardiol (Suppl A):351, 1994.
11. Tan K, Sulke N, et al: Clinical and lesion morphologic determinants of coronary angioplasty success and complications: current experience. J Am Coll Cardiol 25:855–865, 1995.
12. Tuzcu EM, Berkalp B, et al: The dilemma of diagnosing coronary calcification: angiography versus intravascular ultrasound. J Am Coll Cardiol 27:823–838, 1996.
13. Zampieri PA, Colombo A, et al: Results of coronary stenting of ostial lesions. Am J Cariol 73:901–903, 1994.

31. BIFURCATION LESIONS AND TORTUOUS VESSELS

Glenn Barquet, M.D., and Eduardo deMarchena, M.D.

BIFURCATION LESIONS

1. What constitutes a true bifurcation lesion?

A true bifurcation lesion is one that compromises 50% or more of a parent vessel lumen and involves the ostium of a sidebranch. Bifurcation lesions account for 4% to 16% of all interventional procedures. The majority of these bifurcation lesions involve the left anterior descending (LAD) coronary artery–diagonal system. The increased shear stress at vascular bifurcations is considered to be an inciting factor for endothelial dysfunction and initiation of plaque formation.

2. Match the bifurcation lesions illustrated below with the appropriate classification type (types 1 to 4). Note that subclassifying the bifurcation lesion into class A or B merely denotes sidebranch involvement versus sidebranch sparing, respectively.

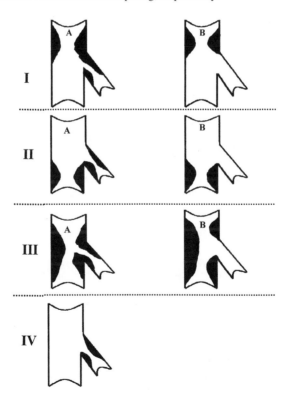

Answer

    I-   Type 2: Parent vessel stenosis proximal to bifurcation

    II-   Type 3: Parent vessel stenosis distal to bifurcation

    III- Type 1: Parent vessel stenosis proximal and distal to bifurcation

    IV- Type 4: Parent vessel normal with sidebranch stenosis (therefore, no subgrouping)

3. What should be the primary goal during an intervention on a bifurcation lesion?

Although bifurcation lesions obviously involve two vessels, both arteries are not, generally, created equally. The ultimate goal should be to assure procedural success within the parent vessel. Overemphasis on the final angiographic appearance of the sidebranch may be counterproductive and increase complications within the parent vessel. For example, successful treatment of the LAD in a patient with a LAD–diagonal bifurcation lesion leaves the patient with single vessel or branch vessel disease, which carries an acceptable prognosis. Conversely, attempts to perfect the final angiographic appearance of the diagonal could jeopardize the LAD and significantly worsen the patient's long-term prognosis.

4. What are the predictors of postintervention sidebranch narrowing and occlusion?

The risk of sidebranch narrowing and occlusion depends on the initial degree of sidebranch narrowing and the proximity of the sidebranch take-off to the parent vessel stenosis. In addition, patients with unstable angina have an increased risk of sidebranch occlusion during percutaneous coronary interventions (PCIs). Development of parent vessel dissection clearly increases the risk of sidebranch occlusion. The risk of jeopardizing sidebranch flow can be divided into low, moderate, and high risk depending on the lesion's morphology (see table below).

Risk of Sidebranch Occlusion and Bifurcation Anatomy

ANATOMY	RISK OF SIDEBRANCH OCCLUSION
Branch not involved by parent vessel lesion but in jeopardy because of transient occlusion during balloon inflation	Low ($< 1\%$)
Normal branch originating from diseased parent vessel	Moderate ($1–10\%$)
Ostium of branch vessel $> 50\%$ stenosis	High ($14–35\%$)

5. Which bifurcation lesions should be intervened upon using a strategy that incorporates sidebranch protection ("double wire")?

Large sidebranches (diameter > 2.0 mm) with or without ostial stenosis that originates from a diseased parent vessel (i.e., type 1A, 1B, 2A, and 3A) should be intervened upon using a guidewire in each vessel. The amount of myocardium served by the sidebranch should also be considered, as in the case of collateral flow to other vascular beds. Small sidebranches with a less than 50% ostial stenosis, serving a limited myocardial mass and distant from parent vessel lesions, do not require sidebranch protection.

6. What are the most commonly observed technical components of performing PCI for the treatment of a bifurcation lesion?

Beginning with guiding catheter selection, a single large (8Fr, if possible) guiding catheter is preferred to accomodate multiple balloons or stents and guidewires. Before large internal diameter guiding catheters, two guiding catheters were used, which increased the risk of ostial injury and requiring dual arterial punctures. A two- or three-way Touhy-Borst catheter is desirable to allow for multiple guidewires and devices. Both the parent and sidebranch guidewires should be advanced simultaneously to the tip of the guiding catheter in order to limit guidewire entanglement (i.e., wrapping around each other). The more difficult lesion should be crossed first (or the larger of the two vessels if both are of equal complexity). While advancing the guidewires, rotation should be limited to less than 180 degrees to limit guidewire entanglement. Initial undersizing of the balloon or stent using a distal disease-free vessel segment as a reference is preferable to oversizing, which engenders a greater risk of distal complications. If needed, further high-pressure inflations (particularly in the proximal segment) may be performed to attain balloon or stent to and artery ratio of 1.0 to 1.2:1.

7. Describe five ways that stents may be used for the treatment of a bifurcation lesion?

a. **Stenting** of main vessel with **side branch rescue** by balloon dilatation through the stent struts as needed

b. **T stent technique:** Initial placement of a stent in the sidebranch followed by a second stent in the parent vessel

c. **Reverse T stenting:** Initial placement of stent in the parent vessel, if sidebranch rescue becomes imperative, a second stent is deployed by crossing through the predilated struts of the parent vessel stent

d. **Kissing stents:** Simultaneous deployment of stents in the parent and sidebranch with side-to-side apposition of stents in the proximal parent vessel (note: This is the only technique that allows for continuous guidewire access to both vessels)

e. **Culotte stenting:** Initial parent vessel stenting followed by dilation of the struts at the sidebranch takeoff; deployment of a second stent within the sidebranch allowing the proximal segment of the stent to be deployed within the parent vessel stent (proximal stent sandwich)

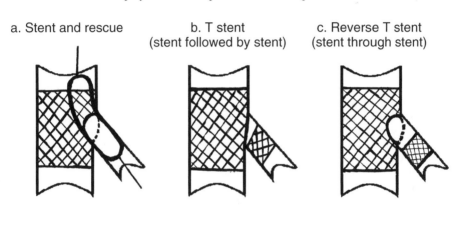

a. Stent and rescue   b. T stent   c. Reverse T stent
(stent followed by stent)   (stent through stent)

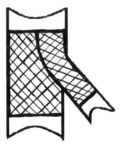 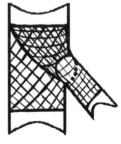

d. Kissing stents   e. Culotte technique

8. What mechanisms jeopardize sidebranch flow during PCI on bifurcation lesions?

a. **Dissection:** As with any coronary intervention, dissection may originate in either the parent vessel or sidebranch and jeopardize blood flow

b. **Plaque shift:** The lateral dislocation of plaque during dilatation therapy, which, if directed toward a sidebranch, may occlude the ostium

c. **Snow-plow injury:** A form of plaque shift that occurs at the carina of a bifurcation where plaque is dislocated from the parent vessel into the ostium of the sidebranch

d. **Spasm:** commonly encountered in both the parent and sidebranch with mixed response to intravenous nitroglycerin

e. **Thrombosis:** rare but potential complication, particularly with incomplete stent deployment

9. Can a stent be safely placed with struts covering the ostium of a sidebranch?

Yes. In experimental studies, the placement of a stent with struts crossing the ostium of a sidebranch has not been shown to significantly affect blood flow to the sidebranch. Parent vessel stenting with ostial sidebranch coverage is safest when the likelihood of sidebranch revascularization is low (see Question 4). Careful case selection is critical in the use of stents for bifurcation lesions because subsequent crossing with a guidewire through the ostial struts (e.g., sidebranch salvage) requires additional expertise.

10. What are the expected success and complication rates with the use of stents for the treatment of bifurcation lesions?

A large number of clinical trials have documented a procedural success rate of 90% to 100% with various stenting techniques for bifurcation lesions. In the STARS trial, a representative bifurcation stenting trial, the sidebranch occlusion rate was 5%. In general, clinical trials comparing differing stenting techniques have shown that the stent and retrieve approach imparts a lower risk of major adverse cardiac events compared with more complex stenting techniques. The longer-term clinical and angiographic results also support the use of a more conservative stent and retrieve approach.

11. How do other interventional techniques compare with stent implantation for the treatment of bifurcation lesions?

Percutaneous transluminal coronary angioplasty (PTCA): Initial procedural success is comparable with stenting in the parent vessel with higher rates of restenosis. The sidebranch procedural success rates are slightly lower because of complications, including\ snow-plow injury, dissection, spasm, and thrombosis. PTCA appears best suited for predilation of both lesions, sidebranch salvage, and final higher pressure dilations.

Rotational atherectomy (RA) is most commonly used to debulk bifurcation lesions before PTCA or stenting. As with all other techniques for bifurcation lesions, significant initial sidebranch stenosis ($> 50\%$) is a powerful predictor of sidebranch occlusion, with rates as high as 42%. If the branch origin is angulated, a smaller burr size is recommended to avoid complications. RA should be avoided if a stent has been deployed because the risk of burr entrapment. Although some centers use RA for the treatment of late ostial side branch stenosis ("stent-jail"), RA should usually be avoided to prevent potential burr entrapment.

Directional coronary atherectomy (DCA): Sidebranch occlusion rates up to 37% have been reported with DCA. These occlusions are generally amenable to salvage using PTCA yielding procedural success rates with DCA between 88% and 100% (comparable to stenting). The restenosis rates with DCA alone are lower than with PTCA but higher than with stenting. The use of nitinol guidewires is recommended for dual guidewire procedures because they are resistant to damage during DCA.

TORTUOUS VESSELS

12. How is coronary tortuosity defined and classified?

There are two major definitions of what constitutes a tortuous coronary artery:
  The presence of two or more bends 75 degrees or greater that are proximal to the target lesion
  At least one proximal bend 90 degrees or more
The degree of vessel tortuosity is classified according to the number of 45-degree bends:
  0: Nontortuous
  1: Mild tortuosity
  2: Moderate tortuosity
  3 or more: Severe tortuosity

13. What technical strategies facilitate procedural success during PCIs involving proximal vessel tortuousity?

Larger guiding catheters and achieving coaxial alignment are essential in order to maximize backup support. The use of smaller (e.g., 0.014 inch), more flexible guidewires is recommended to aid in traversing vessel tortuosity. In addition, hydrophilic wires with tapered cores help to reduce friction but must be used with caution to avoid coronary dissections. For added support, transit catheters or the balloon itself may be used for additional support while traversing tortuous vessels. The guidewire should be advanced and parked as distal as possible to facilitate balloon or stent tracking over the guidewire. Deep inspiration by the patient occasionally helps to elongate the coronaries and diminish tortuosity that may aid in advancing guidewires, balloons, and stents. If over-the-wire or monorail balloon systems fail, a fixed wire–balloon system may be used.

14. How has balloon technology evolved to address lesion tortuosity?

The initial experience with angioplasty of tortuous coronary lesions yielded success rates ranging from 70% to 85%. Improved balloon technology, including improved flexibility, trackability, pushability, and lower profile, has led to procedural success rates in excess of 90%. In general, monorail systems have lower profile, and over-the-wire systems are more trackable and pushable.

15. Which devices are best suited for percutaneous revascularization of highly angulated lesions?

PTCA is a widely used for the treatment of angulated lesions. The procedural success rates range between 85% and 95% with a less than 3% complication rate. The most commonly encountered complications are dissection and abrupt closure. Stents are increasingly used because newer stent designs have allowed for high radial strength with preserved undeployed flexibility. Stent profile has also improved, allowing for navigation across most degrees of proximal vessel tortuosity and lesion angulations. Occasionally, a balloon alone is preferred for highly angulated lesions; retrospective trials have shown that overstraightening of vessel tortuosity caused by stent implantation is a predictor of major adverse cardiac events.

16. What factors account for a greater rate of dissection with balloon angioplasty of angulated lesions? Which balloon design features improve initial outcome?

PTCA of angulated lesions results in two counterproductive forces within the neighboring vessel wall. The first, "straightening forces," may cause stretch of the vessel, particularly at the inner curve, yielding higher rates of dissection. Second, the non-uniform distribution of forces ("dog bone effect") increases the risk of dissection at the proximal and distal ends of the balloon. Although clinical trials have shown inconsistent results, noncompliant balloons are frequently used for angulated lesions to better balance the distribution of forces. Likewise, longer balloons are preferred for angulated lesions because forces are more evenly distributed along lengthier balloons.

17. Are non-balloon and non-stent devices recommended for the treatment of angulated lesions?

No. Debulking instruments including atherectomy and laser devices should generally be avoided for highly angulated lesions. The exception is mild lesion angulation of less than 45 degrees in which atherectomy clinical trials have demonstrated procedural success rates of greater than 90% and complication rates of less than 3% for both rotoblator and DCA. Greater degrees of angulation are associated with increased procedural failure, major ischemic events, dissection, perforation, and mortality. Similar caution-provoking results have been demonstrated with TEC and ELCA.

BIBLIOGRAPHY

1. Abhyankar, AD, Luyue G, Bailey BP: Stent implantation in severely angulated lesions. Cathet Cardiovasc Diagn 40:261–264, 1997.
2. Baim DS, Grossman W: Cardiac Catheterization, Angiography, and Intervention, 6th ed. Philadelphia, Lippincott Williams & Wilkins, 2000.
3. Chevalier B, Commeau P, Favereau X, et al: Limitations of rotational atherectomy in angulated coronary lesions. J Am Coll Cardiol 23:(Suppl A)285, 1994.

4. Ellis SG, De Cesare NB, Pinkerton CA, et al: Relation of stenosis morphology and clinical presentation to the procedural results of directional coronary atherectomy. Circulation 84:644–653, 1991.
5. Gossman DE, Tuzcu EM, Simpfendorfer C, et al: Percutaneous transluminal angioplasty for shepherd's crook right coronary artery stenosis. Cathet Cardiovac Diagn 15:189–191, 1989.
6. Gyöngyösi, M, Yang P, Khorsand A, et al: Longitudinal straightening effect of stents is an additional predictor for major adverse cardiac events. J Am Coll Cardiol 35:1580–1589, 2000.
7. Gray WA, Ghazzai ZMB, White HJ: The effects of balloon length and angle severity on the straightening force developed by polyethylene terephthalate (PET) angioplasty balloons. Circulation 90:I–587, 1994.
8. Iniquez A, Macaya C, et al: Early angiographic changes of side branches arising from a Palmaz-Schatz stented coronary segment: Results and clinical implications. J Am Coll Cardiol 23:911–915, 1994.
9. Leon MB, Baim DS, et al: A clinical trial comparing three antithrombotic-drug regimens after coronary artery stenting. N Engl J Med 339:1665, 1998.
10. Lewis B, Leya F, et al: Acute procedural results in the treatment of 30 coronary artery bifurcation lesions with a double-wire atherectomy technique for side-branch protection. Am Heart J 127:1600–1607, 1994.
11. Lewis B, Leya F, et al: Outcome of angioplasty (PTCA) and atherectomy (DCA) for bifurcation and non-bifurcation lesions in CAVEAT. Circulation 88:I–601, 1993.
12. Meier B, Gruentzig AR, et al: Risk of side branch occlusion during coronary angioplasty. Am J Cardiol 53:10–14, 1984.
13. Safian RD, Freed MS: The Manual of Interventional Cardiology, 3rd ed. Royal Oak, MI, Physicians Press, 2001.
14. Tan K, Sulke N, Taub N, et al: Clinical and lesion morphologic determinants of coronary agioplasty success and complications: current experience. J Am Coll Cardiol 25:855–865, 1995.
15. Walton AS, Pomerantsev EV, et al: Outcome of narrowing related side branches after high-speed rotational atherectomy. Am J Cardiol 77:370–373, 1996.

32. CHRONIC TOTAL OCCLUSIONS

Alan Schob, M.D., and Eric Auerbach, M.D.

1. Should attempts be made attempt to open a chronically totally occluded coronary artery? Isn't that an indication for coronary artery bypass grafting (CABG)?

In the acute setting, when thrombus is fresh, it is soft and generally easy to cross with a guidewire. With time and fibrointimal proliferation, it becomes increasingly difficult to cross a region of an artery that is totally occluded. And even if the lesion is crossed with a guidewire, passage of a balloon through the occlusion and complete balloon inflation may prove impossible. Because of these technical difficulties, chronic occlusion is often cited as a reason not to attempt angioplasty. Indeed, chronic total occlusion is a frequent cause of referral for bypass surgery.

Chronically occluded arteries, however, are commonly identified at angiography, found in 20% to 38% of patients with coronary artery disease (CAD). They are a common cause of angina and left ventricular (LV) dysfunction, both of which may be reversible with percutaneous transluminal coronary angioplasty (PTCA). Although technically difficult to open, they are in some respects safer targets for angioplasty than subtotal occlusions. Moreover, quoted success rates in appropriately selected vessels have been close to 70% in most series. Therefore, attempting angioplasty in the setting of chronic total occlusion is not unreasonable. In fact, these lesions account for at least 10% of angioplasty targets currently, a figure subject to increase with improvements in tools and techniques.

2. What is the natural history of disease progression in patients with a chronic total occlusion? Can this natural history be affected by angioplasty?

Mortality in patients with total occlusion of the left anterior descending (LAD) coronary artery is 10% annually. Mortality in patients with total occlusion of an artery other than the LAD is 4% annually. Such high mortality rates might seem counterintuitive in the setting of a chronic, stable coronary condition. However, adverse events in this patient population occur not from progression of the chronic occlusion but from new obstructions elsewhere in the coronary arteries. Patients with total occlusion of one vessel have a limited ability to withstand new events, because of preexisting LV dysfunction as well as myocardial perfusion that may already rely heavily on collateral circulation. Thus, although restoration of flow in a chronically occluded segment is unlikely to have a dramatic direct impact on the myocardium immediately downstream of the occlusion, it may markedly improve patients' ability to survive future events. Indeed, studies indicate that successfully opening an occluded LAD cuts future event rates in half.

3. What is the rationale for attempting angioplasty in a chronically occluded vessel?

There are six commonly cited justifications for attempting angioplasty to a totally occluded coronary artery:

- For treatment of angina or other symptoms of coronary insufficiency
- In response to abnormal findings on stress testing based on the notion that an improvement in stress test results would be associated with improved prognosis
- To prevent the need for CABG
- To decrease LV remodeling
- To improve LV function
- To improve survival

4. What is "stunned" or "hibernating" myocardium? What benefit can be expected from angioplasty in this setting?

Hibernating myocardium is myocardial tissue that exhibits impaired or absent contractility caused by reduced coronary blood flow and that can be restored to a normal contractile state with the restoration of adequate coronary perfusion. *Myocardial stunning* is transient myocardial dysfunction induced by ischemia. In either state, the dysfunctional myocardium is viable, metaboli-cally active tissue that can be distinguished from infarcted scar tissue by several modalities, in-cluding positron emission tomography scanning, nuclear imaging, and low-dose dobutamine echocardiography. Although chronic coronary occlusion is typically associated with LV dys-function, the demonstration of viable myocardium in the distribution of the occluded vessel is an indication for angioplasty because revascularization in this setting would be expected to restore contractility and improve overall LV function. In fact, angioplasty of chronically occluded coro-nary arteries has been associated not only with improvement in LV ejection fraction (LVEF) but also with prevention of LV remodeling.

5. What is the pathophysiology of a chronically occluded coronary artery, and how does it impact the technical success of angioplasty in this setting?

The two main components of a coronary artery occlusion are atherosclerotic plaque and thrombus. In the chronic setting, the thrombus is likely to be fibrotic because of fibrointimal pro-liferation. However, thrombus may not be uniform in its age and hardness. Rather, multiple lay-ers of thrombus may be present, representing multiple episodes of plaque rupture and thrombus formation leading to partial vessel closure or leading to total occlusion followed by recanaliza-tion. In these cases, older and more fibrosed clot is more difficult to cross and technical success is determined by the ability of the operator to cross the most recent thrombus present.

6. What factors predict technical success in opening a chronic total occlusion?

Factors Negatively Associated with Success in Opening a Chronic Occlusion

1. Duration of occlusion
2. Length of occlusion
3. Absence of a stump or tapered segment for entry
4. Presence of homocollaterals to the distal vessel
5. Occlusion of a bypass graft

The success rate of PTCA declines rapidly during the first 4 weeks after total occlusion. The length of the occluded segment is also a very important factor because it may be impossible to cross a long segment that is totally occluded. Angiographically, a straight segment of a large ves-sel makes a more ideal target for PTCA, and the absence of a stump or other identifying feature of the total occlusion essentially precludes the attempt. Attempts to open chronically occluded vein grafts rarely meet with lasting success, but arterial grafts make better targets.

7. Is it possible to distinguish a chronically occluded artery that has recanalized from an artery with a subtotal stenosis? Does it matter?

There are several mechanisms by which spontaneous recanalization may occur in a totally occluded artery. Early on, spontaneous lysis of clot may result in reperfusion. Later, new chan-nels may form within mature thrombus, resulting in so-called intra-arterial arteries. Finally, dila-tion of the vasa vasorum may allow for reperfusion. A combination of these mechanisms is also possible. Angiographically, the recanalized vessel exhibits antegrade flow, with retrograde filling of the vessel distal to the diseased portion via collaterals. This appearance may be indistinguish-able from that of a subtotal stenosis with development of collaterals. Whereas a subtotal stenosis is generally easily amenable to passage with a guidewire, however, it may be difficult or impos-sible to cross a recanalized vessel, particularly if the antegrade flow seen angiographically is caused by an engorged vasa vasorum or by small passages through a thrombosed segment.

8. Should the presence of collaterals influence the decision to attempt angioplasty? Do col-laterals have implications regarding angioplasty technique?

The presence of collaterals indicates chronicity of a lesion but does not preclude the need for revascularization. In fact, a well-collateralized total occlusion is functionally equivalent to a 90%

stenosis. After a successful PTCA, collaterals instantly and completely disappear. The presence of the collateral network, however, provides a margin of safety, in that collaterals are immediately re-recruited in the setting of restenosis, even years after PTCA.

9. What complications may be expected when attempting angioplasty in the setting of total occlusion?

Complications of angioplasty to totally occluded vessels are similar to those experienced in angioplasty of vessels that are not totally occluded. A more aggressive technique may be necessary to cross a total occlusion; therefore, an increased risk of dissection or perforation would seem likely. However, this risk is offset by the fact that the instrumented vessel is already occluded, as well as by the existence of collateral flow. Overall, the risk of angioplasty in a totally occluded vessel is not significantly different than that in a non-occluded vessel.

10. What special techniques and equipment may be used to improve success in crossing a chronic total occlusion?

In general, use of a stiffer guidewire may enable operators to cross an occlusion that they have failed to cross with a more floppy guidewire. Some wires, such as the Magnum wire and the Athlete wires, have been specifically designed for crossing chronic occlusions. Both of these stiff guidewires have been shown to be of some benefit for crossing occluded vessels in published trials. An alternative approach to increasing stiffness is to advance the balloon catheter close to the tip of whichever guidewire is being used. Finally, it should be noted that some operators prefer a hydrophilic wire (i.e., a coronary Glidewire) when difficulty in crossing an occlusion is encountered.

11. Does stenting TCOs effect outcome?

Multiple moderate-sized, randomized trials have reported improved outcomes with stenting compared with PTCA alone. Minimal lumen diameters (MLDs), restenosis rates, and clinical events were all impacted favorably by the use of stents. This was seen with a variety of stents in the various studies. Part of the beneficial effects of stenting may be caused by the use of larger balloons for stent deployment resulting in higher MLDs. One study found that restenosis when it occurs within a stent tends to be diffuse compared with a more focal lesion in PTCA. The authors conclude that short stents should be used whenever possible.

12. Does debulking improve outcome in total occlusions?

No randomized trials have examined debulking techniques before stent placement for TCOs. However, been numerous reports have used rotational atherectomy (RA), directional atherectomy and laser debulking before stent placement with good short- and long-term results. Whether these techniques are preferable to PTCA is not known. Particularly bulky lesions or heavily calcified lesions (for which RA should be considered) may be suitable candidates for debulking before stent placement.

13. Is restenosis a problem after angioplasty of a totally occluded vessel?

Studies indicate that restenosis occurs in approximately 50% to 60% of angioplasties performed in totally occluded vessels, representing a restenosis rate more than twice that generally found in angioplasty overall. One explanation for this finding may be the high distal coronary pressure that is generated by collateral vessels in the setting of a chronic occlusion. Restenosis, however, need not result in total reocclusion, making a successive angioplasty attempt not only technically easier but also safer given the presence of the collateral network.

14. What factors predict restenosis after successful stenting of a chronic total occlusion?

Sallam, et al, angiographically restudied 56% of 665 patients within 6 months of stent placement for TCO. Restenosis ($\geq$ 50% lumen narrowing) was seen in 37%. 10.6% had complete reocclusion. Univariate analysis showed restenotic lesions, final MLD, number of stents per lesion, and total stent length predicted recurrent complete occlusion. Total stent length was the only multivariate independent predictor of reocclusion (OR = 1.46; 95% confidence interval = 1.12–1.82; $P = 0.0069$).

15. What new technologies are on the horizon for dealing with the challenge of chronically occluded coronary arteries?

Laser energy can be used to debulk tissue with low heat dissipation and has been commercialized in the Prima Total Occlusion System (Spectranetics, Colorado Springs, CO), a steerable guidewire containing a pulsed excimer laser. In published trials, crossing with a laser guidewire was successful in 58% of cases in which prior attempts with conventional guidewires had failed. However, this procedural success was associated with a 21% perforation rate, limiting enthusiasm for this modality.

A more recent technology that has shown promise in treating total occlusions is the use of a fiberoptic guidance system (Safe-Steer TO Crossing System, Intraluminal Therapeutics, Carlsbad, CA), which uses optical coherence reflectometry to distinguish between atherosclerotic plaque and the arterial wall. With this system, the operator is literally provided with a green light signal to advance the guidewire through plaque, and a red light signal when encountering normal arterial tissue. In a small published trial, the system has resulted in a procedural success rate of 86% in treatment of chronic total coronary occlusion.

Finally, the Frontrunner CTO Catheter (LuMend, Inc., Redwood City, CA) is designed for blunt microdissection through atheroma within a coronary artery. The Frontrunner is an intracoronary catheter that be steered and rotated by the operator, with a distal tip that consists of blunt jaws that the operator can open 3 to 4 mm in order to dissect out a passage though the occluded vessel. After such dissection, the Frontrunner catheter is removed and a standard guidewire can be used to cross the lesion. In a prospective, controlled trial of 107 patients with chronic total occlusions that could not be crossed by standard technique, use of the Frontrunner was associated with subsequent success in crossing with a guidewire in 56%, with two associated mild perforations and no cases of hemopericardium or tamponade (unpublished data, courtesy of LuMend, Inc.).

BIBLIOGRAPHY

1. Danchin N, Angioi M, Cador R, et al: Effect of late percutaneous angioplastic recanalization of total coronary artery occlusion on left ventricular remodeling, ejection fraction, and regional wall motion. Am J Cardiol 78:729–735, 1996.
2. Delacretaz, E, Meier, B. Therapeutic strategy with total coronary artery occlusions. am J Cardiol 79: 185–187, 1997.
3. Gruberg, L. Mehran, R. Dangas, G. et al. Effect of plaque debulking and stenting on short- and long—term outcomes after revascularization of chronic total occlusions. J Am Coll Cardiol 35:151–156, 2000.
4. Lotan, C. Rozenman, Y. Hendler, A. et al: Stents in total occlusion for restenosis prevention the multicentre randomized STOP study: the Israeli Working Group for Interventional Cardiology. Eur Heart J 21:1960–1966, 2000.
5. Meier B: Chronic total occlusion. In Topol EJ (ed), Textbook of Interventional Cardiology, 3rd ed. Philadelphia, W.B. Saunders Company, 1999, pp 280–296.
6. Morales PA, Heuser RR: Chronic total occlusions: experience with fiber-optic guidance technology—optical coherence reflectometry. J Intervent Cardiol 14:611–616, 2001.
7. Puma JA, Sketch MH, Tcheng JE, et al: Percutaneous revascularization of chronic coronary occlusions: an overview. J Am Coll Cardiol 26:1–11, 1995.
8. Sallam M, Spanow V, Briguori C, et al: Predictors of re-occlusion after successful recanalization of chronic total occlusion. J Invas Cardiol 13:511–515, 2001.
9. Serruys PW: Total occlusion trial with angioplasty by using laser guidewire (The TOTAL Trial). Eur Heart J 21:1797–1805, 2000.
10. Sievert H, Rohde S, Utech A, et al: Stent or angioplasty after recanalization of chronic coronary occlusin? (The SARECCO Trial). Am J Cardiol 84:386–390, 1999.

33. LONG LESIONS AND SMALL CORONARY ARTERY INTERVENTIONS

Mustafa Ridha, M.D., and Eduardo de Marchena, M.D.

1. What is the relationship between lesion length and translesional flow?

Flow varies inversely as a function of lesion length. This is governed by the **Poiseuille's law**:

$$Flow = \frac{\pi(\Delta P)(r^4)}{8(\eta)X\ (L)}$$

ΔP = Pressure difference across the lesion
r = The minimal lumen radius of the stenotic segment
η = Blood viscosity
L = Length of the lesion

It is necessary to realize that the flow across a lesion varies as a fourth power of the radius but as a first power of the lesion length. It is expected that the lesion length exerts little relative impact for discrete ($<$ 5 mm) lesions. However, as the length of the stenotic lesion increases (e.g., from 5 to 25 mm), a fivefold decrease in blood flow across the lesion could be expected.

2. What is the relationship between lesion length and procedural success and complications?

Lesion length is a powerful predictor of procedural success and complications.

The predicted success rates for Percutaneous transluminal coronary angioplasty (PTCA) for different lengths of lesions are:

$<$ 10 mm: 95%
10–20 mm: 85%
$>$ 20 mm: 78%

The rate of abrupt closure also increases significantly as the lesion length icreases.

3. What is the mechanism behind the association of lesion length and complications of long lesion interventions?

- Longer lesions are usually associated with other adverse morphologic features
- Longer lesions are usually less uniform in term of plaque composition, which results in uneven shear stress during angioplasty and, therefore, with a higher possibility of dissections.

4. How does the lesion length influence the restenosis rate after successful PTCA?

The lesion length was identified as an independent predictor of restenosis rate. For lesions smaller than 5 mm in length, the restenosis rate is less than 33%. For lesions larger than 7 mm, the rate is greater than 48% in some reports.

5. Do longer lesions respond more favorably to longer balloons?

Long lesion angioplasty safety and efficacy are enhanced by the use of longer balloons. This is true by several means:

a. Balloons that cover the entire length of the lesion may distribute pressure more evenly during dilation.

b. Balloons that cover the entire length of a stenotic lesion as well as normal proximal and distal vessel segment may produce less shear stress at the transition points between the diseased and normal vessel, thus reducing the chances of dissection.

c. Long lesions often involve angulated segments that are thought to respond more favorably to the use of longer balloons.

6. How often do coronary arteries taper or change caliber along the length of a treated lesion?

The following are the frequency and pattern of tapering of coronary arteries:

- 50% maintain a uniform or nearly uniform
- Diameter(< 0.5 mm taper)
- 19% show significant taper (0.5–1.0 mm)
- 23% shows marked taper (> 1 mm taper)
- 8% shows reverse taper (proximal segment is smaller than the distal)

7. What effect does the use of decremental balloons (i.e., tapered balloons) have on longer lesions?

Tapered balloons have been shown in some small trials to offer optimal dilation in tapered arterial segments with a low complication rate (2.1% significant dissection) and a high success rate.

8. Compared with balloon angioplasty, how do excimer laser coronary angioplasty (ELCA) and rotational atherectomy (RA) influence early and late outcomes after angioplasty of long lesions?

The ERBAC trial randomized patients with long lesions to treatment with either balloon PTCA, ELCA, or DA. RA was associated with a higher procedural success rate compared with balloon angioplasty and ELCA (89%, 79%, and 77%, respectively). However, the 6-month target vessel revascularization rate was significantly higher with RA and the ELCA group compared with the balloon angioplasty (42%, 46%, and 32%, respectively).

Despite the above, RA continues to play a role in the initial treatment of complex lesion types that respond poorly to balloon dilation, especially calcified long lesions. The restenosis appears to be decreased when the treated segment is covered with a stent after rotoablation, the so-called roto-stent strategy.

9. Does the length of the stented segment influence procedural success, complications, and restenosis rates?

Yes. As the stented segment length increases, the success rate decreases, acute thrombosis increases, and restenosis rate increases.

In a study by Kobayashi et al., in which three groups of patients were studied:

GROUP	STENT LENGTH	PROCEDURAL SUCCESS, %	ACUTE THROMBOSIS, %	RESTENOSIS RATE, %
I	15±3 mm	96	0.2	34±26
II	30±3 mm	98	0	39±26
III	52±16 mm	92	1.2	52±29

10. What is the benefit of additional stent implementation after achieving an optimal result with balloon angioplasty in long lesions (> 20 mm)?

Additional stenting after optimal balloon angioplasty improves early minimal lumen diameter (MLD) and lowers the angiographic restenosis rate. However, the late major adverse cardiac event MACE–free survival does not appear to improve after additional stenting. The bailout stenting strategy, on the other hand, is associated with an increased periprocedural increase in cardiac injury markers.

11. Does intravascular ultrasound (IVUS)–guided stenting of long coronary lesions influence the restenosis rate and long-term MACE?

It appears to. In a study by Colombo et al, IVUS-guided *spot stenting* of predilated long lesions was associated with good acute outcome. In this strategy, stenting is only used after balloon dilatation if a less than an optimal outcome is demonstrated with IVUS. Then only the region of the treated lesion that is identified as being less that optimal is stented using the shortest possible stent to cover this segment. The angiographic restenosis rate using this strategy was 25% for the IVUS-guided group compared with 39% for the traditional stenting group. Moreover, the MACE and target vessel revascularization (TVR) was 22% versus 38% and 19% versus 34%, respectively.

12. What percent of PCIs are performed on vessels smaller than 3.0 mm?

Nearly 50% of all interventions reported in registries report a reference vessel size that's smaller than 3.0 mm.

13. Is PTCA restenosis affected by vessel size?

Yes. There is an inverse relationship between the size of a vessel and the incidence of restenosis. The smaller the vessel, the greater the restenosis.

14. Is it worthwhile to stent small vessels?

Early retrospective analysis of the STRESS I and II trials suggested a continued restenosis benefit for small vessel stenting. Because of this observation, multiple trials have been performed in the past 5 years attempting to prove this finding. Additionally, there has been much interest in developing a stent with design characteristic that would make it perform optimally as a small vessel stent. As a whole, most trials have shown either a statistically significant or a trend to reduction of restenosis and target lesion revascularization in vessels from 2.0 to 3.0 mm. An analysis done by Kastrati suggested that stenting a small vessel only reduced restenosis in procedures in which PTCA alone had been less than optimal. In patients with a post-PTCA residual stenosis of 30%, the addition of a stent reduced restenosis by nearly 30%. However, in patients with post-PTCA residual stenosis of less than 20%, there did not appear to beany significant reduction of restenosis with stenting. To date, there has not been any stent-on-stent trials to prove conclusively whether one stent design is superior to another.

BIBLIOGRAPHY

1. Banka VS, Baker HA III, Vemuri DN, et al: Effectiveness of decremental diameter balloon catheters (tapered balloon). Am J Cardiol 69:188–193, 1992.
2. Berne R, Levy M: Cardiovascular Physiology. St. Louis, Mosby, 1986, pp 109–115.
3. Colombo A, De Gregorio J, Moussa I, et al: Intravascular ultrasound-guided percutaneous transluminal coronary angioplasty with provisional spot stenting for treatment of long cronary lesions. J Am Coll Cardiol 38:1427–1433, 2001.
4. Hirshfeld JW, Schwartz S, Jugo R, Macdonald RG, et al. and the M-HEART Investigators: Restenosis after coronary angioplasty: a multivariate statistical nodel to relate lesion and procedure variables to restenosis. J Am Coll Cardiol 18:647–656, 1991.
5. Kastrati A: Stenting for small coronary vessels: a contestable winner. J Am Coll Cardiol 3815: 1604–1607, 2001.
6. Kobayashi Y, De Gregorio J, Kobayashi N, Akiyama T, et al: Stented segment length as an independent predictor of restenosis. J Am Coll Cardiol 34:651–659 199.
7. Reifart N, Vandormael M, Krajcar M, et al: Randomized comparison of angioplasty of complex coronary lesions at a single center: Excimer Laser, Rotational Atherectomy, and Balloon Angioplasty Comparison (ERBAC) study. Circulation 96:91–98, 1997.
8. Savage MP, Fischman DL, Rake R, et al: Efficacy of coronary stenting versus balloon angioplasty in small coronary arteries: Stent Restenosis Study (STRESS) investigators. J Am Coll Cardiol 31:307–311, 1998.
9. Serruys PW, Foley DP, Suttorp MJ, et al: A randomized comparison of the value of additional stenting after optimal balloon angioplasty for long coronary lesions: final results of the Additional Value of NIR Stents for Treatment of Long Coronary Lesions (ADVANCE) study. J Am Coll Cardiol 39: 393–399, 2002.
10. Sharma SK, Israel DH, Kamean JL, et al: Clinical, angiographic, and procedural determinants of major and minor coronary dissection during angioplasty. Am Heart J 126:39–47, 1993.
11. Tan K, Sulke N, Taub N, Sowton E: Clinical and lesion morphologic determinants of coronary angioplasty success and complications: current experience. J Am Coll Cardiol 25:855–865, 1995.
12. Tenaglia AN, Zider JP, Jackman JD, et al: Treatment of long coronary artery narrowings with long angioplasty balloon catheters. Am J Cardiol 71:1274–1277, 1993.

34. SAPHENOUS VEIN GRAFT INTERVENTION

Javier Jimenez, M.D.

1. What is the short- and long-term vein graft patency rate after coronary artery bypass graft (CABG)?

Early graft failure within 1 week after CABG is between 7% and 10%. During the first year, 15% to 20% of vein grafts fail, and more than 50% fail after 10 years. Multiple reasons, such as surgical technique, poor distal run off, and traditional risk factors for atherosclerosis such as tobacco use and hyperlipidemia may be involved in vein graft failure.

2. What is the most common presentation of vein graft failure after CABG?

In most instances, when graft failure occurs, the patient remains asymptomatic. This is a result of the presence of antegrade flow through native vessels or is caused by recruitment of collaterals supplying the area in jeopardy. Acute early ischemia after CABG may occur because of acute graft thrombosis in 3% to 5% of patients. Subacute ischemia within the first year is commonly related to stenotic lesions at the level of the anastomosis and rarely present as acute myocardial infarction (MI). Ischemia after the first year is more commonly associated with degenerated vein grafts filled with friable atherosclerotic material. Late graft failure can present as acute or subacute ischemia.

3. List the most important prognostic factors for development of vein graft atheroslcerosis.

The most important factors involved in the development of graft atherosclerosis are history MI (OR 1.47; 95% confidence interval [CI] 1.17–1.85), continuing tobacco use (OR 1.47; 95% CI 1.04–2.08), years since CABG (OR 1.18; 95% CI 1.04–1.06), trygliceride elevation (OR 1; CI 1.00–1.00), and mean arterial pressure increase (OR 1.01; CI 1.00–1.02).

4. What is the best approach for the management of patients with acute MI after CABG?

Few data are available on reperfusion therapies after CABG. Although a bypass graft, compared with a native vessel is more likely to be the culprit lesion; patients presenting with graft occlusion are less likely to have ST segment elevation, cardiac enzyme release, or symptoms. Neither thrombolytic therapy nor percutaneous revascularization in post-CABG patients with acute MI has been established as the treatment of choice. Registry data show similar efficacy of PCI versus thrombolyisis; however, early reperfusion results may favor a mechanical approach.

5. Does stenting improve clinical outcome over balloon angioplasty?

Extended use of balloon angioplasty in vein graft occurred in the 1980s after the early experience in the native coronary arteries. Procedural success was reported between 85% and 97%; however, restenosis occurred in up to 60% of cases. Stents were later found to decrease restenosis in native coronary arteries. Since then, stent use has been applied to vein graft intervenion. The SAVED trial (Stent placement Vs. balloon angioplasty for obstructed coronary arteries) revealed that compared with balloon angioplasty, stenting saphenous vein grafts (SVGs) had higher procedural success rates (92% vs. 69%; $P < 0.0001$) and higher freedom form death, MI, repeat CABG, or revascularization (73% vs. 58%; $P = 0.03$) but without significant benefit in restenosis (37% vs. 40%; $P = 0.24$).

6. Describe the results of using glycoprotein (GP) IIb/IIIa inhibitors as adjuvant medical therapy in SVG intervention.

Use of abximicab as adjuvant therapy during percutaneous coronary intervention (PCI) has been shown beneficial in multiple lesion subsets (osteal, calcified, long lesions, and others). However, data on the benefit of abximicab during SVG intervention are limited. Several studies have shown no benefit and possibly a deleterious effect of the use of GpIIbIIIa inhibitors in vein graft

PCI. This result may be due to a greater tendency of embolization in the degenerated, largely thrombotic veing grafts.

7. Is there any advantage of directional atherectomy (DA) over PTCA in vein graft intervention?

Initial results using directional atherectomy were encouraging; however, the CAVEAT II trial, in which DA and PTCA in SVGs were randomized, revealed that DA was associated with higher incidence of complications and no benefits in restenosis (45% DA vs. 50% PTCA; $P = 0.49$). Some authors, however, recommend using DA in combination with stents for aorto-ostial SVG lesions.

8. List the preferred indications for the use of rheolytic thrombectomy during SVG percutaneous revascularization.

Rheolytic thrombectomy is based on the Bernoulli principle, allowing thrombus extraction from degenerated SVGs. Lesions with large, visible, degenerated thrombus located within the proximal two thirds of the vein graft provide the best indications for this device. The VEGAS-2 trial comparing intracoronary urokinase and the Angiojet device showed some benefit from rheolytic thrombectomy but failed to show improvement in distal embolization or no-reflow phenomenon.

9. How common is distal embolization and no reflow during vein graft PCI?

Distal embolization occurs as atherosclerotic or thrombotic material becomes displaces and obstructs distal vessels. This complication, which is less common in native vessels, occurs in up to 15% of SVGs during PCI. No reflow is an angiographic phenomenon in which a column of contrast dye appears static or sluggish during the emptying phase. Microembolization and humoral activation have been attributed to this phenomenon. The incidence of the no-reflow phenomenon parallels that of macroembolization and cannot always be predicted.

10. Describe the use of distal protection devices in SVG interventions.

Distal protection devices can be classified as balloon occluders or as filter devices. The purpose of balloon occluders is to temporarily occlude the vessel during balloon dilatation and stent

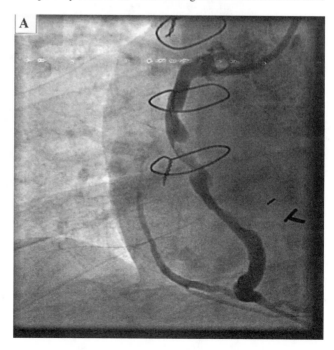

FIGURE 1. PCI of degenerated SVG using GuardWire (temporary occlusion and aspiration system). *A,* Degenerated SVG. (*continued*)

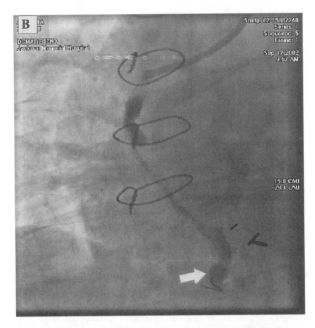

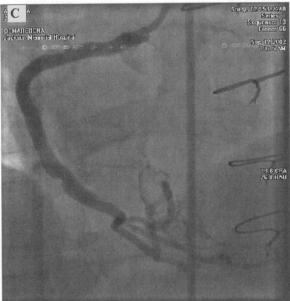

FIGURE 1. (*continued*) *B,* Stent placement after inflation of distal protection ballon (*arrow*). *C,* Final result after deployment of stent, aspiration, and deflation of distal protection ballon.

deployment with aspiration of debris before resumption of blood flow. Filter devices allow filtration of small particles likely to cause embolization but with preservation of flow during the revascularization procedure. The SAFER trial was the first device trial to demonstrate the benefit of balloon occluder in SVG intervention. In this trial using the PercuSurge GuardWire device, there was a 50% in-hospital and 30-day reduction of death, MI, and repeat CABG.

11. Describe the therapeutic alternatives in the management of a thrombosed SVG.

Several methods have been used to diminish or abolish thrombus formation within degenerated SVGs. Use of intragraft urokinase has been described as adjunct to balloon angioplasty in thrombotic lesions; however, urokinase has been withdrawn from the United States market. More recently, intracoronary tissue plasminogen activator (t-PA) administered locally as a continuous infusion or as a small bolus (10–20 mg) has been used as an alternative to facilitate PCI in the setting of thrombotic vein grafts. This strategy, however, is rarely used today. Transluminal extraction catheter (TEC) atherectomy allows simultaneous cutting and aspiration with complete clot removal in most cases. In the TOPITT trial, comparing TEC with PTCA in thrombotic degenerated SVGs, TEC use was associated with less ischemic complications and cardiac enzyme release despite higher risk of dissection. Rheolytic thrombectomy with devices such as the Hydrolyzer (Cordis) and the AngioJet (Possis, Minneapolis, MN) may allow suction of large clots without the associated risk of thombolytic use or TEC catheter disection. More recently, mechanical thrombolysis has also be achieved by delivering ultrasound waves locally at the site of thrombosis with devices such as the Acolysis system (Vascular Solutions, Inc., Minneapolis, MN); however, experience using this device is still limited.

12. Describe the potential advantages and disadvantages of different distal protection devices.

	BALLOON OCCLUDERS	FILTER DEVICES
Ease of use	+ +	+ + +
Ischemia	+ + +	+
Thrombus removal	+ + +	+ + +
Microparticle removal	+ + +	+
Vessel size	3 mm	
Limited imaging	+ + +	+

BIBLIOGRAPHY

1. Baim DS, Wahr Dennis, George B, et al: Randomized trial of distal embolic protection device during percutaneous intervention of saphenous vein aorto-coronary bypass graft. Circulation 105:1285–1290, 2002.
2. Domanski M, Borkowf CB, Campeau L, et al: Prognostic factors for atherosclerosis progession in saphenous vein graftrs: the Post CABG trial. J Am Coll Cardial 36:1877–1883, 2000.
3. Ellis SG, Lincoff AM, Miller D, et al: Reduction in complications of angioplasty with abciximab occurs largerly independently of baseline lesion morphology. J Am Coll Cardiol 32:1619–1623, 1988.
4. Fitzgibbon GM, Leach AJ, Kafka HP, et al: Coronary bypass graft fate: Long-term angiographic study. J Am Coll Cardiol 17:1075–1080, 1991.
5. Holmes D, Topol E., Califf R, et al: A multicenter, randomized trial of coronary angioplasty versus directional atherectomy for patients with saphenous vein bypass graft lesions. Circulation 91:1966–1974, 1995.
6. Kuntz RE, Baim DS, Cohen DJ, et al: A trial comparing rheolytic thrombectomy with intracoronary urokinase for coronary and vein graft thrombus (the vein graft Angiojet study—Vegas 2). Am Med J 89:326–330, 2002.
7. Savage MO, Douglas JS, Fischman DL, et al: Stent placement compared with balloon angioplasty for obstructed coronary bypass grafts. N Engl J Med 337:40–47, 1997.

35. THROMBOTIC CORONARY INTERVENTION

Mustafa Ridha, M.D., and Eduardo de Marchena, M.D.

1. What are the grades of coronary thrombus?

There are six grades of coronary thrombus according to the TIMI (Thrombolysis In Myocardial Infarction) grade system:

Grade 1 = Mural opacities suggestive of possible thrombus

Grade 2 = Small thrombus (< 0.5 times normal lumen diameter) at greatest dimension

Grade 3 = 0.5 to 1.5 times normal diameter

Grade 4 = >1.5 times normal diameter

Grade 5 = Totally occluded culprit vessel with apparently recent thrombotic occlusion ending abruptly with a squared-off or an upstream convex termination creating a stump or arterial cul-de-sac from which dye washout is delayed

Grade 6 = The total occlusion tapers smoothly to supply a terminal side branch with a brisk runoff

2. Does the presence of thrombus seen on a coronary angiogram affect outcome of percutaneous coronary angioplasty?

Yes. Although the in-hospital and 6-month mortality rates of patients with angiographically detected thrombus is not statistically different in than those with no thrombus, there is a higher incidence of in-hospital myocardial infarctions (MIs; 8.2% vs. 5.2%; $P < 0.001$). Moreover, there is a higher rate of in-laboratory abrupt vessel closure among patients with detectable thrombus at baseline (5.9% vs. 3.9%; $P < 0.001$). The 6-month rate of MI is also higher in patients with coronary thrombus.

3. Does the presence of coronary thrombus influence the outcome of percutaneous coronary intervention (PCI) in the recent era with the use of coronary stents?

In a study conducted at Mayo clinic, a comparison was done between patients who had PCI before 1995 (in which only 13% of patients with thrombus received stents) and patients who had PCI after 1995 (in which 82% of patients with thrombus had stents placed). The presence of thrombus in both groups carried similar rates of death (2%), and total MI (9% vs. 11%, $P = NS$). The procedural success rate, however, was higher in the recent era when more stents were used (93% vs. 88%, $P < 0.001$), and abrupt closure was significantly less (4% vs. 7%, $P = 0.01$).

4. Does the presence of coronary thrombus influence the restenosis rate?

Yes. In a study by Violaris et al., the restenosis rate was 43% in patients with detectable thrombus at baseline compared with 34% for patients with no thrombus ($P = 0.028$). This higher restenosis rate was attributed to higher occlusion rate. Moreover, patients with detectable thrombus had more complex lesions, tighter stenoses, greater proportion of dissection after percutaneous transluminal coronary angioplasty (PTCA), higher residual stenosis, and longer duration of inflation during angioplasty. Logistic regression analysis confirmed that the presence of total occlusion before PTCA and total inflation time are positively related and reference diameter after PTCA is negatively related to occlusion rate at follow-up angiogram.

5. Is angioscopy superior to angiography in detecting coronary thrombus?

Yes. Angioscopy has much higher specificity and sensitivity. Moreover, thrombus detection by angioscopy was associated with high adverse outcome. However, angioscopy is highly impracticable and has fallen out of favor as a diagnostic device.

6. What variables were associated with detection of intracoronary thrombus in an angioscopy study?

The two major variables that were associated with detection of intracoronary thrombus are presence of unstable angina (74% vs. 15% for stable angina) and complex coronary lesion (American Heart Association/American College of Cardiology lesion type A = 28%; B1 = 58%; B2 = 68%; C = 68%).

7. Does prophylactic use of thrombolytic therapy during angioplasty for unstable angina reduce clinical events after PTCA?

No. Its use is actually associated with higher adverse angiographic and clinical events. This may be related to an increase in subintimal hematomas after PTCA because thromblytics dissolve fibrin, hampering intimal sealing at the treatment site. Moreover, because the thrombi in acute coronary syndromes are mainly platelet rich, lytic agents have little effect and maybe harmful because of their procoagulant effects and potential activation of platelets.

8. Does pretreatment with platelet glycoprotein (GP) IIb/IIIa receptor inhibitors in patients with acute coronary syndrome (ACS) decrease thrombus burden and adverse cardiac events?

Yes. This was shown in PRISM-PLUS (Platelet Receptor Inhibition for Ischemic Syndrome Management in Patients Limited by Unstable Signs and Symptoms). The patients who were pretreated with tirofiban and heparin had 23% less thrombus burden of the culprit lesion beyond the effect of heparin and aspirin alone. These data were consistent with 32% reduction in the risk of death, MI, and refractory ischemia observed at 7 days and a 43% reduction of death or MI. Moreover, persistent thrombus increased the composite endpoint at 30 days by 2.1-fold and increased each component of the composite endpoint by twofolds. Patients with persistent thrombus had more interventions by 30 days (1.54-fold PTCA; 1.63-fold coronary artery bypass graft surgery, 2.23-fold for any interventions).

9. Do patients with unstable coronary syndrome undergoing coronary intervention derive particular clinical benefit from treatment with platelet GP IIb/IIIa receptor inhibitors?

Yes. A subgroup of patients in the EPIC trial (Evaluation of 7E3 in preventing Ischemic Complications trial) with unstable angina or patients with complex coronary lesions who received a bolus and 12-hour infusion of abciximab, had a 62% reduction in the composite endpoint (12.8% vs. 4.8% for placebo; $P = 0.012$). This was mainly becauase of a reduction in the incidences of death (3.2% vs. 1.2%; $P = 0.164$) and MI (9% vs. 1.8%; $P = 0.004$). This benefit extended to 6 months with the death rate at 1.8% in the treatment arm versus 6.6% in the placebo group. The MI rate was 2.4% versus 11.1% in the placebo group; both being statistically significant. Moreover, the magnitude of risk reduction with abciximab was greater in this trial among patients with unstable angina compared with stable angina for endpoints of death at 30 days and 6 months and for MI at 6 months. This is consistent with the fact that patients with unstable coronary syndromes have a higher burden of intracoronary platelet-rich thrombus, although it may not be all detected by plain angiography. Therefore, potent inhibition of platelets are expected to neutralize the adverse effects of coronary thrombus.

10. Is rheolytic thrombectomy with AngioJet in thrombus-containing lesions safe and effective?

Yes, it is both safe and effective, but with different short- and long-term results in patients with native coronary versus vein graft interventions.

INTERVENTION	RATE
In overall coronary interventions	
Procedure success	93
In-hospital mortality	1.4
In-hospital death or MI	4.2
In-hospital death, MI, or TVR	5.6
One-year mortality	10.0
One-year death or MI	13.3
One-year death, MI, or TVR	35.5
In vein graft intervention	
Procedural success rate	91.0
One-year mortality	16.0
One-year death or MI	19.0
One-year death, MI, or TVR	46.0

Therefore, AngioJet thrombectomy was both effective and safe in native coronary and vein graft interventions. However, the long-term outcome of patients with vein graft interventions was worse.

BIBLIOGRAPHY

1. Ambrose JA, Almeida OD, Sharma SK, Torre SR, et al: for the TAUSA investigators: Adjunctive thrombolytic therapy during angioplasty for ischemic rest angina: results of the TAUSA trial. Circulation 90:69–77, 1994.
2. Lincoff AM, Califf RM, Anderson KM, et al: for the EPIC investigators. Evidence for prevention of death and myocardial infarction with platelet membrane glycoprotein IIb/IIIa receptor blockade by abciximab (c7E3 Fab) among patients with unstable angina undergoing percutaneous coronary revasculariztion. J Am Coll Cardiol 30:149–56, 1997.
3. Singh M, Berger PB, Ting HH, et al: Influence of coronary thrombus on outcome of percutaneous coronary angioplasty in the current era (the Mayo Clinic experience). Am J Cardiol 88:1091–1096, 2001.
4. Singh M, Reeder GS, Ohman EM, et al: Does the presence of thrombus seen on a coronary angiogram affect the outcome after percutaneous coronary angioplasty? An angiographic trials pool data experience. J Am Coll Cardiol 38:624–630, 2001.
5. Singh M, Tiede DJ, Mathew V, Garratt KN, et al: Rheolytic thrombectomy with angiojet in thrombus containing lesions. Cathet Cardiovasc Intervent 56:1–7, 2002.
6. Violaris AG, Melkert R, Herrman JR, Serruys PW. Role of angiographically identifiable thrombus on long-term luminal renarrowing after coronary angioplasty: a quantitative angiographic analysis. circulation 93:889–897, 1996.
7. White CJ, Ramee SR, Collins TJ, et al: Coronary thrombi Increases PTCA risk: angioscopy as a clinical tool. Circulation 93:253–258, 1996.
8. Zhao XQ, Theroux P, Snapinn SM, Sax FL for the PRISM-PLUS Investigators: Intracoranary thrombus and platelet glycoprotein IIb/IIIa receptor blockade with tirofiban in unstable angina or non-Q-wave myocardial infarction: angiographic results from the PRISM-Plus Trial (Platelet Receptor Inhibition for Ischemic Syndrome Management in Patients Limited by Unstable Signs and Symptoms). Circulation 100:1609–1615, 1999.

36. TRANSRADIAL CORONARY INTERVENTIONS

Ramon Quesada, M.D., Margaret Kovacs, Ed.D., M.S.N.,
and Linda Mourant, R.N.

1. What essential assessment must be completed before transradial access is attempted, and how is it done?

The Allen test is the essential assessment. The operator compresses both the radial and the ulnar arteries simultaneously until blanching of the patient's hand occurs. He or she then releases the ulnar artery and assesses the rapidity of flow return (hyperemia within 5 to 7 seconds), which indicates dual circulation to the hand.

2. What are the contraindications to transradial access?

An abnormal Allen test result is caused by implied single artery circulation to the hand. When the ulnar pressure is released, the hand remains pale until radial pressure is released. In the case of postprocedure thrombosis of the radial artery, circulation to the hand is compromised.

3. Who is the ideal candidate for transradial access?
- 90% of the population who have dual circulation to the hand
- Obese individuals who are at increased risk of complications from transfemoral access
- Individuals with severe peripheral artery disease

4. What are the disadvantages of transradial access? Which patients are not ideal candidates?
- Transradial access often requires special catheter shapes for coronary cannulation for more inexperienced operators. It is associated with a physician learning curve.
- Elderly hypertensive patients may have increased tortuousity of the radial and subclavian arteries, which makes the procedure more challenging because stiffer guidewires are needed.

5. What are the five important steps for a successful transradial cannulation?
- Use local anesthesia. Use a generous amount in this sensitive area and allow time for it to take effect.
- Enter the artery with a 21-gauge, thin-wall needle.
- After the artery is cannulated, advance a 0.025-inch guidewire through the needle.
- A 4-, 5-, 6-, 7, or 8-Fr introducer sheath is inserted.
- A "cocktail" (i.e., verapamil 2 mg, lidocaine 2% (1 cc) diluted in normal saline followed by heparin 40 u/kg IV bolus [in addition to the usual use of nitrates, and so on]) is injected through the catheter side arm to reduce vessel spasm.

6. What are the advantages of transradial access?
- Decreased incidence of major entry site complications
- Easier vascular access and hemostasis for obese patients
- Decreased time to ambulation
- Decreased postprocedural cost
- Increased patient movement

7. What are the potentially serious complications of transradial access and what is the cause?
- Radial occlusion, which is usually asymptomatic, is one complication (reported incidence of 4.7%). This is related to catheter size; the use of an 8-Fr catheter imposes double the risk of a 6-Fr catheter

- Symptomatic radial occlusion occurs in 0.2% of patients.
- Significant hematoma occurs in 0.2% of patients.
- Compartment syndrome occurs in 0.07% of patients.

Barbeau et al. (1996) reported on these complication rates based on a series of 1372 interventions.

8. In Figure 1, identify the complication of transradial access, indicate the probable cause, and describe the steps in the management of the patient.

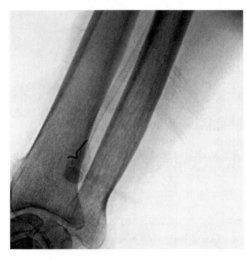

FIGURE 1

This complication is wire fracture. It is caused by excessive manipulation or torquing of the guidewire through the needle. Patient management by interventional cardiologist: Make a small superficial incision with a scalpel. Then under fluoroscopy, use a hemostat to remove the fractured wire. Close the incision with absorbable suture. Proceed with the transradial intervention via a more proximal cannulation of the artery.

9. A 69-year-old male with hypertension, severe coronary artery disease (CAD), and a prior transradial coronary intervention is now undergoing a repeat diagnostic cardiac catheterization via right radial access. After placing the introducer and advancing the diagnostic catheter over the guidewire, you encounter resistance. To overcome this, you choose to attempt advance of a more flexible guidewire (i.e., Benson wire or Wholey wire). Despite this, you are unable to overcome the resistance. After pulling back the wire and injecting contrast dye, you note an area of extravasation of contrast. What is the complication, what should the patient management be, and how should this be avoided?

Complication: Perforation of a small branch of the radial artery caused by tortuosity or angulation of the radial artery and overconfidence of the operator.

Patient management: To avoid continuous bleeding and potential compartment syndrome, surgery is the standard treatment. Because of the small size of the perforated artery, a covered stent is not suitable. However, surgery can be avoided by using the following intervention:

Using an infusion catheter, advance to the exact site of perforation.

Embolize the perforation with Trufill n-Butyl Cyanoacrylate (n-BCA) Liquid Embolic System. You must make certain that you are at the exact point of perforation and that the flow of the main artery is not compromised.

Lesson learned: In cases of extreme tortuosity as evidenced by both resistance and angio-

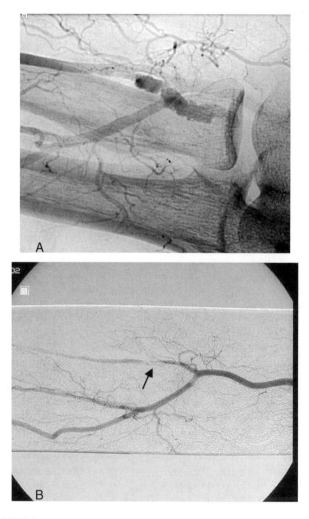

FIGURE 2. *A,* Injection of nBCA. *B,* Filling defect is glue overlying the artery.

graphic visualization, do not risk perforation; instead, use a very flexible guidewire with maximum torquing ability and proceed cautiously. Sometimes a 0.14- or 0.18-inch coronary guidewire is very useful in overcoming tortuousity.

10. The use of a new method or technique often meets administrative (operational) and clinical resistance from both the center and fellow physicians. What arguments could be made based on randomized trials for the use of the transradial technique?

Operational arguments: Fewer complications, faster discharge, cost reduction, equal success rate, improved patient satisfaction, decreased staffing needs. Mann et al. compared radial to femoral approach in a prospective study. There were significant differences ($P = < 0.01$) favoring the radial approach for fewer vascular complications, shorter length of stay (LOS), and decreased cost for catheterization laboratory and total hospital charges. There was a 19% reduction in hospital charges when comparing the radial to the femoral approach.

Clinical arguments: Despite learning curve, the decrease in puncture site complications is of benefit to the patient and the operator.

A randomized comparison of three different approaches for coronary angioplasty (i.e., radial, brachial, and femoral) by Kiemeneij et al. found that the success rate by the radial approach was more successful than the other methods. There were no entry site complications for the radial approach, seven for the brachial and six for the femoral.

11. Dr. Smith has cautioned you never to attempt a transradial intervention on elderly, diabetic, frail patients. However, you believe that you can successfully overcome these challenges by using a variety of techniques. What steps would increase success in these elderly patients?

- Using a small introducer (5- or 6-Fr), advance the diagnostic or guiding catheter over a Benson or Wholey wire into the ascending aorta.
- If there is significant tortuosity in the subclavian artery, switch to a stiff exchange 0.035- or 0.038 inch Cook or Amplax guidewire.
- Pull the wire into the shaft of the catheter in order to facilitate the manipulation (torquing) of the catheter.
- After the coronary is cannulated, remove the guidewire, aspirate to make sure there are no bubbles, and proceed with diagnostic or coronary intervention.

In a series of 300 procedures, 232 elderly patients older than age 75 years (125 men and 66 women) the transradial access was used successfully in 92% of the patients with no local complications and two cardiac complications (one related to the intervention) and one case of gastrointestinal bleeding secondary to the use of abciximab. This success rate does not differ significantly from the success rate in younger patients (Javier et al., 2001).

12. It is well documented that women have high complication rates associated with coronary interventions because of their small body size and smaller vessels; symptomatic CAD develops at an older age in women, and their symptoms are atypical. Aggressive intervention for women is becoming the standard rather than the exception. How can you ensure successful interventions for female patients?

- Access techniques applicable to the elderly are well suited to female patients (see question 11).
- Because their arteries are smaller and are more prone to radial spasm, the patient needs to be premedicated with appropriate sedation and well hydrated before the procedure.
- The use of intraarterial calcium channel blockers and nitrates after placing the introducer and before removing the introducer is extremely important to prevent radial spasm.

It is well known that the standard transfemoral approach is associated with higher complications in women than in men. There is increasing documentation of the success of the transradial access in women. In a series of 279 procedures in women (mean age, 67 years, range, 34–90 years), the success rate was 97% (Ardid et al., 2001).

13. When you are performing a coronary procedure via the femoral approach using the standard Judkins technique, the manipulation of catheters to get into the left coronary artery is minimal. That is not the case for the right coronary artery. What modifications, in general, would you need to make to properly cannulate the coronary arteries from when using the transradial access?

- If you are using the left radial artery, you can use the same catheters that are used for the femoral Judkins technique.
  You may need to downsize the left coronary catheter (e.g., for example if you would use a JL4 for the femoral artery, you would use a JL3.5 for the radial artery).
  The right coronary artery can be cannulated with a standard JR4.
- If you are using the right radial artery, then for the left coronary a special Kimny or right brachial catheter, which is also good for the right coronary artery, is preferred.

- There are other conventional catheters that can be used for either right or left transradial access:

LEFT RADIAL ACCESS	RIGHT RADIAL ACCESS
For lesions in LCA	**For lesions in LCA**
XB 3.5	XB 3.0
JL 4	JL 3.5
	Kimny
For lesions in RCA	**For lesions in RCA**
JR 4	JR 4
AL I or Al II	AL I or AL II
MP	MP
	Kimny

14. Aside from the obvious equipment differences needed for transradial access, what other differences are there in preparing, intervening, and caring for patients?

- Position the patient on the table with the procedure arm extended with adequate support with the palmar surface up.
- Prepare the arm from mid forearm to fingertips, front and back.
- Rather than taping the hand to a board, use a sterile towel folded and wrapped over the palm and clipped under the board. Experience using this method shows that the sensation of immobilization is adequate for the patient and minimizes discomfort.
- More anesthetic is needed proportionately for this area than for the femoral artery, and adequate time for the local anesthetic to take effect is important for patient comfort.
- During the intervention, the only difference may be in the type of catheters used.
- Remove the sheath and place a Hemoband.
- Gradually loosen per protocol and observe for hematoma formation and bleeding and that there is good circulation to the hand; gradually wean off.
- Educate the patient that there may be discomfort from the Hemoband. The use of analgesics postprocedure can usually help with this discomfort.

15. How would you approach a 75-year-old man after coronary artery bypass graft (CABG) surgery with severe peripheral arterial disease and no femoral access but a good bilateral Allen test result? What specific considerations would you have in planning and performing this intervention?

Planning: Investigate previous surgery so that you know what conduits were used for the bypass grafts. If you have left internal mammary artery grafts and vein grafts, the choice for access is the left radial artery. If you have to cannulate both the right and left internal mammary arteries, the choice for access could be either the right or left radial arteries.

Performing: The Kimny catheter is usually the catheter of choice because you can cannulate both mammaries and saphenous vein grafts if using the left radial approach. The special maneuver needed to make the catheter enter the right mammary is to approach the aortic valve, rotate the catheter toward the arch, and advance the guidewire into the right subclavian artery, as shown in Figure 3A. You can also use the internal mammary catheter when approaching from the left. Then pull back the guidewire, and the tip of the catheter will engage the right mammary. For the left internal mammary artery (LIMA) and vein grafts, you can use conventional catheters (Fig. 3B).

16. The patient is a 74-year-old woman with a history of CAD, CABG 15 years ago, with severe peripheral arterial disease, crescendo angina, with an ejection fraction of 40%. The patient has a totally occluded saphenous vein graft to the obtuse marginal branch (OMB), a small nondominant right coronary artery, patent LIMA to the LAD, and has a high grade stenosis of the distal left main and proximal circumflex artery. What approach do you use?

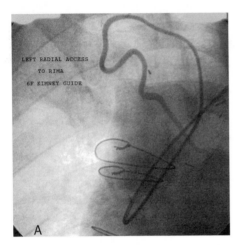
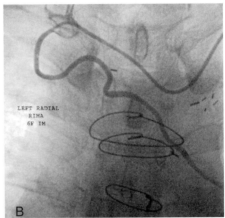

FIGURE 3.

Because of the complexity of the lesions to be treated, you would anticipate the need for adequate guide support. You are also considering debulking before stenting because of the calcification, but you have the limitation of severe peripheral arterial disease and poor femoral access. Transradial access is the alternative of choice in this case despite its complexity (Fig. 4).

Procedure considerations:

- Because the patient is small and has small size arteries, you should use a 6-Fr introducer.
- For cannulation of the left coronary artery system, you can use the XB3.5 or you may choose to use a special shaped left fajadet guide catheter. Then proceed to advance your 0.14-inch coronary guidewires. In this particular case, we elected to proceed with a rotational atherectomy and advanced our roto wire.
- After debulking we proceeded with conventional PTCA and stenting.

Conclusion: Despite the complexity of the case secondary to the patients' coronary anatomy, the use of the transradial access was a viable means of treating this patient.

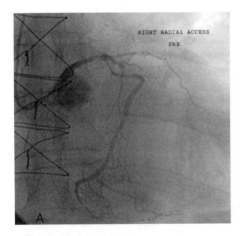
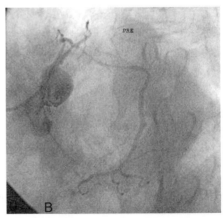

FIGURE 4. *A,* Preprocedure. *B,* Preprocedure. (*continued*)

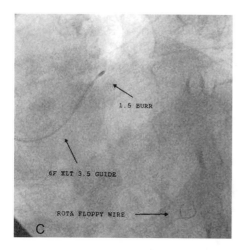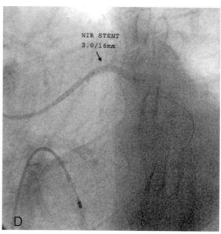

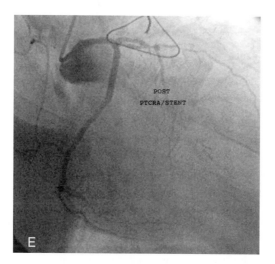

FIGURE 4. (*continued*) *C*, Procedure. *D*, Postprocedure. *E*, Postprocedure.

17. A 65-year-old morbidly obese man presented with an acute inferior wall MI within 3 hours after onset of chest pain. The patient received thrombolysis in the emergency department with initial relief of chest pain and improvement of ST changes. You have been called because the patient is having recurrent chest pressure 1 hour after thrombolysis and worsening of ST elevations in inferior leads. His blood pressure is 90/60 mmHg, heart rate is 110, and he is diaphoretic. The catheterization laboratory is available, and you elect to take the patient for coronary angiography and rescue intervention. Detail your approach, management, and treatment of this patient considering these factors.

The patient's obesity makes the use of the femoral approach problematic because he is at high risk for bleeding complications after thrombolysis. The use of transradial access offers the advantage of no bleeding complications despite the use of thrombolysis and heavy anticoagulation (Fig. 5).

• The disadvantage of transradial access in acute MI is the learning curve and degree of com-

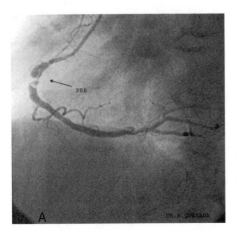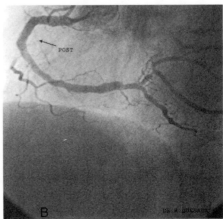

FIGURE 5. *A,* Preprocedure. *B,* Postprocedure.

fort you feel with this approach. For experienced operators, transradial access is ideal for this patient.

- With a large thrombus burden in this patient's proximal RCA, the use of a protection device to prevent distal embolization should be considered. This was followed by eximer laser thrombectomy, but other thrombectomy devices can be used. The procedure was completed with conventional angioplasty and stenting.

Conclusion: In our experience, transradial access is the first choice for the interventional management of patients with acute coronary syndromes, specifically for acute MI going for direct PCI.

BIBLIOGRAPHY

1. Ardid, MI , Javier JJ, Mourant, L, Quesada, R: Is transradial rotational atherectomy feasible and safe? Presented at the Society for Cardiac Angiography and Interventions, Annual Meeting, Houston, TX, May 16–19, 2001.
2. Barbeau GR, Carrier G, Ferland S, et al: Right transradial approach for coronary procedures: preliminary results. J Invas Cardiol 8(suppl D):19–21, 1996.
3. Javier JJ, Ardid MI, Mourant L, Quesada R: Is the transradial technique feasible for elderly patients? Presented at the Society for Cardiac Angiography and Interventions, Annual Meeting, Houston, TX, May 16–19, 2001.
4. Kiemeneij F, Laarman GJ, Odekerken D, et al: A randomized comparison of percutaneous transluminal coronary angioplasty by the radial, brachial and femoral approaches: the access study. J Am Coll Cardiol 29:1269–1275, 1997.
5. Lotan C, Hasin Y, Mosseri M, et al: Transradial approach for coronary angiography and angioplasty. Am J Cardiol 76:164–167, 1995.
6. Mann JT III, Cubeddu MG, Schneider JE, Arrowood M: Right radial access for PTCA: a prospective study demonstrates reduced complications and hospital charges. J Invas Cardiol 8(suppl D):40–44, 1996.
7. Mathias DW, Bigler L: Transradial coronary angioplasty and stent implantation in acute myocardial infarction: initial experience. J Invas Cardiol 12:547–549, 2000.
8. Ochiai M, Isshiki T, Toyoizumi H, et al: Efficacy of transradial primary stenting in patients with acute myocardial infarction. Am J Cardiol 83:966–968, A10, 1999.
9. Yokoyama N, Takeshita S, Ochiai M, et al: Direct assessment of palmar circulation before transradial coronary intervention by color Doppler ultrasonography. Am J Cardiol 86:218–221, 2000.

VII. Coronary Vascular Complications

37. CORONARY DISSECTION AND VASOSPASM

Joshua Purow, M.D., and Alexandre C. Ferreira, M.D.

1. What are the most common causes of periprocedural ischemic-related chest pain?
- Coronary dissection
- Intracoronary thrombus
- Guide or balloon catheter damping
- Vasospasm
- Side branch occlusion
- Distal embolization

2. What is the incidence of coronary dissection after a coronary intervention, and how often do these dissections lead to complications?

Because the process of balloon dilatation requires fracturing and splitting of the atherosclerotic plaque, this often results in tearing of the intima and media as well. Differentiating between a therapeutic dissection and a complication of the procedure is difficult. Despite this, angiographic evidence of coronary dissection is present in approximately 20% to 50% of patients after angioplasty. With intravascular ultrasound (IVUS), the incidence has been shown to be even higher. Dissections occur more frequently with certain interventional techniques, such as excimer laser surgery and atherectomy. Also, weak contrast dye injections may cause streaming in the vessel and give the false angiographic impression of a dissection.

Coronary dissections can be caused by overly aggressive attempts at passing a guidewire. However, the majority of dissections are caused by "controlled injury" induced by inflation of the balloon.

Coronary dissection is the leading cause of acute closure and can result in ischemic complications, such as death, myocardial infarction (MI) and emergent coronary bypass graft surgery (CABG). The risk of developing a severe ischemic complication was fivefold greater in patients with a complicated dissection. Nevertheless, the majority of dissections are not associated with complications, and the incidence of complications has been greatly reduced in the stenting era. Most untreated dissections heal themselves over the next 3 to 6 months. Additionally, dissections have no impact on the risk of restenosis.

3. What is the National Heart, Lung and Blood Institute's (NHLBI) classification system for coronary dissections?

TYPE	DESCRIPTION	RATE OF ACUTE CLOSURE, %
A	Mild luminal haziness	0
B	Intraluminal linear dissection	3
C	Extraluminal contrast dye staining or extraluminal cap (with persistence of dye after dye clearance)	10
D	Spiral dissection	30
E	Dissection with filling defects	9
F	Dissection with limited or no flow	69

Type A and B dissections are considered minor dissections because they rarely result in ischemic complications. Types C to F are complicated dissections and are much more likely to result in ischemic complications.

4. What types of lesion have a higher risk for dissection during angioplasty?

- Long lesions
- Eccentric lesions
- Calcified lesions
- Diffuse disease
- American Heart Association/American College of Cardiology type B or C lesions
- Tortuous vessels

5. Are certain procedural techniques more or less likely to result in dissection?

More likely

- Balloon oversizing: Powerful independent predictor of dissection if the balloon-to-artery ratio is > 1.2.
- Deflation rate: Gradual deflations may possibly result in more dissections.
- Type of intervention: Excimer laser and atherectomy have higher incidences of dissection.

Less likely

- Duration of inflation: Fewer dissections are seen with more prolonged inflations rather than multiple short inflations.
- Inflation rate: Gradual inflations may possibly result in fewer dissections.
- Predilation: May result in fewer dissections.

No effect

- Balloon compliance: Most studies showed no significantly better outcome with compliant balloons. Noncompliant balloons may reduce dissections when they are used for calcified or angled lesions.
- Inflation pressures: There is no difference between low versus high pressures except when exceeding the maximum recommended pressure. High pressures with compliant balloons may increase the risk of dissection.
- Balloon catheter system: There is no difference between the over-the-wire versus the monorail system.

6. After a dissection has occurred, what angiographic and clinical factors suggest a higher risk of progression to a major ischemic event?

- NHLBI dissection types C to F
- Long dissection length > 15 mm
- Residual stenosis > 70%
- Thrombolysis in myocardial infarction flow 0 to 2
- Unstable angina
- Transient in laboratory occlusion
- Chronic total occlusions

7. How should a dissection be managed?

The management of dissections depends heavily on its classification. Most non–flow-limiting dissections without high-risk features should be treated conservatively without additional mechanical or pharmacologic intervention. These dissections rarely lead to ischemic complications and often heal themselves. Nevertheless, many interventionalist stent these dissections because of the ease of stent placement.

The prognosis and management of patients with complicated coronary dissections have changed radically since the development of stents. As mentioned previously, the risk of ischemic complications after these dissections is high. This includes types C to F dissections or those with any of the other high-risk features even if flow is not impaired. The placement of stents at the point of dissection serves to tack up the wall of the vessel and dramatically reduces the incidence of acute closure. With the widespread use of coronary stents, ischemic complications after a coronary dissection are rare. In addition, the intimal tear exposes the vessel wall components, such as collagen and tissue factor, and may lead to an increased risk of thrombosis. Therefore, therapy with antiplatelet agents, heparin, glycoprotein (GP) IIb/IIIa receptors, and direct thrombin inhibitors should also be strongly considered.

8. Can a dissection occur with stent placement?

Even though stents are used to treat dissections, stent placement can cause a dissection, usually at the edges of the stent. This is called an "edge dissection" and usually results from inappropriate sizing of the stent, overexpansion, or balloon overhang. The struts of the stent are responsible for the intimal tear. These edge dissections can be treated with additional stent implantation.

9. List some of the nonprocedural causes of coronary dissection.
- Peripartum spontaneous dissection
- Chest trauma
- Aortic root dissection
- Vasculitis
- Coronary spasm
- Cystic medial necrosis
- Systemic hypertension
- After cardiac surgery
- Cocaine use
- Intense excercise
- Idiopathic

10. Describe the features of spontaneous coronary artery dissection.

Spontaneous coronary dissection, also known as dissecting aneurysm, is a rare condition that commonly occurs in the third trimester of pregnancy or in the immediate postpartum period. It can result in ischemia, MI, or sudden death. Mostly, middle-aged women are affected who are otherwise healthy without any significant coronary stenoses. This diagnosis must be considered in patients who have a low cardiovascular risk and present with a MI, especially young women who are pregnant or have recently given birth. The incidence may be underestimated because of the high incidence of associated sudden death, the lesions may angiographically mimic atherosclerotic disease, and the low referral rate for angiography in this population. The left anterior descending coronary artery (LAD) is overwhelmingly the affected artery with occasional involvement of the right coronary artery. The dissection usually occurs in the outer media with pushing of the inner media toward the opposite wall, causing luminal obstruction. Histopathologic evaluations have associated spontaneous dissections with eosinophilic inflammation of the adventita.

The overall prognosis for patients with this condition is poor with a very high mortality rate. Medical treatment has been mostly successful in uncomplicated infarctions and includes aspirin, nitrates, beta blockers, and calcium antagonists. Both (CABG) and percutaneous coronary intervention (PCI) with stenting have also been performed successfully for this condition. Surgical techniques are complicated by difficulty in differentiating between the true and false lumen. Percutaneous techniques are also complicated by selective cannulation of the false lumen. The decision to treat spontaneous dissections medically, percutaneously, or surgically remains unclear and depends heavily on symptoms and hemodynamic stability.

11. Classify the various types of vasospasm by location along the artery.
- Proximal epicardial spasm: Often catheter induced
- Intralesional spasm: Caused by endothelial dysfunction or a result of PCI
- Distal epicardial spasm: Also common after PCI; may be induced by the guidewire
- Microvascular spasm: Part of the no-reflow phenomenon

12. What is the pathophysiology of vasospasm after PCI?

There are a number of factors responsible. Percutaneous devices result in denudation of the vascular endothelium, resulting in an inability to produce nitric oxide. The vasomotor tone is thus unable to counteract the affects of localized vasoconstrictors. Numerous platelet-derived vaso-constrictors are produced, including thromboxane, serotonin, and platelet-activating factor. There is also a decreased sensitivity to other vasodilators. The effects of vasospasm are most common during the procedure but may last for many months afterwards.

13. What is the incidence of vasospasm after angioplasty?

Although some degree of vasoconstriction exists after every intervention, the incidence of clinically significant coronary artery spasm is approximately 1% to 5%. These can infrequently result in ischemic complications and, rarely, in acute closure. Predisposing factors for postproce-dure spasm include noncalcified lesions, eccentric lesions, and younger age. Excimer laser and atherectomy had a high rate of severe spasm, as high as 15% to 35%, associated with their use, but this has been significantly reduced with the current saline infusion techniques.

14. What are the therapeutic options to treat refractory vasospasm?

Refractory vasospasm refers to postprocedure spasm not responsive to nitrates. Most patients with procedure-related vasospasm respond to the administration of intracoronary nitroglycerin. The usual dosing is 50 to 100 μg, although higher doses may occasionally be required.

If vasospasm persists, a number of therapeutic options are available:

1. Intracoronary calcium antagonists, including verapamil, 100–400 μg boluses up to 1.0–1.5 mg, diltiazem, 0.5–2.5 mg boluses up to 5–10 mg, and nicardipine, 100–200 μg boluses.

2. Removal of interventional dilation catheters; the guidewire should absolutely not be removed

3. Repeat PTCA with prolonged, low-pressure balloon dilatations

At this point, if the spasm remains refractory, there is a high likelihood of coronary dissec-tion or thrombus. This possibility should be investigated thoroughly and treated appropriately. If the spasm continues or if dissection is present, then coronary stenting should be performed. This often relieves episodes of severe refractory spasm. Stents should also be considered earlier if ev-idence of active persistent ischemia or hemodynamic instability exists. The other possible me-chanical option is circulatory support with an intraaortic balloon pump. This should be reserved for cases associated with hypotension.

15. What is vasospastic angina, and how can it be diagnosed in the catheterization laboratory?

In 1959, Prinzmetal first described an ischemic syndrome, which he called variant angina be-cause the angina was not provoked by the usual precipitating factors. The syndrome manifests with typical chest pain not necessarily occurring with exertion or stress and is associated with ST segment changes on the electrocardiogram (ECG). Coronary blood flow obstruction occurs, at least partially, as a result of coronary vasospasm and can result in MI and sudden death. The va-sospasm often occurs at the site of a fixed stenosis but may occur with angiographically normal or mildly obstructive coronary arteries.

The intravenous administration of ergonovine maleate or acetylcholine can be used diagnos-tically to induce vasospasm. Various protocols are used for the administration of ergonovine. One commonly used protocol requires ergonovine to be administered at increasing doses of 0.02, 0.18, and 0.2 mg at 3-minute intervals. Repeat angiograms should be obtained after each interval. The dignosis of vasospastic angina is made with the angiographic presence of spasm associated with ST segment changes on the ECG or the recurrence of symptoms. Variant angina responds med-ically to nitrates and calcium antagonists in the majority of cases.

16. Is there a role for PCI for noncritical fixed stenoses and symptomatic vasospastic angina?

Although not an accepted indication, both PTCA and stenting have been performed to treat vasospasm superimposed on a fixed atherosclerotic lesion, which is refractory to medical therapy.

This treatment has often achieved symptomatic relief. However, the restenosis rate is high at approximately 35% to 50%. Vasospasm can also recur often at previously unaffected coronary segments. This therapy should be limited to fixed lesions with a focal discrete segment of superimposed spasm. Procedure-induced spasm does not occur at any increased frequency in patients with variant angina.

BIBLIOGRAPHY

1. Bell MR, Reeder GS, Garratt KN, et al: Predictor of major ischemic complications after coronary dissection following angioplasty. Am J Cardiol 71:1402–1407, 1993.
2. Fischell TA: Coronary artery spasm after percutaneous transluminal coronary angioplasty: pathophysiology and clinical consequences. Catheter Cardiovasc Diagn 19:1–3, 1990.
3. Freed MS: Coronary artery spasm. In Safian RD, Freed MS (eds): The Manual of Interventional Cardiology, 3rd ed. Royal Oak, MI, Physician's Press, 2001, pp 381–386.
4. Freed MS, O'Neill WW, Safian RD: Dissection and acute closure. In Safian RD, Freed MS (eds): The Manual of Interventional Cardiology, 3rd ed. Royal Oak, MI, Physician's Press, 2001, pp 387–412.
5. Ilia R, Bigham H, Brennan J, et al: Predictors of coronary dissection following percutaneous transluminal coronary balloon angioplasty. Cardiology 85:229–234, 1994.
6. Mohamed HA, Abdulhamid E, Habib N: Spontaneous coronary artery dissection: a case report and review of the literature. Angiology 53:205–211, 2002.
7. Rabinowitz A, Dodek A, Carere RG, Webb JG: Stenting for treatment of coronary vasospasm. Catheter Cardiovasc Diagn 39:372–375, 1996.
8. Sharma SK, Israel DH, Kamean JL, et al: Clinical, angiographic and procedural determinants of major and minor coronary dissection during angioplasty. Am Heart J 126:39–47, 1993.

38. ACUTE CLOSURE AND NO REFLOW

V.S. Srinivas, M.B., B.S., and Suleiman M. Kharabsheh, M.D.

1. What are the different types of vessel closure that can complicate percutaneous coronary intervention (PCI)?

   a. Threatened closure: Angiographic appearance of dissection or thrombus resulting in more than 50% residual stenosis and associated with thrombolysis in myocardial infarction (TIMI) 3 flow.

   b. Imminent closure: Acute worsening of intervened lesion with TIMI 2 flow

   c. Acute closure: Total occlusion with TIMI 0 flow.

2. What are the common causes of acute closure?

Coronary dissection is most common cause of acute closure on histopathologic studies. It is noted in 20% to 40% of cases on angiography and in 60% to 80% of cases by intravascular ultrasound after balloon angioplasty. The incidence of acute closure increases as the dissection becomes more complex (see Table 1). Thrombus and coronary artery spasm are other causes.

3. What is the incidence and timing of acute closure after PCI?

In the pre-stent era, acute closure occurred in 2% to 11% of patients after percutaneous transluminal coronary angioplasty (PTCA); 50% to 80% of the occlusions occurred with the patient in the catheterization laboratory, and the rest occurred within the next 6 hours. Most of these events were related to the presence of severe dissections or newly developed thrombus at the PTCA site. Late acute closure (> 24 hours after PTCA) occurred mostly after primary PTCA for acute myocardial infarction (MI) and after PTCA for chronic total occlusions, often related to new thrombus formation.

In the current era of stenting, acute stent thrombosis is rare (< 1%) and almost always results from incomplete stent expansion, uncovered dissection, or residual clot. Subacute stent thrombosis that occurs between 2 and 11 days after the procedure has been largely eliminated with routine high-pressure inflation of the stent and more effective antiplatelet regimens.

4. What are the major clinical and angiographic predictors of dissection after PTCA?

- Calcified lesions
- Eccentric lesions
- Long and intermediate lesion length
- Diffuse disease
- Complex lesion morphology (type B or C)
- Vessel curvature
- Unstable angina

5. Does pretreatment with aspirin help prevent acute closure after PCI?

Aspirin reduces the risk of abrupt vessel closure and acute MI in patients undergoing angioplasty. Baranathan et al. conducted a review of antiplatelet therapy among 300 patients after initial successful PTCA. Patients were classified into three groups: the no aspirin group ($n = 121$) who did not receive aspirin or dipyridamole any time before PTCA; the standard treatment group ($n = 110$) who received aspirin with or without dipyridamole before admission but not before PTCA; and the maximal treatment group ($n = 32$) who received both aspirin and dipyridamole at both time periods. The presence of angiographic thrombus was assessed before, immediately after, and at least 30 minutes after the last balloon inflation at the PTCA site. New thrombi were detected at 15% of the PTCA sites, of which one third were considered clinically significant (defined as causing 100% occlusion or requiring emergency surgery or streptokinase therapy).

The no aspirin group had the highest incidence of both angiographic thrombi and clinically significant thrombus (10.7%); standard treatment reduced both angiographic thrombus and clinically significant thrombus (1.8%). Patients who received maximal treatment had neither angiographic thrombus ($P = 0.001$) nor significant thrombus ($P = 0.04$).

Stepwise logistic regression analysis demonstrated that the lack of effective antiplatelet therapy was the most discriminatory variable for the presence of any thrombus, followed by current smoking, higher percent diameter stenosis, and dissection. However, only the lack of pretreatment with effective antiplatelet therapy was predictive for clinically significant thrombus.

6. Is there a relationship between activated clotting time (ACT) during angioplasty and abrupt closure?

Several studies have demonstrated an inverse relationship between the degree of anticoagulation during angioplasty and the risk of abrupt closure. Although a minimum target ACT has not been identified, it has been observed that the higher the intensity of anticoagulation, the lower the risk of abrupt closure. Intraprocedural ACT measurements in 62 cases of in- and out-of-laboratory abrupt closure after non-emergency coronary angioplasty were compared with a matched control population of 124 patients without abrupt closure. Patients who experienced abrupt closure had significantly lower initial ACT levels of 350 seconds versus 380 seconds ($P = 0.004$). In addition, minimum ACT levels during the procedure were lower, 345 seconds versus 370 seconds ($P = 0.014$) compared with control subjects. Significantly, higher ACTs were not associated with a higher likelihood of major bleeding complications. A strong inverse linear relationship between the ACT and the probability of abrupt closure was identified. However, it is unclear how these results are to be interpreted in the current era of widespread stenting.

7. What is the optimal ACT that should be achieved during coronary interventions to achieve the least acute closures?

According to the recently published American College of Cardiology/American Heart Association guidelines, the target ACT for PCI should be 250 to 300 seconds with the HemoTec device and 300 to 350 seconds with the Hemochron device.

Chew et al. performed a pooled analysis of more than 5000 patients from six randomized, controlled trials in which unfractionated heparin constituted the control arm. Patients were divided into 25-second intervals of ACTs, from 275 to 476 seconds. The incidence of death, MI, revascularization, and major or minor bleeding at 7 days was lowest with ACTs in the range of 350 to 375 seconds (6.6% or a 34% relative risk reduction) compared with ACTs between 171 and 295 seconds ($P < 0.001$).

8. Are there any long-term sequelae after uncomplicated in-laboratory coronary artery closure?

Transient, uncomplicated, in-laboratory acute closure does not have any adverse long-term effect. However, a concomitant elevation of postprocedure cardiac enzymes has an important and significant adverse effect on long-term outcomes. In a study of more than 4000 consecutive patients who underwent successful PTCA or directional coronary atherectomy (DCA), 85 patients had an uncomplicated, successfully reversed transient in-laboratory vessel closure. These 85 patients were then compared with 4775 patients without in-laboratory closure. Successfully treated, uncomplicated transient vessel closure did not have an adverse effect on long-term prognosis (i.e., death, MI, or coronary interventions). However, increase in creatine kinase–myoglobin (CK-MB) was associated with a significant adverse effect on long-term outcome. By multivariate logistic regression, an increase in postprocedure CK-MB was the most significant correlate for cardiac death (risk ratio [RR], 1.25; $P < 0.0001$). It was also the strongest correlate of major ischemic complications (i.e., death, MI, or coronary interventions) on follow-up (RR, 1.08; $P = 0.0005$).

In a recent combined analysis of more than 8000 patients by Ellis et al., postprocedural elevations of CK-MB more than five times were associated with a greater short-term risk for mortality without any additional long-term risk. It appears that the long-term sequelae of acute closure are related more closely to the presence or absence of associated myocardial necrosis.

9. What is the best treatment for dissection or threatened or acute closure after PTCA?

Acute occlusion after balloon coronary angioplasty is associated with an increased risk of angina, emergency coronary artery bypass grafting (CABG), periprocedural MI, and death. The incidence of acute closure after PTCA alone is 4% to 12%. Initial approaches to treat and reverse acute closure (e.g., repeat PTCA, vasodilators, and thrombolytics) reduce the need for emergency surgery, however, both morbidity (40%) and in-hospital mortality (5%) remain high.

DCA is useful in excising focal dissection flaps. Currently, intracoronary stenting is the most reliable way to restore patency and avoid these complications; the use of stents has decreased the incidence of acute closure to less than 1%. As a bailout, numerous studies have demonstrated a success rates of more than 95%. Given the high success rates and excellent profile, stents has become the standard treatment for significant dissections (NHLBI C–F) and acute vessel closure after PTCA (Table 1). If stenting fails, emergency CABG should be considered.

Table 1. Relationship of Coronary Artery Dissection (NHLBI Grade)
and Acute Closure

TYPE	DESCRIPTION	ACUTE CLOSURE, %
A	Minor radiolucencies within lumen without persistence after contrast clearance	—
B	Angiographically defined parallel tracts or double lumen without persistence of contrast	3
C	Extraluminal cap with persistence of contrast	10
D	Spiral luminal defects	30
E	New persistent filling defects	9
F	Non-A–E types with impaired flow or total occlusion	69

10. What is no reflow or slow flow?

No reflow is a reduction in coronary blood flow (TIMI 0 or 1 flow) through the coronary artery without angiographic evidence of mechanical vessel obstruction. No reflow has been documented in more than 30% of patients after thrombolysis or mechanical intervention for acute MI. During coronary interventions, no reflow has been reported in 0.6% to 2.0% of cases. The incidence is highest with atherectomy (7.7%), PTCA or stenting of thrombus-containing lesions, primary or rescue PTCA for acute MI, and saphenous vein graft interventions.

Slow flow is a lesser degree of impairment in coronary flow (usually TIMI 2 or 3 flow grade). Lesser degrees of "slow-flow," especially those associated with TIMI 3 flow, may be difficult to identify unless a Doppler flow wire is used. Using Doppler flow wires, patterns of no relow or slow flow are described as the presence of systolic retrograde flow, diminished systolic antegrade flow, and rapid deceleration of diastolic flow.

11. What are the different types of no reflow?

    a. Experimental no reflow (induced in experimental animals)
    b. No reflow after reperfusion in acute MI
    c. Angiographic no reflow, flow deterioration after successful percutaneous reperfusion, often in the setting of PCI on thrombus-laden lesions or vein grafts

Although all refer to the same phenomenon, different mechanisms may mediate each.

12. What are the proposed mechanisms for no reflow?

No clear-cut, single mechanism for no reflow has been identified. It appears to result from a complex interplay between lesional characteristics and myocardial capillaries. However, it is conceptually important to determine the important components of the no-reflow phenotype so that therapies may be tailored to the particular clinical situation.

- **Experimental no reflow:** This often follows the release of experimentally induced coronary obstruction (when applied for 40 minutes). It is often characterized by persistent subendocardial perfusion defects. On pathology, endothelial damage, tissue edema, and local platelet and fibrin activation within the myocardium are associated with no reflow. Pheresis of platelets and neutrophils appears to attenuate this reaction, suggesting an inflammatory role.

- **After MI:** Recent data indicate that cardiac sympathetic reflex with resulting α-adrenergic micro- and macrovascular constriction and reperfusion injury mediated by platelets and macrophages play an important role in the MI no-reflow phenomenon
- **Angiographic no reflow:** In thrombus-laden lesions, degenerated saphenous vein grafts (SVGs), and after atherectomy procedures, angiographic no reflow is predominantly related to atheroembolism.

13. What are the proposed therapies for no reflow?
Pharmacologic agents:
- Anecdotal reports have shown normalization of flow with intracoronary (IC) administration of papaverine, adenosine, nicorandil, nitroprusside, verapamil, and systemic abciximab.
- Intracoronary sodium nitroprusside (direct nitric oxide donor) at doses of 50 to 1000 μg is one of the most effective therapies for no reflow.
- Rapid high-velocity IC delivery of adenosine boluses using small syringes (3 mL) at doses of 24 to 48 μg improved TIMI flow in SVG-related no reflow.
- IC verapamil (500 μg) bolus injections
- Glycoprotein (GP)IIb/IIIa failed to provide microvascular protection in patients with SVG disease (in the EPIC and EPILOG studies) and, therefore, may not be an effective therapeutic agent when used alone.

Distal protection devices: In the recent multicenter randomized SAFER trial, using the PercuSurge system for protection from distal embolization in SVGs, no reflow was reduced from 8.0% to 3.4%. Current studies are underway to determine if the device can be used in other clinical situations such as acute MI and in native coronaries.

No reflow after rotational atherectomy: The following techniques have been proposed to reduce the incidence of no reflow:
- Low burr-to-artery ratio (0.6–0.8)
- Low rotational speed (, 140,000 rpm), less platelet aggregation
- IC adenosine boluses (24–48 mg)
- IC cocktail of verapamil (10 μg/mL) + nitroglycerin (4 μg/mL) + heparin (20 IU/mL) to be infused through the sheath of the Rotablator.

BIBLIOGRAPHY

1. Abdelmeguid AE, Whitlow PL, Sapp SK, et al: Long-term outcome of transient, uncomplicated in-laboratory coronary artery closure. Circulation 91:2733–2741, 1995.
2. Barnathan ES, Schwartz JS, Taylor L, et al: Aspirin and dipyridamole in the prevention of acute coronary thrombosis complicating coronary angioplasty. Circulation 76:125–134, 1987.
3. Chew DP, Bhatt DL, Lincoff AM, et al: Defining the optimal activated clotting time during percutaneous coronary intervention: Aggregate results from 6 randomized, controlled trials. Circulation 103:961–966, 2001.
4. Ellis SG, Chew D, Chan A, et al: Death following creatine kinase-MB elevation after coronary intervention. Circulation 106:1205–1210, 2002.
5. Hilleglass WB, Dean NA, Liao L, et al: Treatment of no-reflow and impaired flow with nitric oxide donor nitroprusside following percutaneous coronary interventions: Initial human clinical experience. J Am Coll Cardiol 37:1335–1343, 2001.
6. Narins CR, Hillegass WB Jr, et al: Relation between activated clotting time during angioplasty and abrupt closure. Circulation 93:667–671, 1996.
7. Rezkalla SH, Kloner RA: No-reflow phenomenon. Circulation 105:656–662, 2002.

39. CORONARY PERFORATION AND EMERGENT CORONARY BYPASS

Hooshang Boolooki, M.D., and H. Michael Boolooki, B.S.

1. What are the indications for urgent surgical intervention during percutaneous transluminal angioplasty of coronary arteries?

Urgent surgical intervention during percutaneous transluminal coronary angioplasty (PTCA) is indicated when a coronary artery that perfuses a large segment of the myocardium suddenly occludes. The cause is acute dissection or luminal closure due to intimal plaque rupture or particle embolization. The incidence of this complication is less than 2%. Angiogram clearly shows the obstruction to coronary blood flow. The initial studies, prior to angioplasty, most likely had indicated the significance of the target coronary artery, and a surgical team should have been alerted to the planned PTCA.

Upon development of the complication, immediate electocardiographic changes of ischemia may appear and cardiac dysfunction may develop (generally in the form of tachycardia, hypotension, and segmental wall motion abnormalities) associated with chest pain. Immediate remedies include administration of coronary vasodilators and anticoagulants, along with attempts at re-opening of the obstructed coronary artery with balloon angioplasty. In the majority of cases, these maneuvers are successful in eliminating evidence of ischemia especially when the artery can be kept open with the use of a stent. Failure to achieve a TIMI III flow and hemodynamic deterioration are indications for prompt consultation with a cardiac surgery team while circulatory assistance with an intra-aortic balloon pump through the opposite femoral artery is initiated. Arrangements may be made for immediate transfer of the patient to the operating room or as soon as a room becomes available.

If repeat angiography shows satisfactory blood flow, surgical intervention may be delayed or cancelled. Otherwise, the steps indicated above with emergency use of IABP and urgent surgical intervention should be implemented.

There are extensive case reports of instances in which complications in the course of PTCA have been successfully managed with emergent coronary bypass operation. In most of these patients, the operation was performed in the form of single or double coronary bypass frequently with the use of the internal thoracic artery and by using the beating heart technique. Few large series of patients have been reported; specifically, the long-term follow up and the graft patency rates are not known.

Very few cases with follow-up echocardiograms or studies of left ventricular function have been reported. Most of the reports include an overall complication rate of 1.5–3.5% in the course of PTCA. The risk factors for failure of surgical treatment include obesity, comorbidity such as renal and pulmonary disease, need for pressor therapy in the cardiac catheterization laboratory to maintain the blood pressure, requirement for the use of percutaneous cardiopulmonary bypass for cardiac standstill or cardiac arrest, prolonged respiratory support, and prolonged period of cardiopulmonary resuscitation. It is not known if patients operated with beating heart technique or with the use of cardiopulmonary bypass have different outcomes. No early or late data have been presented comparing these two types of operative interventions. There is no doubt that long acting antiplatelet therapy for a number of days (as prophylactic therapy in preparation for PTCA) would increase the incidence of postoperative bleeding. In those patients, we believe beating heart technique for myocardial revascularization is probably associated with less bleeding. However, any methodology used for securing the coronary bypass grafts should consider complete myocardial revascularization of all major coronary arteries that are affected with precise grafting and satisfactory conduit utilization. The mortality rate of patients who have been operated emergently after PTCA complications ranges between 10 and 15%. This mortality rate in recent years (since

1994) has in fact increased somewhat in spite of a marked decrease in the incidence of compli-cations associated with PTCA. The increase in operative mortality has been attributed to comor-bidities, older age patients, and female patients.

2. What types of circulatory support can be urgently employed to reverse the course of myocardial ischemia and cardiac failure in the catheterization laboratory?

The most frequently used circulatory support device that is available in all cardiac catheter-ization laboratories is the **intra-aortic balloon pump (IABP).** The device is utilized because of its salutary effect on cardiac function by systolic unloading and by improvement in coronary blood flow. Most importantly, with IABP there is a marked decrease in myocardial oxygen con-sumption (MVO^2) simultaneous with an increase in myocardial oxygen supply. This change re-sults in a significant improvement in myocardial oxygen balance and decreases the damage from the ischemic insult. The balloon catheter can be inserted through the femoral artery used for car-diac catheterization or through the opposite femoral artery. The counterpulsation process is initi-ated and continued while diagnostic cardiac catheterization is halted for a few minutes. Once counterpulsation is successful and adequate diastolic augmentation is achieved, cardiac catheter-ization process may proceed. Diagnostic catheter advancement in the aorta is done while the intra-aortic balloon is on stand-by (deflation) mode for a few seconds. Once the catheter is engaged in the coronary artery orifice, balloon pumping can be resumed.

Percutaneous cardiopulmonary bypass (PCPB) is a helpful but highly invasive device. It is utilized when there is cardiac arrest unresponsive to cardiac massage or when there is evidence of electromechanical dissociation with minimal stroke volume. Percutaneous femoral (inflow) line is established by cannulating the femoral artery and venous (outflow) line by cannulating the femoral vein. The arterial and the venous cannulae are inserted with great care over guidewires and are advanced beyond the iliac bifurcation of the aorta and high into the inferior vena cava, respec-tively. Care must be exercised when the venous cannula is advanced. Fluoroscopic control should always be used. The guidewire at times may enter a small branch vessel and may cause perfora-tion of the iliac vein or artery with subsequent retroperitoneal hemorrhage if the cannula is threaded over it into the vein branch. When the proximal end of the venous catheter reaches the right atrium, it is secured to the thigh distally with sutures. Excellent blood flow return to the heart-lung machine can be established if the tip of the venous catheter is in the lower right atrium. A blood flow of ap-proximately 3.5–4.5 liters (for a normal adult) can be maintained with an extracorporeal membrane oxygenator (ECMO) system. During cardiac arrest, these patients require tracheal intubation and sedation. Cannula insertion in these patients should be managed by a resuscitation (CPR) team, a cardiac anesthesiologist, a cardiac surgery circulating nurse, and two physicians (or a cardiac sur-geon and a physician assistant). Both the intra-aortic balloon pump and the PCPB system are tem-porary assist devices. If the reason for diagnostic studies is correctable organic cardiac disease (valvular or coronary artery disease) and the pathology is defined, the patient should be transferred to the operating room for definitive surgical management once a stable condition is achieved.

3. Describe the pathologic anatomy and management of acute coronary occlusions (dis-section and perforation) during diagnostic catheterization and PTCA.

Coronary artery occlusions are generally in the form of acute dissection or obstruction due to lacerations caused by a catheter or guidewire passage, or because of balloon inflation or stent placement. In the operating room, depending on the extent of the lesion, hemopericardium may be present. This is due to extravasation of blood from the site of coronary perforation and dis-section. Coronary artery dissection may not be obvious immediately over the epicardial coronary arteries, although surface discoloration with a purple hue or intra-epicardial hematoma may be observed, which suggests coronary dissection. Opening the suspected coronary artery distally would show a double lumen vessel indicating acute coronary dissection. The hematoma should not be explored, and surgical endarterectomy should not be done.

Proper surgical management is coronary bypass grafting to a suitable area with acceptable diameter (> 1.5 mm) with precise anastomosis of the graft to all layers of the coronary artery wall to establish central blood flow. In urgent cases, a venous graft is appropriate; otherwise, the internal thoracic or the radial artery should be harvested and used. The coronary artery should not be probed for the fear of causing additional intimal tears. Generally, the intimal entry is high near the coronary take off and the dissection is always antegrade. There is usually only one entry point, somewhat different from acute dissection of the thoracic aorta, which may have multiple tears and reentries along its course. Establishment of blood flow within 4–6 hours of coronary occlusion via the true lumen, in majority of patients, results in a satisfactory myocardial revascularization. In these patients, acute, gross changes of the myocardium due to ischemia may be reversed as soon as revascularization is complete.

The operation may be performed with the aorta cross-clamped and by using cardioplegic infusion (by retrograde technique) or without cross-clamping the aorta. In my opinion, attempts at continuing to perfuse a coronary artery that is already dissected and is ischemic by using the beating heart technique would yield a less precise anastomosis of the graft to the coronary artery. Furthermore, attempts at placement of an intracoronary shunt within the dissected lumen of a coronary artery that has limited blood flow may cause further intimal injury and laceration of thin wall intima. Retrograde cardioplegia provides satisfactory myocardial preservation, especially of the left ventricle.

Acute coronary dissection, without luminal obstruction, may go unnoticed. Clinical presentation and symptomatology are dependent on the extent of coronary blood flow. Significant decrease in coronary flow presents clinically with hypotension and sudden changes in cardiac rhythm. Chest pain may precede these findings. Upon observation of electrocardiographic changes of myocardial ischemia, contrast injection would show a marked decrease in coronary blood flow in the affected artery. Generally, the guidewire that is already in place is used to dilate the vessel if possible and to secure the area of dissection with a stent. If this is not possible, however, and if the patient's hemodynamic condition deteriorates with hypotension (systolic pressure < 80 mmHg), immediate consideration should be given to use circulatory assist with an intra-aortic balloon pump. In the acute phase, cardiac massage and cardiopulmonary resuscitation (CPR) may be needed to maintain systemic perfusion.

It is important to note that **spontaneous coronary dissection** can occur especially in hypertensive patients (women > men). The diagnosis is made after an aortic root or left coronary artery injection. It is difficult to conclude if dissection was the cause of the clinical symptoms (chest pain, acute ECG changes and hemodynamic instability) or the presentation was due to rupture of an unstable plaque and the actual dissection was a consequence of cardiac catheterization. In any case, circulatory assist with IABP and emergency myocardial revascularization are the proper management. If the patient reaches the operating room with a stable cardiac function, there is a high chance for survival. Need for vasopressor therapy, renal and respiratory failure, as well as development of cardiac arrest and need for CPR longer than 10 minutes are risk factors for poor outcome.

Acute coronary perforation occurs when aggressive manipulation of a significantly occluded coronary artery is undertaken, especially in hypertensive patients with calcified or tortuous coronary artery. Coronary perforation generally occurs during passage of the guidewire through the coronary artery wall that goes undetected followed by enlargement of perforation during contrast angiography.

The clinical presentation may be similar to coronary dissection with electrocardiographic changes of ischemia, hypotension, chest pain, cardiac tamponade, or cardiac arrest. Free perforation of the coronary wall into the pericardial cavity will result in pericardial tamponade. Accumulation of more than a 100 cc of blood within the pericardial cavity may result in interference in right atrial filling and right ventricular contraction. Echocardiography shows external pressure over the right atrium and hindrance to the function of the right ventricle. With acute hemorrhage, some of the intra-pericardial blood will clot. The nonclotted blood is amenable to pericardial aspiration to alleviate the hemodynamic instability. Removal of a small amount of blood (20–30 cc) from the pericardial sac in a patient with tamponade may result in marked improvement in blood pressure. A soft catheter (pig-tail) may be inserted from the subxiphoid area into the pericardial cavity to decrease the intra-pericardial pressure and in preparation for transfer of the patient to the operating room. It is best that the cardiac (diagnostic) catheter and the guidewire are not pulled out from the coronary perforation, since this results in additional bleeding. The catheter can be pulled back from the groin entry site in the operating room under direct vision.

Frequently, patients who have a small coronary perforation respond to conservative management if no signs of pericardial tamponade have appeared and intra-coronary injection of contrast material has not shown extravasation into the epicardial layer or pericardial cavity. Conservative management may be associated with a short period of stability followed by catastrophic deterioration of the patient's condition. Circulatory assist with IABP may be considered but may not be helpful. In the case of active bleeding, counterpulsation with balloon assist may cause additional bleeding as a result of increase in intra-aortic pressure in the course of balloon inflation.

Generally, we prefer to correct the initial cardiac pathology (valvular and coronary disease, etc.) during the emergency procedure. However, in certain patient groups, this plan should be modified. These patients include Jehovah's Witness patients who have had a large amount of blood loss (to Hbg < 8 g/L) and patients who have developed cardiac arrest and have required more than 10 minutes of external cardiac massage. Another group are patients who have received a long acting antiplatelet agent (clopidogrel) before the coronary artery pathology was defined. In these situations, pericardial drainage is done urgently and the other cardiac pathology is dealt with after a few weeks of recovery.

The perforated coronary artery usually seals by clots and may not be bleeding at the time of pericardial exploration. Since the epicardial layer of the pericardium covering the coronary arteries is a very strong tissue, after the initial perforation and bleeding, it may prevent further extravasation of blood. The site of coronary perforation rarely needs surgical exploration or suturing unless it is actively bleeding with an expanding hematoma.

4. Do decisions for surgical intervention and use of circulatory support depend on which coronary artery is damaged?

The significance of the obstruction of a coronary vessel is directly dependent upon the extent of the myocardium that it perfuses. **The left anterior descending coronary artery (LAD)** generally perfuses the entire anterior (and with the diagonal artery the lateral) wall of the left ventricle and (with the septal perforators) close to 90% of the ventricular septum. Sudden occlusion of this artery high at its take-off results in approximately a 40% decrease in the left ventricular function acutely and may lead to cardiogenic shock and cardiac arrest.

Sudden obstruction of **the left main coronary artery** also may result in sudden death or cardiogenic shock. For these reasons, significant (>70%) obstructions at the take-off of LAD coronary artery or within the left main trunk have the highest priority in receiving coronary bypass grafts and in urgent situations with signs of acute coronary syndrome in use of temporary circulatory assistance. Significant obstruction of LAD high at its take-off necessitates immediate surgical intervention. Intravascular manipulation (PTCA) of a non-supported left main coronary artery or LAD is considered a high risk undertaking and at times is performed with elective use of an intra-aortic balloon pump.

A dominant **right coronary artery** that is injured by dissection or perforation or is occluded suddenly may cause bradyarrhythmia or cardiac standstill, especially when the proximal section of the artery is involved. Placement of an intravenous pacemaker lead (to treat bradyarrhythmia) and counterpulsation support with IABP may alleviate the problem temporarily. PCP bypass may be needed if cardiac arrest does not quickly respond to CPR.

Sudden occlusion of a large **dominant circumflex coronary artery** that supplies the left lateral wall and the posterior septum may cause acute hemodynamic instability and mitral valve incompetence leading to pulmonary edema and need for circulatory assist with an intra-aortic balloon pump or percutaneous cardiopulmonary bypass. The clinical presentation of mild congestive heart failure in these patients may become aggravated during left ventriculography.

In general, when such vessels are considered for percutaneous intravascular revascularization, an intra-aortic balloon setup should be readily available (on standby) and at times should be used electively prior to intra-coronary manipulation and angioplasty. The surgical team should be notified prior to high-risk angioplasty. Emergency myocardial revascularization (within 4 hours of coronary occlusion) is necessary to alter the course of an evolving myocardial infarction due to acute occlusion of a major coronary artery. Therefore, surgical intervention and use of circulatory assist devices are dependent on the anatomy and functional significance of the coronary artery.

5. Should hemopericardium due to coronary artery perforation be managed by needle aspiration or by surgical drainage (pericardial window)?

Needle aspiration of the hemopericardium (due to coronary artery perforation or cardiac injury) is preserved for patients with large pericardial effusions with clinical signs of pericardial tamponade. The feasibility and rapid preparation for needle aspiration of the pericardial fluid make this the procedure of choice in emergent situations. In acute cases, pericardial aspiration serves only as a temporary evacuation measure lasting no more than a few minutes or hours. Leaving a drainage catheter (pig-tail) in the pericardial cavity with a syringe (for aspiration purposes) attached to it and transferring the patient immediately to the operating room are the method of management that we use. The operation is performed using various incisions, frequently limited in size. A small subxiphoid incision and tube drainage (window) are adequate for large effusions that are chronic in nature. In acute situations, a small left anterior thoracotomy and/or median sternotomy is performed depending on the location of injury. Circumflex coronary and its marginal branches and the anterior descending artery injuries may be managed with a left thoracotomy incision, which leads directly over the injury site. However, in patients in whom a definitive surgical procedure has to be done (such as multiple coronary bypass operations and/or valvular heart surgery), a median sternotomy incision is needed.

BIBLIOGRAPHY

 1. Andreasen JJ, Mortensen PE, Andersen LI, et al: Emergency coronary artery bypass surgery after failed percutaneous transluminal coronary angioplasty. Scand Cardiovasc J 34:242–246, 2000.
 2. Bolooki H: Clinical Application of Intra-aortic Balloon Pump, 3rd ed. Armonk, NY, Futura Publishing, 1998.
 3. Bonacchi M, Prifti E, Giunti G, et al: Emergency management of spontaneous coronary artery dissection. JCV Surg 43:189–193, 2002.
 4. Boylan MJ, Lytle BW, Taylor PC, et al: Have PTCA failures requiring emergent bypass operations changed? Ann Thorac Surg 59:283–287, 1995.
 5. Carcagni A, Camellini M, Maiello L, et al: Percutaneous transluminal coronary revascularization in women: higher risk of dissection and need for stenting. Ital Heart J 1:536–541, 2000.
 6. Fukutomi T, Suzuki T, Popma JJ, et al: Early and late clinical outcomes following coronary perforation in patients undergoing percutaneous coronary intervention. Circulation J 66:349–356, 2002.
 7. Gruberg L, Pinnow E, Flood R, et al: Incidence, management, and outcome of coronary artery perforation during percutaneous coronary intervention. Am J Cardiol 86:680–682, 2000.
 8. Lazar HL, Jacobs AK, Aldea GS, et al: Factors influencing mortality after emergency coronary artery bypass grafting for failed percutaneous transluminal coronary angioplasty. Ann Thorac Surg 64:1747–1752, 1997.
 9. Mitsui N, Koyama T, Marui A, et al: Experience with emergency cardiac surgery following institution of percutaneous cardiopulmonary support. Artif Organs 23:496–499, 1999.
10. Reinecke H, Fetsch T, Roeder N, et al: Emergency coronary artery bypass grafting after failed coronary angioplasty: What has changed in a decade? Ann Thorac Surg 70:1997–2003, 2000.
11. Singh M, Nuttall GA, Ballman KV, et al: Effect of abciximab on the outcome of emergency coronary artery bypass grafting after failed percutaneous coronary intervention. Mayo Clin Proc 76:784–788, 2001.

VIII. Medical and Peripheral Complications

40. RENAL INSUFFICIENCY AND ATHEROEMBOLISM

Cesar Jara, M.D.

1. How does renal insufficiency affect percutaneous coronary intervention (PCI) outcome?

Patients with renal insufficiency have a poor outcome after PCI. There is a direct relationship between renal insufficiency and mortality after PCI, as high as 25% after 1 year in diabetic patients. There is also a higher incidence of restenosis, with a reported 50% in some series.

Patients with contrast-induced nephropathy (CIN) and acute renal failure have the worst outcome, with an in-hospital mortality of 25%. Therefore, careful selection of patients for PCI is mandatory when renal failure is present.

2. What is the most common cause of renal insufficiency after PCI?

The leading cause of renal insufficiency after PCI is CIN. Other important causes are hypovolemia (from bleeding, fasting, diuresis), low cardiac output, aortic dissection, malposition of intraaortic balloon pump, drugs, atheroembolism, and bladder obstruction.

3. What is CIN?

CIN is the new onset or exacerbation of renal dysfunction after contrast administration (absent other causes) with an increase of greater than 0.5 mg/dL or by greater than 25% from baseline serum creatinine.

4. What causes CIN?

There are several mechanisms for contrast media to induce renal damage, such as direct injury to the renal tubular cell and intrarenal vasoconstriction, affecting especially the renal medulla, with subsequent hypoxemia, free radicals, oxidative stress, and apoptosis. Diabetic patients particularly show exaggerated vasoreactivity responses to contrast media. A high osmotic load with increased blood viscosity produces diuresis and more medullary injury.

5. How long does it take between a coronary intervention and the onset of CIN?

CIN usually occurs 24 to 48 hours after contrast exposure, with creatinine peaking 5 to 7 days later and returning to normal within 7 to 10 days in most patients. Oliguria can be present in 30% of patients and carries a worse prognosis.

6. How common is CIN after PCI?

The overall incidence is 3%. However, the incidence of CIN is clearly determined by the patient population undergoing PCI. In the general population, it is less than 1%; it increases to 5% in patients with prior renal insufficiency. In diabetics with creatinine levels between 2 to 4 mg/dL, it is approximately 25% and it is up to 80% in diabetic patients if the preprocedure creatinine is greater than 4 mg/dL.

7. List the risk factors for CIN after PCI.
- Chronic renal insufficiency
- Diabetes mellitus with renal insufficiency
- Intravascular volume depletion
- Congestive heart failure
- Nephrotic syndrome
- Myeloma
- Hypotension
- Nephrotoxic drugs
- Large volume of contrast

8. How can CIN during PCI be prevented?
First any modifiable risk factor for CIN (e.g., treat decompensated heart failure, hypovolemia; remove nephrotoxic drugs such as nonsteroidal antiinflammatory drugs) should be corrected.

Second, in patients with a creatinine of greater than 2.0 mg/dL, especially if diabetes mellitus is present, infusion of saline and fenoldopam should be started. Other agents used are N-acetylcysteine and non-ionic, low osmolar dye, although the benefits are controversial (Table 1).

Third, during PCI, contrast load should be minimized and adequate hemodynamic status (i.e., avoid hypotension, arrhythmias, heart failure) should be maintained. There are several definitions for "low" contrast volume, 100 cc being the most acceptable cutoff point.

There is no role for the routine use of mannitol, furosemide, calcium channel blockers, or low-dose dopamine; these could actually be deleterious.

Table 1. Prevention of Contrast-induced Nephropathy

DRUG	COMMENT
IV saline	1.0–1.5 cc/kg/h 0.45% NS 6–12 hours before PCI or 0.5 cc/kg/h 0.45% NS 6–12 hours before PCI if EF < 30% Maintain hydration for 12 hours after PCI
Fenoldopam	Start 1 to 2 hours before PCI, titrate from 0.05 μg/kg/min up to 0.1 μg/kg/min every 20 min. Discontinue if SBP < 90 mmHg despite reducing dose to one half or one third. Maintain infusion for 4–12 hours after PCI. Can be abruptly discontinued (half-life is 5 min). This is a specific dopamine-1 receptor agonist that prevents vasoconstriction.
N-acetylcysteine	600 mg PO bid the day before and on the day of PCI. This is an antioxidant with controversial benefit.

9. What is the risk of metformin in CIN?
Metformin does not cause CIN. If renal failure develops after PCI, metformin use is associated with lactic acidosis, with a high mortality, up to 30% to 50%; therefore, it is recommended to withhold its use for 48 hours after intervention, until renal failure has been ruled out.

10. What is the incidence of aortic atheroembolism during coronary intervention?
The true incidence is unknown. Retrieval of atheroembolic material from catheters and incidental autopsy findings of cholesterol embolization are reported to be as high as 10% to 25%. Clinically important atheroembolism is rare (< 0.2%) and includes stroke (0.07%); atheroembolic renal failure (occurs > 1 week after procedure, unlike CIN); and peripheral manifestations (e.g., livedo reticularis, petechiae, digital infarction or gangrene, purple toe, Hollenhorst plaques [cholesterol crystals in retinal artery], and splinter hemorrhage).

Blood tests suggestive of atheroembolism are eosinophilia (> 3% or > 350 eosinophil absolute count), eosinophiluria, high sedimentation rate, and elevation in creatinine 1 week after intervention.

Another form of atheroembolic disease is distal coronary atheroembolization. Frequently overlooked, it is of clinical importance because damage to the coronary microcirculation reflected by troponin or creatine phosphokinase (CPK) release is associated with an adverse late outcome.

Although seen more often with debulking techniques, elevation in markers of myocardial necrosis has been reported in up to 20% of patients after PCI.

11. Which patients are at risk of aortic atheroembolization during PCI?

Every patient is at risk! A meticulous technique should be always used to prevent it. Certainly, some patients are at higher risk of atheroembolism; these include patients with a history of embolic event; severe peripheral vascular disease, especially aortic disease (e.g., aneurysm); very tortuous aorta; transesophageal echocardiography (TEE) findings of protruding aortic atheromas; and indication of procedure for acute coronary syndrome. This last factor illustrates the presence of a systemic hypercoagulable state, which affects unstable plaques in different vascular regions.

12. How is aortic atheroembolism prevented?

The use of long wires (260 cm) to exchange catheters, allowing backbleeding after wire removal, advancing catheters over the wire to minimize "scraping" of the aorta, avoiding long catheter or wire manipulation at the aortic arch, and adequate anticoagulation are some recommended measures. Radial or brachial approach still carries a risk of embolic cardiovascular accident, especially in the vertebrobasilar bed.

13. Is there any treatment for atheroembolic stroke?

Acute stroke during PCI can also be hemorrhagic from antiplatelet and antithrombotic therapy. After this condition has been excluded with a plain brain computed tomography scan, expeditious catheter-based therapy with neurovascular angiography, gentle mechanical fragmentation of the embolus, and careful dosage of lytic or antiplatelet agent has been reported to be associated with a favorable outcome.

BIBLIOGRAPHY

1. Al-Mubarak N, Vitek J, Mousa I, et al: Immediate catheter-based neurovascular rescue for acute stroke complicating coronary procedures. Am J Card 90:173–176, 2002.
2. Briguori C, Manganelli F, Scarpato P, et al: Acetylcysteine and contrast agent-associated nephrotoxicity. J Am Coll Cardiol 40:298–303, 2002.
3. Ellis S: Elective coronary angioplasty: technique and complications. In Topol E (ed): Textbook of Interventional Cardiology, 3rd ed. Philadelphia, W.B. Saunders Company, 1999, pp 147–162.
4. Hill J: Radiographic contrast agents. In Pepine C, Hill J, Lambert C (eds): Diagnostic and Therapeutic Cardiac Catheterization, 2nd ed. Baltimore, Williams & Wilkins, 1994, pp 183–194.
5. Kini A, Mitre C, Kamran M, et al: Changing trends in incidence and predictors of radiographic contrast nephropathy after percutaneous coronary intervention with use of fenoldopam. Am J Cardiol 89: 999–1002, 2002.
6. Lepor N, Maydoon H, McCullough P, et al: Radiocontrast Nephropathy: Managing the High-risk Patient. CD Program/Monograph. Los Angeles, Institute of Medical Education, 2001.
7. Rihal C, Textor S, Grill D, et al: Incidence and prognostic importance of acute renal failure after percutaneous intervention. Circulation 105:2259–2264, 2002.
8. Saklayen M, Gupta S, Suryaprasad A, et al: Incidence of atheroembolic renal failure after coronary angiography: A prospective study. Angiology 48:609–613, 1997.
9. Scanlon P, Faxon D, Audet A, et al: ACC/AHA Guidelines for coronary angiography. J Am Coll Cardiol 33:1756–1824, 1999.
10. Shmuely H, Zoldan J, Sagie A, et al: Acute stroke after coronary angiography associated with protruding mobile thoracic aortic atheromas. Neurology 49:1689–1691, 1997.
11. Tumlin J, Wang A, Murray P, et al: Fenoldopam mesylate blocks reductions in renal plasma flow after radiocontrast dye infusion: A pilot trial in the prevention of contrast nephropathy. Am Heart J 143: 894–903, 2002.

41. HEMATOMA, BLEEDING, AND INFECTION

Juan C. Sotomonte, M.D.

1. What are the possible bleeding complications related to a percutaneous cardiac catheterization?

Local vascular complications at the site of catheter insertion are the most commonly seen complications after cardiac catheterization. Most of the time, they are related to poorly placed punctures, vessel lacerations, excessive anticoagulation, and poor technique. Because the femoral approach is most often used, bleeding in this particular case can be seen as a free hemorrhage, femoral hematoma, or retroperitoneal bleeding, most of which become evident within the first 12 hours after the procedure. With brachial and radial approaches, bleeding can also be free or into the surrounding soft tissues. Of particular concern is the development of compression syndromes, which can lead ultimately to limb loss, one of the most feared complications.

2. How do the American College of Cardiology (ACC)/American Heart Association (AHA) practice guidelines define procedure-related bleeds?

A revised guideline from the ACC/AHA establishes vascular site complications as one of the possible six basic categories of complications from cardiac interventional procedures. According to the guidelines, bleeding is defined as blood loss at the site of vascular access caused by a transverse artery or vein requiring transfusion or prolonged hospital stay or a decrease in the hemoglobin level of more than 3 mg/dL.

3. What are the possible types of bleeding related to percutaneous cardiac catheterization?

Bleeding can be classified as free if there is poor vascular access control at the site of puncture during or after the procedure. These complications occur more frequently while obtaining access and positioning sheaths or early after removal when local pressure can not be applied and hemostasis is not properly achieved. Bleeding can also occur into the surrounding soft tissues; this situation is the most common vascular event and is not considered a significant complication unless it has a diameter of more than 10 cm. The incidence of local hematomas varies from 1% to 7%, and most of them require no further intervention. Approximately 7% require blood transfusion either because of local bleeding or retroperitoneal expansion or gastrointestinal bleeding. Especially with high punctures above the inguinal ligament, where initial hemostasis is difficult to achieve, retroperitoneal accumulation of blood can occur. Most frequently, retroperitoneal hematomas localize in the pelvic and paracolic spaces.

4. When may a retroperitoneal hematoma occur?

When the front or back arterial wall is punctured above the inguinal ligament, blood can spread into the retroperitoneal space because the inguinal ligament serves as an anatomical barrier between the pelvic and infrainguinal spaces. It is usually not evident on the surface but should be considered when a patient has new onset of hypotension, flank pain, or decreased hematocrit level. Ultrasound or computed tomography (CT) scan, usually localizing hematomas in the pelvic or pararenal recesses, can confirm diagnosis. Treatment is usually expectant and supportive rather than surgical unless major hemodynamic compromise is present. Peripheral balloon angioplasty can also be used to occlude the site of bleeding.

5. How can retroperitoneal bleeding be prevented?

Careful identification of the puncture site to avoid entry at the common femoral near or above the inguinal ligament is the most successful way to prevent retroperitoneal hematomas. Pseudoaneurysms may form or coexist. Fluoroscopic localization of the skin nick to overlie the inferior border of the femoral head avoids misplacement of the puncture site; this prevents vascular complications, especially aneurysm formation secondary to puncture of the superficial femoral artery or profunda because only soft tissue surrounds these structures and the vessel cannot be adequately compressed when the sheaths are removed. Localization of the puncture site by the inguinal crease is a particularly poor way of obtaining adequate access because it is inaccurate in more than 60% of patients. The best way to localize the optimal site of puncture is to identify the mid segment of the common femoral artery (i.e., where the femoral pulse is felt with more intensity).

6. How does the site of vascular access influence the incidence of bleeding complications?

Most interventional procedures are performed via femoral access; the overall incidence of complications from this site is approximately 1% to 3%. Other approaches such as the radial or brachial approaches have a much lower incidence of bleeding complications. Recent trials have reported no bleeding complications from radial access; however, most centers perform as much as 90% of the interventions from the femoral site, which has a higher procedural success rate and allows the usage of broader interventional technologies.

7. What are the most frequent complications after the femoral approach?

Initial extensive free bleeding occurring around the artery suggests laceration of the artery. If this complication takes place during the procedure, a larger size sheath should be inserted. The site can be compressed and heparin reversed. More common than free bleeding is the occurrence of local hematoma, a collection of blood within the soft tissues, which usually resolves in the first 2 weeks as blood spreads and reabsorbs. Occasionally, femoral nerve compression and accompanying limb weakness may occur and may take more than 2 weeks to resolve.

8. What are the advantages of the transradial approach?

Although technically challenging and somewhat more time consuming than femoral techniques, radial approaches allow earlier ambulation times and sooner discharges for ambulatory procedures. Patient predilection could be as high as 75% for the radial approach. Also, it is important to recognize that there is a significant decrease in workload for hemostasis achievement. The feasibility of intervention is excellent, approaching 90% for diagnostic procedures. As a result of lower need for hospital stay and lower rates of complications, a significant reduction in cost is also a factor to consider, having close to a 15% decrease in hospital charges. The rate of complications and cost effectiveness remains higher when radial or brachial approaches are compared with femoral access even if arteriotomy closure devices are used.

9. What factors predispose patients to vascular access site bleeding?
Patient-related factors
  Older age
  Obesity
  Calcified vessels
  Hypertension
  High blood pressure
  Female gender
  Early ambulation
  Use of multiple antiplatelets agents, use of anticoagulants, coagulopathy, thrombocytopenia
Procedure- or operator-related factors
  Back wall puncture
  Low or high puncture
  Multiple attempts to obtain vascular access
  Larger sheath size
  Angulation of sheath

Prolonged procedures
Prolonged in-dwelling sheath time
Higher ACT levels
Operator inexperience
Poor hemostasis or pressure

10. What is the incidence of vascular complications with the use of antiplatelet agents such as glycoprotein IIb/IIIa inhibitors?

Earlier studies, such as the EPIC trial, a randomized trial of the use of abciximab in percutaneous coronary interventions (PCIs), showed that the incidence of vascular complications (i.e., major vascular access site bleed with a decrease in hematocrit level > 15%, minor bleeding, or the need for surgical repair) occurred in 12% of patients receiving bolus plus abciximab infusion as opposed to 1.4% in the placebo group. All types of bleed occurred in 21.8% of patients treated with abciximab as opposed to 9.1% in the placebo group. Predictors of bleeding were the use of abciximab, acute myocardial infarction (MI) at the time of enrollment, higher baseline hematocrit level, duration of procedure, higher body weight, female gender, and maximum ACT reached in the catheterization laboratory. This results have been attributed mainly to the use of unadjusted doses of heparin; if the heparin dose is reduced to 70% of the usual, maintaining a prothrombin time 1.5 to 2.5 times normal, the incidence of vascular complications is significantly lower, although it is still higher compared with unfractionated or low molecular weight heparin alone. Other factors contributing to the decrease in bleeding complications are the fact that heparin is usually discontinued right after intervention is performed, vascular sheaths are removed only when ACT values are below 150, and there has been a trend to increase use of arteriotomy closure devices. Fatal bleeding or intracranial hemorrhage is very infrequent in this setting, and bleeding complications tend to be transient and well tolerated in most cases.

11. What is the incidence of bleeding complications with the use of other antiplatelet agents such as the thienopyridines?

Results from earlier experience in the CAPRIE trial did not show a significant difference in bleeding complications when aspirin was compared with clopidogrel in the setting of recent atherosclerotic vascular disease. In the CURE trial, a randomized trial of the use aspirin and clopidogrel in acute coronary syndromes, the incidence of bleeding not related to coronary artery bypass graft surgery was significantly increased when both agents were used; the rates of major bleeding were 2.7% versus 3.7%, respectively. Minor bleeding occurred twice as frequently when newer antiplatelet agents were used. It is important to clarify that in these trials, bleeding was not necessarily restricted to those related to cardiac catheterization procedures; hence, direct assumptions cannot be made, but because it was clear that all type of bleeding were increased, caution should be taken when performing interventional procedures in this particular setting.

12. Are hematomas related to other vascular complications?

Hematomas are the most frequent complication after PCI; although some are related to the formation of a pseudoaneurysm, most are isolated hematomas that will resolve and reabsorb spontaneously. Hematomas may be difficult to recognize in obese patients, but other signs of vascular compromise such as nerve palsy or vagal reactions from bleeding may occur earlier and point to the diagnosis of hematomas. Nerve compression should be suspected when pain is out of proportion to the size of the hematoma because nerve compression is more likely to occur when a pseudoaneurysm is present.

13. Is there a difference in bleeding complications between coronary interventions and diagnostic procedures?

The overall incidence of complications related to percutaneous transluminal coronary angioplasty (PTCA) has been reported from 0.9% to 9.0%. Most authors report an incidence ranging from 1% to 3%. After adjustment for multiple variables, the performance of intervention seems not to increase the incidence of bleeding complications by itself. In most instances, the usage of larger sheath sizes and higher levels of anticoagulation account for the difference in bleeding complications from diagnostic as opposed to interventional procedures. During earlier experience, bleeding was more frequent during intracoronary stenting than standard balloon angioplasty or extraction atherectomy (14.0%, 3.2%, and 12.5%, respectively). These results probably reflect the mandatory use of Coumadin anticoagulation after stent deployment, which is not currently considered standard therapy.

14. How do vascular complications influence general hospital outcomes?

Peripheral vascular complications defined as pulse loss, hematoma, or pseudoaneurysm have an important correlation with death, myocardial infarction (MI), emergent CABG, or abrupt vessel closure after PCI. If vascular complications are present, the incidence of such outcomes is more frequent. Predictors of higher risk are older age, female gender, postprocedural use of heparin, and intraaortic balloon pump use. In-hospital costs are greatly affected by the occurrence of vascular complications. There is an additional increase in long-term mortality in this group, suggesting that these patients require a closer long-term follow-up.

15. Is there any advantage to the use of arteriotomy closure devices (ACDs)?

Although earlier hemostasis is achieved with the use of these devices, vascular complications, including hematoma, decrease in hematocrit level, or need for surgical repair, tend to occur more frequently when ACDs are used. This was much more pronounced in earlier reports when experience with this type of devices was limited; currently, there is a tendency toward a decrease in vascular complications compared with other hemostasis-achieving devices, and the rate of complications is almost comparable to those occurring when manual compression is used for hemostasis achievement. Independent predictors of vascular complications in this particular setting are increasing age, smaller body size, and female gender.

16. What are the differences in vascular complications with the use of different vascular closure devices?

Vascular closure devices offer a tempting option when anticoagulation or antiplatelet therapy cannot be interrupted or when earlier ambulation is desired for improvement of patient comfort. Most devices (e.g., biosealants, collagen plugs, percutaneous sutures, and compression devices) have similar safety profiles and effectiveness when achieving hemostasis. Of note is the fact that no major differences in outcomes have been demonstrated among different devices and that although they have many potential beneficial effects (e.g., allowance of earlier ambulation), a new spectrum of complications can be introduced, such as device embolization, entrapment, and vascular injuries.

17. What is the optimal length of bedrest after arterial puncture?

The optimal time for bedrest after femoral catheterization has not been well established; however, traditionally, the minimal amount of time required is at least 6 hours after hemostasis has been achieved. A recent study showed that reducing the time to 2 hours had no difference in major vascular complications compared with 4 or 6 hours. Most authors agree that at least 1 hour per French size of the arterial sheath is required for higher safety; therefore, the minimal time is usually 4 hours. Although dual access (i.e., venous and arterial) predisposes patients to a higher risk of bleeding, it does not require further delay in time to ambulation.

18. What is the incidence of bacteremia after invasive cardiac procedure?

Because PCIs are such a successful way of revascularization, an increasing number of procedures are performed every day. Infectious complications, although infrequent, may account for significant morbidity and mortality. The overall incidence of bacteremia after any type of nonsurgical invasive cardiac procedure is 0.11%. If the procedure is a diagnostic cardiac catheterization, infection rates approach 0.6%; it is 0.8% for electrophysiologic studies and 0.24% after

PTCA. The time to detection is usually 1.7 days after the procedure is performed, and the hospital stay is significantly prolonged if infection is present.

19. What are the possible bacterial complications of PCI?

The incidence of PTCA-related bacteremia ranges from 0.1% to 0.6% of cases with no particular clustering of events in time. Approximately 20% of patients will have more than one organism identified, and when single blood cultures are positive for organisms, coagulase-negative *Staphylococcus aureus* is the most frequently identified organism. Most of the organisms are not classified as active infection but are the result of local contamination. It was initially reported that access via the brachial artery could be related more frequently to infections because the possibility of cut down and open exposure implied a higher risk of infection. Infection can be local at the site of puncture and present as cellulitis, endarteritis, phlebitis, or mycotic aneurysms. Local dissemination can lead to septic arthritis, osteomyelitis, or epidural abcess formation, and hematogenous spread can present as septic emboli, endocarditis, endophthalmitis, or metastatic infections. There is no significant difference in infection rate whether the procedure is a diagnostic catheterization or an interventional procedure.

20. What are the most frequent organisms encountered in PCI-related infections?

MICROORGANISM	FREQUENCY, %
Staphylococcus aureus	51.0
Coagulase-negative staphylococci	33.0
Klebsiella pneumoniae and *K. oxytoca*	4.0
Group B streptococci	2.2
Pseudomonas aeruginosa	2.0
Enterococci	1.0
Escherichia coli	<1.0
Proteus mirabilis	<1.0
Diphtheroids	<1.0

21. What are the risk factors for bacteremia after coronary angioplasty?

RISK FACTOR	OR	95% CI	P
Congestive heart failure	43.3	4.2–447.4	0.002
Catheterizations at same site, n	4.0	1.3–12.4	0.015
Difficult vascular access	14.9	2.1–108.4	0.007
Sheath in place > 24 hours	6.8	1.3–35.9	0.025
Duration of procedure, hours	2.9	1.0–8.1	0.040
In-dwelling bladder catheter	2.0	N/A	0.010
History of valvular disease	N/A	N/A	N/A

CI = confidence interval; OR = odds ratio.

22. How can infection be diagnosed?

Diagnosis is based on clinical, microbiologic, and radiographic evidence. Patients may manifest fevers or local inflammatory signs such as purulence, hematoma, erythema, tenderness, leukocytosis, or band forms. Detection time varies from 24 hours to 20 days. It is important to note that when fever occurs within a few hours (< 6 hours) after a cardiac catheterization has been performed, other causes for a pyrogenic reaction should be considered such as various allergic reactions to latex products, contrast agents, medications, and other chemicals used during the procedure.

23. Is antibiotic prophylaxis recommended before PCI?

The ACC/AHA does not recommend antibiotic prophylaxis for cardiac catheterization in any given circumstances. Some authors advocate that patients requiring repeat catheterization ipsilaterally may benefit from it, but experts' opinions and consensus meetings have recommended against it.

BIBLIOGRAPHY

1. American College of Cardiology: Cardiology Board Certification Review Guide for Interventional Cardiology, Vascular Access Complications and Bleeding Complications. Bethesda, MD, ACC, pp 102–109a.
2. Baim D, Grossman W (eds): Cardiac Catheterization: Angiography and Intervention, 5th ed. Philadelphia, Williams & Wilkins, 1996, pp 17–38.
3. Clopidogrel in Unstable Angina to Prevent Recurrent Events Trial investigators: Effects of clopidogrel in addition to aspirin in patients with acute coronary syndromes without ST segment elevation. N Eng J Med 345:494–502, 2001.
4. Culver D, Chua J, Rehm S, et al: Arterial infection and Staphylococcus aureus bacteremia after transfemoral cannulation for percutaneous carotid angioplasty and stenting. J Vasc Surg 35:576–579, 2002.
5. Dangas G, Menran R, Kokolis S et al: Vascular complications after percutanues coronary interventions following hemostasis with manual versus arteriotomy closure devices. J Am Coll Cardiol 83:638–641, 2001.
6. Kiemeneij F, Jan Laarman G, Odekerken, D et al: A randomized comparison of percutaneous transluminal coronary angioplasty by the radial, brachial and femoral approaches: the Access study. J Am Coll Cardiol 29:1269–1275, 1997.
7. Mann T, Cubeddu G, Bowen J, et al: Stenting in acute coronary syndromes: a comparison of radial versus femoral access sites. J Am Coll Cardiol 32:572–576, 1998.
8. Munoz P, Blanco J, Rodrigues-Creixems M, et al: Bloodstream infections after invasive nonsurgical cardiological procedures. Arch Intern Med 161:2110–2115, 2001.
9. Rosenfield K, Goldstein J, Safian R, et al: Medical and peripheral complications. In Safian R, Freed M, (eds): The Manual of Interventional Cardiology, 3rd ed. Royal Oak, MI, Physicians Press, 2001.
10. Samore M, Wessolossky M, Lewis S, et al: Frequency, risk factors, and outcome for bacteremia after percutaneous transluminal coronary angioplasty. Am J Cardiol 79:873–877, 1997.
11. Schulman S, Goldschmidt-Clermont P, Topol E: Effects of integrelin, a platelet glycoprotein IIb/IIIa receptor antagonist, in unstable angina. Circulation 94:2083–2089, 1996.
12. Smith SC, JR, Dove JT, Jacobs AK, et al: ACC/AHA guidelines for percutaneous coronary intervention: a report of the American College of Cardiology/American Heart Association Task Force on Practice Guidelines (Committee to Revise the 1993 Guidelines for Percutaneous Transluminal Angioplasty). J Am Coll Cardiol 37:2239i–2239lxvi, 2001.
13. TCT abstracts and oral presentations. Am J Cardiol 31G–33G:111G–113G, 2001.

42. PSEUDOANEURYSM, ARTERIOVENOUS FISTULA, DISSECTION, AND OTHER VASCULAR COMPLICATIONS

Neerav Shah, M.D., and Eduardo de Marchena, M.D.

1. What are the incidences for pseudoaneurysms and arteriovenous (AV) fistulas during cardiac catherization?

For diagnostic catheterization procedures, the incidence ranges from 0.05% to 0.8% and increases to 0.4% to 3% for interventional procedures.

2. What is a pseudoaneurysm, and how does one differentiate it from a hematoma?

A pseudoaneurysm is a hematoma that remains in continuity with the arterial puncture site, allowing flow in and out of the hematoma during systole and diastole. It has no true arterial wall structures (adventitia or media) and is therefore not considered a true aneurysm. It can be differentiated from a simple hematoma by the presence of a bruit and a palpable pulsatile mass.

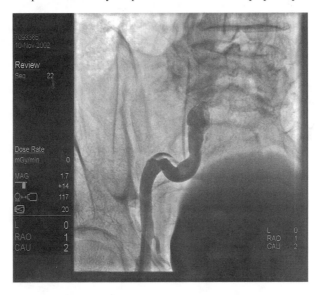

FIGURE 1. Anteroposterior projection of right iliac arteriogram demonstrating a non-flow limiting dissection caused by vascular sheath.

3. What factors increase the likelihood of a vascular complication during cardiac catheterization?

- Older age
- Obesity
- Female gender
- Larger sheath size
- Increased time duration of sheath in place
- Low arterial puncture below the common femoral bifurcation
- Peripheral vascular disease

4. What are the key factors in limiting the formation of a pseudoaneurym?
- Accurate puncture in the common femoral artery $\rightarrow$ Low punctures such as in the superficial femoral artery and profunda femoralis increase the likelihood of complications, because they are smaller caliber vessels and they are below the pelvis, making compression more difficult
- Effective hemostasis

5. What treatment options exist for pseudoaneurysms?
- Surgery
- Ultrasound-guided compression
- Direct thrombin injection
- Observation
- Endovascular placement of a covered stent

6. Name the factors that decrease the likelihood of a pseudoaneurysm being closed by ultrasound-guided compression.
- Size > 8 cm
- Presence of AV fistula
- Anticoagulation

7. How can ultrasound-guided compression be used to treat a pseudoaneurysm?
The principle is to convert the pseudoaneursym to a thrombosed hematoma by compressing the neck under direct visualization, thus stopping flow. After selected intervals, flow can be reassessed and if flow persists, further compression can be performed. If unsuccessful or only partial thrombosis is achieved, the patient can return for additional sessions. Because the pseudoaneurysm is not repaired only thrombosed, follow-up ultrasound should be performed to evaluate for recurrence.

8. Can some pseudoaneurysms be watched? What is the risk if nothing is done?
Only the smallest pseudoaneurysms (those measuring $< 2–3$ cm) should be watched. These may spontaneously thrombose. However, most pseudoaneurysms can become larger and ultimately rupture if they become large enough.

9. Is the incidence of vascular complications higher with closure devices?
Early studies showed a high rate of vascular complications with closure devices ranging from 9% to 16%. As the technology has improved, the incidence of vascular complications has decreased to the range of 2–3%. Furthermore, some studies in the setting of percutaneous coronary intervention with glycoprotein IIb/IIIa inhibitors have shown a lower incidence of complications compared with manual compression. This may be a result of more effective initial hemostasis.

10. What is the management of guidewire-associated iliac or femoral dissection?
Although guidewire dissection can result in pain, it is often not flow limiting. This is because antegrade flow is in the opposite direction of the dissection plane, allowing flow to continue forward. If necessary, contralateral access can be obtained and balloon angioplasty or stenting can be performed on the dissected vessel. If conservative management is planned, close monitoring of distal pulses should be performed, and, if necessary, vascular surgery consultation should be obtained.

11. After sheath removal for a cardiac catheterization, a patient complains of ipsilateral leg pain and on physical examination has a cool extremity and a diminished pulse. What is the diagnosis, and what is the next step in management?
The likely diagnosis is arterial thrombosis at the access site. The incidence is less than 1% after intervention. Typical presentation includes complaints of pain or numbness with diminished pulse, a cool extremity, and possibly cyanosis or pallor. The initial management is heparinization,

duplex scan of the lower extremity, pain control, and vascular surgery consultation. Angiography may also be required to confirm and guide therapy.

12. What are risk factors for thrombotic occlusion at a vascular access site?

- Older age
- Peripheral vascular disease
- Hypercoagulable states (e.g., lupus, protein C or S deficiency, PCV, myeloma, paraneoplastic syndrome, thrombocytosis)
- Small body habitus
- Female gender
- Small caliber vessels

13. What complications can be attributed to atheroembolic phenomena from a cardiac catherization?

- "Blue toe syndrome" (i.e., embolization into the peripheral vascular bed)
- CVA
- Livido reticularis or necrotizing fasciitis (cutaneous manifestions of atheroemboli)
- Arterial ischemia
- Renal failure (usually insidious with an onset of weeks or months after catheterization)

14. What are the clinical manifestations of AV fistulas?

AV fistulas can present days after a cardiac catheterization (Fig. 2). A continuous bruit at the access site can be heard. Arterial insufficiency can be seen if the fistula is large enough to cause a "steal" phenomenon. A swollen and tender extremity can be seen because of venous dilatation. AV fistulas that are significantly large enough can result in high-output congestive heart failure. Because these fistulas tend to get progressively larger, all but the smallest fistulas should be treated with ultrasound-guided compression, endovascular stenting, or surgical repair.

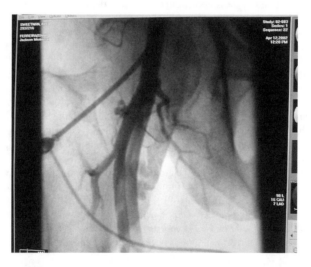

FIGURE 2. Anteroposterior projection of right iliac arteriogram demonstrating an AV fistula. Blood flow is seen filling the femoral vein during femoral artery injection. The patient had a previous vascular sheath inserted one week prior during a diagnostic catheterization.

43. DRUG-INDUCED THROMBOCYTOPENIA AND NEUTROPENIA

Joshua Purow, M.D., and Eduardo de Marchena, M.D.

1. Which medications commonly used during percutaneous coronary intervention (PCI) cause thrombocytopenia?

Although most drugs have been associated with thrombocytopenia, two commonly used drugs in interventional cardiology, heparin and the glycoprotein (GP) IIb/IIIa receptor antagonists, are frequently associated with thrombocytopenia.

2. Differentiate between the two types of heparin-induced thrombocytopenia (HIT).

The non-immune form of HIT (type 1 HIT) causes modest thrombocytopenia by increasing the aggregation of platelets that have been cross-linked by the negatively charged heparin molecules. In this more common form, the decrease in platelet count occurs within 2 days after heparin exposure and is rarely of any major clinical significance. The platelet counts decrease below normal but rarely less than 50% of their initial value. The thrombocytopenia often resolves despite continued heparin exposure.

The immune mediated form of HIT (type 2 HIT) is much less common, yet the thrombocytopenia is much more severe, with levels often below 75,000 cell/cm^3 and rarely below 20,000 cell/cm^3. The average platelet count is approximately 60,000 cell/cm^3. The thrombocytopenia typically occurs 4 to 10 days after the initiation of heparin and rarely after 2 weeks. The syndrome can manifest with both bleeding and thrombosis, including arterial thrombosis.

Heparin-induced Thrombocytopenia: Type 1 vs. Type 2

	TYPE 1	TYPE 2
Incidence	10–20%	0.3–3.0%
Mechanism	Non-immune	Immune
Average platelet count	~100,000 cells/cm^3	~60,000 cells/cm^3
Timing of onset	~ 2 days	4–10 days
Thrombotic events	0%	~50%
Hemorrhage	Very rare	rare
Heparin cessation	Usually not necessary	Necessary

3. What is the incidence of HIT?

The incidence of the non-immune–mediated form, HIT type 1 ranges between 10% and 20%. The incidence of the more severe immune form, HIT type 2, is between 0.3% and 3.0% in patients exposed to heparin for more than 4 days. The incidence varies widely depending on the on the type of patient, the heparin preparation, and the criteria used for diagnosing HIT. **Even small amounts of heparin such as heparin flushes can cause HIT**!

4. What is the mechanism of type 2 HIT?

The negatively charged heparin polysaccharide chains bind to a positively charged GP, produced and released by platelets, known as platelet factor 4 (PF4). The PF4 then undergoes conformational changes, after which it serves as an antigen to which antibodies are produced. The HIT antibody–PF4–heparin complex then binds to platelets via the Fc portion of the IgG molecule. Multimolecular complexes form on the platelet surface, leading to platelet activation. The activated platelets release additional PF4, thereby amplifying the process. The activated platelets aggregate and are subsequently removed from the circulation, resulting in thrombocytopenia. The platelet activation may also lead to thrombosis. In addition, the heparin–PF4 complexes bind to endothelial cell receptors and stimulate the release of tissue factor, which also contributes to the risk of thrombosis.

5. How is type 2 HIT diagnosed?

Because HIT is a clinical syndrome, the initial diagnosis must be suspected clinically. A decrease in platelet count by 50% and the occurrence of thrombotic events should raise the suspicion for type 2 HIT in a patient recently exposed to heparin. A number of serum assays, can test for the HIT antibody. The most sensitive assays include a serotonin release assay, a platelet aggregation assay, and a solid phase immunoassay. The solid phase immunoassay is used most commonly. Treatment decisions are often made on clinical grounds alone because the results of these assays are often not quickly available.

6. Do the low molecular weight heparins (LMWHs) carry the same risk of HIT as does unfractionated heparin?

No. The incidence of LMWH causing immune sensitization resulting in HIT is extremely rare. Patients treated with LMWH have also less commonly been found to have the anti-PF4 antibody, even without the presence of thrombocytopenia. This results in fewer thrombotic events occurring with LMWH and is just another of the many advantages of LMWH over unfractionated heparin. **However, after HIT is diagnosed, all forms of heparin should be avoided in the future.**

7. In the catheterization laboratory, what can be used as a substitute for heparin in patients with HIT?

In patients with HIT, the first step is to carefully avoid all heparin exposure, including heparin flushes. Patients taking LMWH, as already discussed, have a much lower incidence of HIT, but LMWH has nevertheless demonstrated some cross-reactivity in patients already diagnosed with HIT. The LMWHS should be avoided but may be used if absolutely necessary. The direct thrombin inhibitors, such as hirudin and argatroban, have been used safely in patients with HIT who require interventional procedures or anticoagulation (see Chapter 11). These are managed by following the activated clotting time (ACT) or activated partial thromboplastin time (aPTT) in a manner similar to that used for heparin. In patients undergoing a PCI, the dose of argatroban is higher than for treating patients with typical HIT. The hirudin analogue bivalirudin has been approved by the Food and Drug Administration for use in PCIs, although the experience with its use for the treatment of HIT is unclear. Another anticoagulant, danaparoid, is a heparinoid that has also been used safely in patients with HIT. However, up to 10% cross-reactivity exists, so it should be used cautiously. Danaparoid requires measuring antifactor Xa to monitor its anticoagulant effect.

8. What is the incidence of GP IIb/IIIa–inhibitor associated thrombocytopenia?

The incidence of severe thrombocytopenia from exposure to the GP IIb/IIIa antagonists varies depending on the type of agent. The incidence with the chimeric monoclonal antibody, abciximab, is approximately 0.5–2.0% but is much lower with the small molecule agents tirofiban and eptifibitide (~0.2–0.6%). Although thrombocytopenia is infrequent with GP IIb/IIIa inhibition, when it does occur, the platelet count decrease may be severe. And even though the thrombocytopenia adds to the risk of bleeding, the episodes of major bleeding are few. Overall, the benefit of using GP IIb/IIIa inhibitors, especially in thrombotic lesions, is greater than the risk caused by bleeding, with or without thrombocytopenia (see Chapter 13).

9. My patient has received both heparin and a GP IIb/IIIa antagonist. How do I know which one is responsible for the thrombocytopenia?

This is a common problem because many patients receive both agents. Determining which is the responsible agent is often difficult. Thrombocytopenia occurring with the GP IIb/IIIa antagonists usually occurs within the first day after starting the medication. For this reason, a platelet count should always be obtained at baseline before starting the medication and again within 6 hours after starting the infusion. In contrast, HIT usually does not occur until at least 4 days after exposure. In addition, serologic testing for the presence of anti-PF4 antibodies may be helpful. Nevertheless, in this clinical scenario, both agents usually need to be stopped as soon as a significant decrease in platelet count is noted.

10. What is the mechanism of GP IIb/IIIa antagonist–associated thrombocytopenia?

The exact mechanism is unclear, but several mechanisms have been suggested. One mechanism, known as the "innocent bystander" mechanism, suggests that antibody production, which is induced after administration of a drug, also causes destruction to the platelets. The platelet is destroyed as an "innocent bystander" by either complement-induced lysis or splenic removal of the platelet because of opsonization. Another mechanism states that the binding of the GP antagonist to the receptor causes conformational changes in the receptor, unveiling a previously covered epitope. This new receptor epitope stimulates antibody production and binding and allows for platelet destruction by immune-mediated mechanisms. Another mechanism is specific to that of the chimeric antibody, abciximab, and suggests that the monoclonal antibody retains mouse sequences, which can initiate an immune response. It is not possible that the binding of abciximab results in acute platelet removal directly by the macrophages of the reticuloendothelial system because these molecules do not contain the Fc portion to bind to the Fc receptors on the macrophages. One additional hypothesis proposes that some naturally occurring antibodies exist against this newly revealed epitope. The presence of preformed antibodies, without the need for *de novo* antibody production, could explain the rapid occurrence of platelet loss after medication exposure.

11. Should platelet transfusion be used to treat GP IIb/IIIa inhibitor–induced thrombocytopenia?

Platelet transfusion can be used for profound thrombocytopenia but should be reserved for patients with evidence of significant bleeding. Most minor bleeds, such as from an arteriotomy site, stop with cessation of the GP inhibitor and with adequate compression, even in the presence of thrombocytopenia. After discontinuation of the medication, there is little ongoing platelet destruction.

The effect of platelet transfusion varies based on the type of agent used. The large molecule abciximab binds with high affinity to the platelet receptors and can be found bound to circulating platelets for up to 21 days. The molecules left in the plasma are then cleared rapidly. Thus, platelet transfusion is beneficial by providing new uninhibited platelets and assuming the drug is discontinued; then is no longer be any circulating drug molecules to deactivate these new platelets. On the other hand, the small molecules are competitive inhibitors that antagonize the receptor in a reversible, dose-dependent fashion. Therefore, any circulating drug can continue to bind to the freshly transfused platelets, limiting the efficacy of this therapy. Fortunately, because of the short half-life of these drugs, their thrombocytopenic effects resolve much sooner (2–4 hours after discontinuation).

12. What hematologic abnormalities are associated with ticlopidine?

Ticlodipine is a thienopyridine antiplatelet agent that has been used widely in the treatment of patients with atherosclerotic disease. It has been especially successful in aspirin-allergic patients in preventing acute cardiovascular ischemic events and after coronary stent placement to prevent acute stent thrombosis. Activated platelets release multiple chemical mediators, including adenosine diphosphate (ADP). Ticlopidine then binds to the ADP receptor, inhibiting further platelet activation.

Hematologic adverse effects associated with the use of ticlopidine include thrombotic thrombocytopenic purpura (TTP) and granulocytopenia. The incidence of ticlopidine -associated granulocytopenia is approximately 2.5%. The incidence of the much more serious TTP is much lower, approximately one in 1600 patients treated. TTP is characterized by thrombocytopenia, microangiopathic hemolytic anemia, fever, renal dysfunction, and neurologic changes. When this rare complication occurs, the fatality rate is very high, occurring in up to one third of patients. Plasma exchange therapy is the first-line therapy and should be instituted immediately. This therapy can markedly improve the mortality rate.

The drug is thought to induce an autoantibody against a metalloproteinase that degrades von Willebrand factor (vWF). This results in an increase in the quantity of vWF, which subsequently forms large multimers. These large multimers effectively cause platelet binding and aggregation, leading to the development of platelet microthrombi, which characterize the TTP syndrome.

13. How should granulocytopenia be monitored when prescribing ticlopidine?
The use of ticlopidine after coronary stenting requires that a white blood cell (WBC) count be checked at baseline and then every 2 weeks up to 3 months. After 3 months, the risk is significantly decreased. If the drug is stopped during the 3 months, the WBC count should still be monitored for an additional 2 weeks.

14. Clopidogrel has largely replaced ticlodipine for the prevention of stent thrombosis after stent placement. Do I still need to worry about granulocytopenia and TTP?
Clopidogrel is another member of the thienopyridine family and differs from ticlopidine by just one carboxymethyl group. Phase III clinical trials monitoring more than 20,000 patients treated with clopidogrel showed a much improved side effect profile, including no reported episodes of adverse skin or gastrointestinal effects, granulocytopenia, or TTP. For this reason, ticlopidine has mostly been replaced by clopidogrel. However, because of its widespread use, a few sporadic episodes of clopidogrel-induced TTP have been reported. The incidence remains far less than with ticlopidine. Most of the patients responded to plasma exchange therapy; however, some patients required an excessive number of exchanges.

15. What other cardiac drugs cause granulocytopenia?
Other cardiac medications that have been associated with leukopenia or granulocytopenia include procainamide, angiotensin-converting enzyme inhibitors, propranolol, dipyridamole, digoxin, and nifedipine. Procainamide-induced leukopenia is independent of its lupus-like syndrome.

BIBLIOGRAPHY

1. Bennett CL, Weinberg PD, Rozenberg-Ben-Dror K, et al: Thrombotic thrombocytopenic purpura associated with ticlodipine: a review of 60 cases. Ann Intern Med 128:541–544, 1998.
2. Bennett CL, Connors JM, Carwile JM, et al: Thrombotic thrombocytopenic purpura associated with clopidogrel. N Engl J Med 342:1773–1777, 2000.
3. Berkowitz SD, Harrington RA, Rund MM, et al: Acute profound thrombocytopenia after c7E3 Fab (abciximab) therapy. Circulation 95:809–813, 1997.
4. Lincoff AM, Califf RM, Topol EJ: Platelet glycoprotein IIb/ IIIa receptor blockade in coronary artery disease. J Am Coll Cardiol 35:1103–1115, 2000.
5. Stone RM, Bridges KR, Libby P: Hematological-oncological disorders and cardiovascular disease. In Braunwald E, Zipes DP, Libby P (eds): Heart Disease: A Textbook of Cardiovascular Medicine, 6th ed. Philadelphia, W.B. Saunders, 2001, pp 2237–2243.
6. Tsai HM, Lian EC: Antibodies to von Willebrand factor cleaving cleaving protease in thrombotic thrombocytopenic purpura and the hemolytic-uremic syndrome. N Engl J Med 339:1585–1594, 1998.
7. Warkentin TE, Levine MN, Hirsh J, et al: Heparin-induced thrombocytopenia in patients with low molecular weight heparin or unfractionated heparin. N Engl J Med 332:1330–1335, 1995.
8. Warkentin TE: Heparin-induced thrombocytopenia, Part 1. J Crit Illness 17:172–178, 2002.
9. Warkentin TE: Heparin-induced thrombocytopenia: clinical course and treatment. J Crit Illness 17: 215–221, 2002.

IX. Restenosis

44. CORONARY RESTENOSIS

Eduardo de Marchena, M.D., and Alexandre C. Ferreira, M.D.

1. What percentage of patients develop restenosis after percutaneous transluminal coronary angioplasty (PTCA)?

The restenosis rate in patients undergoing balloon angioplasty ranges from 30% to 50% depending on patient characteristics and lesion location. The rate is also greatly influenced by the definition of restenosis. Clinically the most conventionally accepted definition is a recurrence in luminal narrowing of more than 50%.

2. What are the clinical subgroups that predict restenosis?

Several studies have tried to define the clinical characteristics that predict higher restenosis rates. They include male gender, diabetes mellitus, insulin requirement, tobacco use, unstable angina, and variant angina.

3. What are the angiographic predictors of restenosis?

The following angiographic characteristics predict a higher restenosis rate:
- Proximal left anterior descending (LAD) coronary artery location
- Saphenous vein graft (SVG) lesions, especially older grafts and ostial lesions
- Totally occluded vessels
- Ostial lesions of native coronary arteries
- Calcified lesions
- Bifurcation lesions
- Long lesions
- Lesions in small vessels

One of the greatest predictors of restenosis is post-angioplasty residual stenosis. The larger the minimal luminal diameter after intervention, the less the restenosis.

4. What are the main mechanisms of coronary restenosis?

Coronary restenosis is the complex response that occurs after vascular stretch injury. It involves a delicate interplay between changes in coronary geometry and a cellular vascular response to injury. The causes of restenosis can be broken down into two simple mechanisms: mechanical response to injury and cellular response to injury.

1. **Mechanical response (Fig. 1):** After the balloon stretches the artery and atherosclerotic plaque, there is a major change in the local geometry of the vessel. Along with the artherosclerotic plaque, all the vascular components are stretched, fractured, compressed, and remodeled. Immediately after angioplasty, fissuring of the plaque can provoke plaque prolapse into the vessel lumen. Large flaps of plaque can cause acute vessel closure. Smaller amounts of plaque prolapse can, with time, be re-endothelialized, partially encroaching on the vessel diameter. Additionally, immediately after the angioplasty, the vessel's elastic components can recoil, causing the balloon-stretched vessel to return toward its original vessel size.

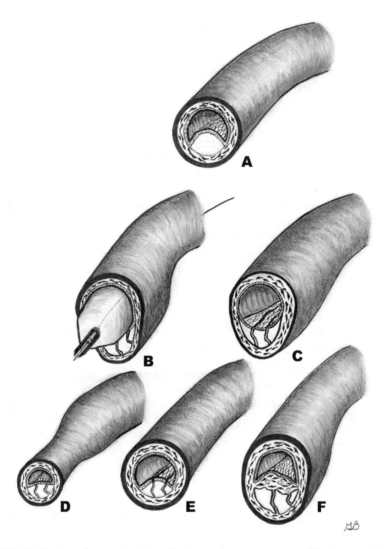

FIGURE 1: Mechanisms of restenosis. *A,* Baseline image of a coronary artery with atheroma critically encroaching on the vessel lumen. *B,* Balloon angioplasty causing compression and fracture of the atheroma with overall vessel expansion. *C,* Immediate result after balloon angioplasty. *D,* Negative remodeling with vessel encroachment at the original angioplasty site caused by scarring and late remodelling. *E,* Immediate vessel recoil with return to original vessel dimension and lumen compromise by atheroma. *F,* Neointimal hyperplasia demonstrating subintimal migration and proliferation of SMC and inflammatory cells, causing lumen loss. (Courtesy of Glenn Barquet, M.D.)

The major mechanism of restenosis is called *negative remodeling*. In a subset of patients, the healing response of the vessel after stretch injury leads to an encroachment of all the vessel layers. At the completion of this process, the vessel appears to have a waist at the site of injury. This process was first recognized with intravascular ultrasound (IVUS) studies.

2. **Cellular Response:** The cellular response to injury is also complex. Initially after plaque rupture and exposure of blood elements to the thrombotic arteriosclerotic material, rich in tissue factor and collagen, there is intense platelet activation and a stimulus for thrombosis. If extreme, platelet and fibrin deposition at the injury site can also lead to acute vessel closure. In more modulated response, however, this process can partially occlude the vessel, which with time can be re-endotheolized, resulting in loss of the vessel lumen.

The cellular response to injury includes the release of multiple chemical mediators, which stimulate a proliferative healing process at the sight of injury, leading to myointimal thickening. Myointimal thickening is a result of cellular proliferation and migration, as well as matrix deposition at the site of injury. Over time, this process can engulf the residual lumen. This is the dominant process for stent restenosis because the mechanical mechanisms are muted by the metal scaffolding offered by the stent.

5. What drug therapies have been shown to decrease restenosis in humans?

Many drugs have been studied for the prevention of restenosis. Although many drugs have shown benefit in animal trials of arterial injury, nearly all have failed in randomized trials in humans. The only studies that have have shown clear benefits have been with the antioxidant and antihyperlidemic agent probucol and a B vitamin combination. Studies with **probucol** show a significant decrease in restenosis in patients pretreated with the drug for 1 month before PTCA. The mode of action of this drug appears to be caused by an improvement in compensatory remodeling after balloon arterial injury. This drug had been used as an antilipemic drug in the United States but was withdrawn by the Food and Drug Administration because of QT prolongation. Recently, a randomized trial showed a benefit of the combination of **folic acid, vitamin B$_{12}$,** and **pyridoxine** in reducing restenosis when therapy was begun on the day of PTCA. Early trials with the antiinflamatory and antiproliferative drug **tranilast** suggested a potential benefit. However, the largest angiographically controlled clinical trial, the PRESTO trial, failed to duplicate the results. Studies with **trapidil** and **cilostazol** are underway after a small trial showed promise.

6. Do atherectomy devices reduce restenosis?

Thorough debulking (i.e., removal of atherosclerotic plaque) with directional atherectomy (DA) has been shown to reduce restenosis to near comparable rates as stenting. Rotational atherectomy and laser ablation of plaque before PTCA have shown to increase subsequent restenosis in trials.

Small trials have suggested that pretreating lesions with either DA or rotational atherectomy (RA) improves the outcome of subsequent stenting and reduces restenosis. Overall, the additional value appears modest and requires a more complex and expensive strategy than stenting alone. Presently, debulking before stenting is reserved predominantly for the treatment of lesions with large plague burden, bifurcation lesions, and some ostial lesions (to minimize plaque shifting), and for highly calcific lesions (to facilitate vessel dilation).

7. How much do bare metal stents reduce restenosis?

Bare metal stents have been show to decrease restenosis in large angiographic trials by about 25%, from a restenosis rate with PTCA of approximately 30% to 40% to a stent restenosis of 20% to 30%. As with PTCA, certain lesions such as long stenosis, small vessels, and SVG lesions have a higher restenosis rate. Stent restenosis is a major problem to treat in that in-stent restenostic lesions have a higher recurrent restenosis rate than PTCA restenotic lesion.

8. In what percent of percutaneous coronary interventions (PCIs) done in the United States are stents used?

Approximately 80%.

9. What percent of procedures done in the United States are performed for the treatment of in-stent restenosis?

Approximately 20% of all procedures are currently performed to treat stent restenosis.

10. Describe the types of in-stent restenosis.

Mehran et al. have proposed a classification of in-stent restenosis that helps predict the recurrence of restenosis after a second treatment at the affected site.

Type I: Focal restenosis within the stent
Type II: Diffuse intra-stent restenosis
Type III: Proliferative restenosis in the stent and adjacent vessel
Type IV: Diffuse total in-stent restenosis

11. What is the rate of target lesion revascularization for each in-stent restenosis type after treatment with repeat PCI?

IN-STENT RESTENOSIS TYPE	TARGET LESION REVASCULARIZATION AT 12 MONTHS, %
Type I	19
Type II	35
Type III	50
Type IV	83

12. Should atherectomy devices be used in the treatment of in-stent restenosis?

Although there was early enthusiasm for attempting to debulk in-stent restenostic segments with atherectomy devices, randomized trials have failed to show substantial benefit. The largest of these trials, the ARTIST trial, randomized PTCA versus RA for the treatment of in-stent restenosis. The trial failed to show superiority of the RA strategy but rather found a more favorable recurrent restenosis rate with PTCA alone. Debulking with atherectomy or laser devices may still be helpful at times in very resilient, elastic, "rubbery" lesions and in large-vessel restenosis in which the restenotic myointimal cap is thick and difficult to compress.

13. Does cutting ballon angioplasty decrease in-stent restenosis?

Although small trials had suggested reduction of restenosis with the use of the cutting balloon, a recent larger randomized trial has failed to confirm this finding. However, it has become a favorite tool for the treatment of in-stent restenosis because of the ease with which this device dilates the "rubbery" restenostic segment. During inflation, conventional balloons frequently slide forward or backward from this resilient, slippery treatment site, "the watermelon seed effect" (much like a wet watermelon seed slips out when squeezed tightly between two fingers). This slipping from the intended treatment site potentially damages the adjacent "normal" vessel segment. The cutting balloon, as it is slowly inflated, cuts into the thick myointimal layer, preventing its displacement from the treatment site and giving a more controlled angioplasty of the treatment site.

14. What is the main mechanism by which brachytherapy reduces restenosis?

Both gamma and beta radiation have been shown to dramatically reduce the proliferation of cells. In so doing, it nearly eliminates the myointimal proliferation that is seen after vascular injury.

15. Why is brachytherapy predominantly used in the treatment of in-stent restenosis?

Brachytherapy has been particularly helpful for the treatment of in-stent restenosis because it is nearly totally caused by a dense sheet of myointimal thickening. In vessels treated with PCI but not stented, other mechanical mechanisms (e.g., plaque prolapse, recoil, and negative remodeling) also come into play, reducing the efficacy of this therapy.

16. Do radiation-emitting stents reduce restenosis?

Stents that emit beta radiation have been tested with the goal of reducing restenosis. Although the therapy largely eliminates the myointimal thickening within the stent segment, there is a paradoxical increase in restenosis at the stent edges, the "candy wrapper effect." Apparently, prolonged low-dose radiation at the stent margins provokes enhanced myointimal proliferation. This strategy has been abandoned for now.

17. How do drug-eluting stents work in reducing restenosis?

For the past 2 decades, interventional cardiologists have been waiting for a tool that could both effectively and safely allow for optimal angioplasty, prevent acute closure, and have nearly no restenosis. The drug-eluting stent offer this potential. A drug-loaded polymer coating enveloping a standard bare metal stent allows a given drug to be released at the site of deposit for an allotted time. This gives a high local drug concentration with negligible systemic drug levels. Multiple drugs and polymers are being tested. Drug-eluting stents with sacrolimus and paclitaxel (Taxol) have already been shown to nearly eliminate myointimal thickening in the stented segment and dramatically reduce restenois and target vessel revascularization. Although this therapy will only be helpful in vessels that can be stented, it appears that the Holy Grail of interventional cardiology has been found.

18. What is the potential clinical application for antisense c-Myc therapy for restenosis prevention?

One of the potential clinical applications of antisense therapy is the prevention or treatment of restenosis after PCI. Vascular smooth muscle cells (SMCs) within the normal vessel wall are quiescent and have a low mitotic rate. After the blood vessel has been injured, the SMCs enter the cell cycle and a series of genes are expressed, including c-Myc. Expression of c-Myc is necessary for cell cycle progression in vascular SMCs. The inhibition of c-Myc *in vitro* or *in vivo* arrests vascular SMCs. In addition, c-Myc expression may also be required for vascular SMC migration, further enhancing the restenotic process.

19. What are the limitations of antisense therapy?

The clinical applicability of antisense technology is limited because of a relative lack of specificity, slow uptake across the cell membrane, and rapid intracellular degradation of the oligonucleotide. Clinical studies are underway to investigate the safety and efficacy of local delivery of antisense therapy to reduce restenosis after coronary stenting.

20. What is the role of vascular endothelial growth factor (VEGF) in restenosis prevention?

VEGFs can be used for their arterioprotective endothelial functions and for prevention of postangioplasty restenosis and bypass graft arteriopathy. The endothelial cell growth properties of VEGF promote endothelial regeneration. On the other hand, VEGF-induced endothelial production of nitric oxide and prostacyclin inhibits vascular SMC proliferation, which may lead to reduced restenosis.

Gene therapy in cardiovascular disease has an exciting future, but further advances in gene transfer vector technology and the identification of additional target genes are yet to achieved.

21. How much will drug-coated stents eliminate the need for CABG?

Although one would intuitively predict that the effect would be monumental, a recent analysis at the authors' center forecasts that it will be more modest, decreasing the need for surgery by about 20%. It is important to note that drug-eluting stents will nearly eliminate restenosis but will not improve the outcome in other challenging anatomic lesions such as diffuse vessel disease, chronic total obstruction, very tortuous vessels, and bifurcation lesions. Further engineering of PCI devices and stents will be required to reduce the need for CABG more substantially.

BIBLIOGRAPHY

1. Bailey S: Coronary restenosis: a review of current insights and therapies. Cathet Cardiovasc Interv 55:265–271, 2002.
2. Cannon RO: Restenosis after angioplasty. N Engl J Med 346:1182–1183, 2002.
3. Dietz U: Angiographic analysis of the angioplasty versus rotational atherectomy for the treatment of diffuse in-stent restenosis trial (ARTIST) Am J Cardiol 90:843, 2002.
4. Kipshidze N: Perspectives on antisense therapy for the prevention of restenosis. Curr Opin Mol Ther 3:265–277, 2001.
5. Mauri L: Cutting balloon angioplasty for the prevention of restenosis: results of the Cutting Balloon Global Randomized Trial. Am J Cardiol 90:1079, 2002.
6. Mehilli J, Kastrati A, Dirschinger J, et al: Comparison of stenting with balloon angioplasty for lesions of small coronary vessels in patients with diabetes mellitus. Am J Med 112:13–18, 2002.
7. Mehran R: Angiographic patterns of in-stent restenosis: classification and implications for long-term outcome. Circulation 100:1872–1878, 1999.
8. Mehta SR: Coronary stenting reduced the rate of restenosis in patients with a first or subsequent restenosis. Evidence-based Cardiovasc Med 3:13, 1999.
9. O'Sullivan M: Gene therapy for coronary restenosis: is the enthusiasm justified? Heart 86:491–493, 2001.
10. Poon M: Overcoming restenosis with sirolimus: from alphabet soup to clinical reality. Lancet 359:619–622, 2002.
11. Tanguay JF: In-stent restenosis: experimental and clinical results. Am J Cardiol 88(Suppl 5A):50, 2001.
12. Vom Dahl J: Rotational atherectomy does not reduce recurrent in-stent restenosis: results of the angioplasty versus rotational atherectomy for treatment of diffuse in-stent restenosis trial (ARTIST). Circulation 105:583–588, 2002.

45. CORONARY BRACHYTHERAPY

Cristiane Takita, M.D.

1. What is the incidence of coronary restenosis?

It is estimated that more than 800,000 percutaneous coronary interventions (PCIs) are performed annually in the United States, with 80% of the procedures involving the use of a stent. About 20% of these patients develop in-stent restenosis.

2. Describe the mechanisms involving the process of restenosis.

Elastic vessel *recoil* happens within 24 to 48 hours after arterial injury. The *neointimal hyperplasia,* the migration of smooth muscle cells (SMCs) from the media to the intima, begins within 24 to 48 hours from the time of injury, changing from the contractile and regulatory function to a proliferative state. The constrictive arterial *remodeling* (negative remodeling) occurs between 1 and 6 months after injury.

3. What are the effective therapies used to prevent coronary restenosis?

A number of trials using pharmacologic approaches to prevent restenosis have evaluated several drugs, including antiproliferative and antiplatelet and antithrombotic agents, but the results have been disappointing (see Chapter 44). Coronary stenting has shown a 30% to 50% reduction in the rates of restenosis by preventing the constrictive remodeling and recoil of the artery but at the cost of an increase in the neointimal hyperplasia. Coronary brachytherapy has reduced restenosis rates by 40% to 70% in patients with in-stent restenosis by decreasing the neointimal hyperplasia and the late constrictive vascular remodeling. Most recently, rapamycin-coated stents showed promising results in preventing restenosis in a short-term follow-up study.

4. What is the rationale for using radiation to prevent restenosis?

Radiation has been succesfully used to treat patients with benign proliferative disorders (e.g., keloids, heterotopic ossification, and gynecomastia) using low doses of radiation ranging from 8 to 12 Gy, with treatment delivered within 24–48 hours from the time of injury. Animal studies showed efficacy of radiation in inhibiting intimal hyperplasia after arterial injury, leading to clinical trials.

5. What is coronary brachytherapy?

Coronary brachytherapy is the use of radioactive sources after percutaneous transluminal coronary angioplasty (PTCA) to decrease the incidence of restenosis.

6. Who are the professionals involved in the coronary brachytherapy procedure, and what are their roles?

Coronary Brachytherapy Team and Their Roles

TEAM MEMBER	DUTIES
Interventional cardiologist	Performs PTCA
	Inserts the intravascular brachytherapy catheter at the site of procedure
	Gives important treatment information concerning vessel diameter after PTCA and length of PTCA injury
Radiation oncologist	Prescribes and delivers the treatment using radioactive sources through the intravascular brachytherapy catheter placed by interventional cardiologist
Medical physicist	Calculates and measures the appropriate radiation dose to be delivered to the patient
	With the radiation oncologist, responsible for safe handling of radiation sources and radiation safety of the patient and staff

7. Describe the physics characteristics of the radioisotopes most commonly used for coronary brachytherapy.

*Physics Characteristics of Isotopes Most Commonly Used
for Coronary Brachytherapy*

ISOTOPE	EMISSION TYPE	MAXIMUM ENERGY (KEV)	AVERAGE ENERGY (KEV)	HALF-LIFE
Ir-192	Gamma	612	375	74 days
P-32	Beta	1710	690	14 days
Sr/Y90	Beta	2270	970	28 years

8. Compare gamma and beta radiation for coronary brachytherapy.

Comparison between Gamma and Beta Radiation

CHARACTERISTIC	GAMMA RADIATION	BETA RADIATION
Depth of penetration	Penetrates deeper	Shallower depth of penetration
Radiation exposure to personnel	Staff needs to leave the room during treatment delivery	No need to leave the room; minimal radiation exposure
Dose distribution in the coronary artery wall	Ideal dose distribution, less dose variation within vessel wall	Greater variation caused by rapid dose fall off
Ability to treat larger vessels (peripheral arteries)	Can be used to treat larger vessels	Limited use as vessel diameter increases
Treatment time of coronary brachytherapy	15–20 minutes	3–5 minutes
Efficacy to prevent in-stent restenosis	Both types of radiation have shown to reduce in-stent restenosis in randomized trials	

9. Which patients benefit from the use of coronary brachytherapy?

In several randomized trials, coronary brachytherapy has been shown to decrease the incidence of in-stent restenosis after a PTCA in about 40% to 70% (refer to questions 10 and 11). A recent multicenter study used coronary brachytherapy for patients with in-stent restenosis of a saphenous venous graft (SVG). There was a decrease in the restenosis rate in the irradiated group compared with placebo (21% vs. 44%; $P = 0.005$). The rate of major adverse cardiac events (MACE) was 49% lower, with a 70% reduction in the rate of revascularization of the target lesion. The Beta-Cath trial used 1456 patients to assess the role of coronary brachytherapy in *de novo*, nonstented and stented lesions. No benefit from the addition of radiation was noted, possibly because of geographic miss (i.e., radiation treatment did not fully cover the coronary injured area).

10. What are the clinical data to support the use of coronary brachytherapy using gamma radiation?

See Table on page 249.

11. What are the clinical data for beta radiation in coronary brachytherapy?

See Table on page 250.

12. What are the complications for coronary brachytherapy?

Subacute thrombosis rate was about 6% to 9% of patients in the initial coronary brachytherapy studies and was found to be increased in patients who had stents placed at the time of brachytherapy. The use of prolonged antiplatelet therapy for more than 6 months after the procedure combined with the avoidance of placement of stents at the time of brachytherapy led to a significantly decreased rate of subacute thrombosis.

Coronary Brachytherapy Clinical Trials Using Ir-192 Gamma Radiation

TRIAL	NUMBER, TYPE, AND LENGTH OF LESION	DOSE	FOLLOW-UP	% MACE		% TLR		% IN-STENT RESTENOSIS		COMPLICATIONS
				RT	PLACEBO	RT	PLACEBO	RT	PLACEBO	
Scripps I	55 Restenosis (native vessels) or SVG ≤ 30 mm length	≥ 8 Gy furthest media < 30 Gy closest media by IVUS	3 years	23	55	15	48	33	64	None
Gamma I	252 in-stent restenosis in native vessel lesions ≤ 45 mm	Same as Scripps I	9 months	28	44	24	45	22	51	Late subacute thrombosis (SAT) 5.3%, associated with stent placement at time of treatment
Gamma II	125 in-stent restenosis in native vessel lesions ≤ 45 mm	14 Gy at 2 mm radius	6 months	30		23		25		Late SAT 4%
Wrist	130 in-stent restenosis 100 native vessels 30 SVGs	15 Gy at 2 mm depth (3–4 mm vessel diameter) 15 Gy at 2.4 depth (> 4 mm)	6 months	29	68	14	63	19	58	None
Long wrist	120 patients lesions length ~ 36–80 mm	18 Gy to 2 mm depth				17		24		None

Coronary Brachytherapy Clinical Trials Using Beta Radiation

TRIAL	NUMBER, TYPE, AND LENGTH OF LESION	DOSE	FOLLOW-UP (MONTHS)	% TLR		% IN-STENT RESTENOSIS		COMPLICATIONS
				RT	PLACEBO	RT	PLACEBO	
START (Sr/Y-90) 30mm source	476 in-stent restenosis lesion ≤ 20 mm length	18 Gy at 2 mm radius (vessel ≥ 2.7 < 3.35 mm/ 23 Gy at 2mm radius (Vessel >3.35 − ≤ 4mm)	8	13	22	14	41	One case of SAT
START 40/20 (Sr/Y-90) 40-mm source	207 in-stent restenosis lesions ≤ 20 mm length	Same doses as START trial	8			16		None
Prevent (P32)	105 lesions 70% *de novo* lesions ≤ 25 mm length	16–20–24 Gy at 1 mm from source	6	6	24	8	39	None
Inhibit (P32)	332 in-stent restenosis lesion ≤ 40 mm length	20 Gy at 1 mm from source	9	11	29	16	49	None
Beta Wrist	50 in-stent retenosis		6	16		22		None

13. Describe the available systems to deliver coronary brachytherapy.

The Food and Drug Administration (FDA) has approved two systems: the Cordis Checkmate System (Best Medical International, Springfield, VA) and the Beta-Cath System (Novoste Corp., Norcross, GA). The Galileo/Guidant System (Guidant Corp., Houston, TX) is awaiting FDA approval. The Cordis Checkmate system uses gamma radiation from iridium-192 seed train (6, 10, 14, 18, and 22 seeds) with a manual delivery system, noncentered catheter, fixed dosimetry based on intravascular ultrasound (IVUS), and a treatment time of about 15 to 20 minutes. The Beta-Cath system uses beta radiation from strontium/ytrium-90 seed train, 30 to 40 mm source train length, a hydraulic delivery system, a noncentered catheter, a fixed dose prescription of 2 mm depth, dose depending on the vessel diameter after PTCA, and a treatment time of about 3 to 5 minutes. The Galileo/Guidant system uses beta radiation from phosphorus-32 source wire, with a computerized afterloading system, allowing centering catheter, with a fixed prescription at 1 mm depth into the vessel wall or balloon surface, with treatment time of about 2 to 4 minutes.

14. Does coronary brachytherapy increase the radiation exposure to catheterization laboratory personnel?

A single-institution study analyzed the radiation safety issues associated with iridium-192 coronary brachytherapy in the cardiac catheterization laboratory environment. Radiation exposures were measured in more than 500 cases. Personnel were carefully monitored over 5 years of procedures. The results showed that with a prudent radiation safety program in place, there was no significant additional dose to staff. Regular staff training was vital to the safety of staff. The use of beta sources for coronary brachytherapy is less concerning with regard to radiation exposure because of the rapid fall off and shallower depth of penetration. In order to reduce radiation exposure, ALARA (*as low as reasonably achievable*) principles should be followed: use the least *time* you can spend close to the radiation source, at the longest *distance* possible, with appropriate *shielding*.

BIBLIOGRAPHY

1. Amols HI: Review of endovascular brachytherapy physics for prevention of restenosis. Cardiovasc Radiol Med 1:64–71, 1999.
2. Crocker I, Robinson KA: Rationale for coronary artery radiation therapy. Semin Radiol Oncol 12:3–16, 2002.
3. Grise MA, Masullo V, Jani S, et al: Five-year clinical follow-up after intracoronary radiation: results of a randomized clinical trial. Circulation 105:2737–2740, 2002.
4. Jani SK, Steuterman S, Huppe GB, et al: Radiation safety of personnel during catheter-based Ir-192 coronary brachytherapy. J Invas Cardiol 12:286–290, 2000.
5. Leon MB, Teirstein PS, Moses JW, et al: Localized intracoronary gamma-radiation therapy to inhibit the recurrence of restenosis after stenting. N Engl J Med 344:250–256, 2001.
6. Suntharalingam M, Laskey W, Lansky AJ, et al: Clinical and angiographic outcomes after use of strontium90/yttrium90 beta radiation for the treatment of in-stent restenosis: results from the Stents and Radiation Therapy 40 (START 40) registry. Int J Radiat Oncol Biol Phys 52:1075–1082, 2002.
7. Tripuraneni P: Coronary artery radiation therapy for the prevention of restenosis after percutaneous coronary angioplasty, II: outcomes of clinical trials. Semin Rad Oncol 12:17–30, 2002.
8. Verin V, Popowski Y, de Bruyne B, et al: Endoluminal beta-radiation therapy for the prevention of coronary restenosis after balloon angioplasty: the Dose-Finding Study group. N Engl J Med 344:243–249, 2001.
9. Waksman R, Ajani AE, White RL, et al: Intravascular gamma radiation for in-stent restenosis in saphenous-vein bypass grafts. N Engl J Med 346:1194–1199, 2002.
10. Waksman R, Robinson KA, Crocker IR, et al: Endovascular low dose irradiation inhibits neointima proliferation after coronary artery baloon injury in swine: a possible role for radiation therapy in restenosis prevention. Circulation 91:1533–1539, 1995.
11. Waksman R: Vascular Brachytherapy, 2nd ed. New York, Futura Publishing Company, 1999.
12. Waksman R, Raizner AE, Yeung AC, et al: Use of localised intracoronary beta radiation in treatment of in-stent restenosis: the INHIBIT randomised controlled trial. Lancet 359:551–557, 2002.

46. DRUG-ELUTING STENTS

Fausto Feres, M.D., Ph.D., Amanda Sousa, M.D., Ph.D.,
Alexandre Abizaid, M.D., Ph.D., and J. Eduardo Sousa, M.D., Ph.D.,

1. How common is coronary restenosis?

Randomized, multicenter clinical trials comparing balloon angioplasty with intracoronary stenting have demonstrated a reduced probability for restenosis after coronary stenting. At present, intracoronary stenting is the most commonly used percutaneous catheter-based strategy for treatment of symptomatic coronary arterial obstructions. It is estimated that at least 800,000 procedures are performed annually in the United States. The long-term clinical efficacy of intracoronary stenting, however, is limited by restenosis, which occurs in 15% to 30% of patients.

2. What are the mechanisms of coronary restenosis?

Intracoronary stenting decreased restenosis because of the scaffolding properties of a stent to inhibit the chronic constrictive vascular remodeling. In-stent restenosis (ISR) is caused solely by neointimal hyperplasia. Stent-induced mechanical arterial injury and a foreign body response induce acute and chronic inflammation in the vessel wall. The subsequent elaboration of cytokines and growth factors induces multiple pathways to activate smooth muscle cell (SMC) migration and proliferation. The expression of inflammatory cytokines from proliferating T cells is associated with the release of growth factors, which induces SMC proliferation and migration as well as secretion of matrix proteins. The long-term effects of smooth muscle cell migration, proliferation, and matrix formation are the development of neointimal hyperplasia that may obstruct the stent lumen, resulting in restenosis.

3. What is the definition of ISR, and which patients should be considered for treatment?

At follow-up stent implantation, ISR is considered whenever the in-stent lesion is greater than 50% by coronary angiography. Patients with ISR may present with or without symptoms and be associated with the presence or absence of objective evidence of ischemia. In order to decide the need for a new revascularization, it is imperative to assess the presence of myocardial ischemia.

4. How can we treat patients with ISR?

ISR remains the major limitation of percutaneous coronary interventions (PCIs). The treatment of ISR with balloon angioplasty has been doomed with rates of ISR and need for new revascularizations greater than 50%. In addition, ablative techniques such as rotational atherectomy (RA) or laser also failed to reduce those rates. However, the treatment of patients with ISR with balloon angioplasty with the adjunctive use of intracoronary radiation (beta and gamma) has been reported to be successful and safe. Several clinical trials comparing balloon angioplasty with and without the adjunctive use of brachytherapy have been reported, showing a reduction from 45% to 20% (a 50% relative reduction) of new ISR in favor of brachytherapy. Because of the latter, approximately 30,000 patients are undergoing brachytherapy for the treatment of ISR. However, brachytherapy has shown to have some important limitations such as late thrombosis caused by delayed endothelization (partially resolved with prolonged use of clopidogrel), edge effect caused by geographic miss (partially resolved with longer sources), and the additional personnel required to perform the techniques and the special training needed for these cumbersome devices.

5. What is the rationale for drug-eluting stents to prevent in-stent restenosis?

Recent advances in the understanding of the vascular biology of restenosis coupled with the development of stents as local delivery vehicles of therapeutic agents have generated enthusiasm for the application of drug-coated stents in the prevention of restenosis. The rationale for stent-based drug therapy is based on the physical properties, the mechanism of action, and the experimental data of some drugs (e.g., sirolimus and paclitaxel) that document their efficacy in preventing neointimal formation.

6. Which drugs are used, and what is the mechanism of action for inhibiting neointimal formation after stent implantation?

An antirestenotic agent should be one that inhibits the multiple components of the complex restenosis process. Uncontrolled neointimal tissue accumulation shows some parallels to tumor growths; thus, the usage of antitumor strategies seems to be a logical consequence. Numerous pharmacologic agents with antiproliferative properties have been tested for their potential to inhibit restenosis, with mostly disappointing results. Antimitotic compounds such as metrotexate and colchicinae have failed to inhibit SMC proliferation and intimal thickening. There is a great variety of potential drugs; however, only a few show convincing preclincal results, a prerequisite of clinical testing. Two of them, sirolimus and paclitaxel, have been tested in large, randomized clinical studies. Sirolimus (Rapamycin) is approved by the Food and Drug Administration for the prophylaxis of renal transplant rejection; it was approved in 1999. It is a naturally macrocyclic lactone with immunosuppressive properties that blocks G1 to S cell cycle progression by interacting with a specific target protein mTOR (mammalian target of rapamycin) and inhibits its activation. The latter results into inhibition of proliferation and migration, conferring a cytostatic characteristic to the drug.

Paclitaxel is a cytotoxic antineoplasic agent that is currently used to treat patients with several types of cancers. It exerts its pharmacologic effects through formation of numerous unorganized microtubules. This enhances the assembly of unstable microtubules, interrupting proliferation, migration, and signal transduction. The therapeutic mechanism of action is shown in Figure 1.

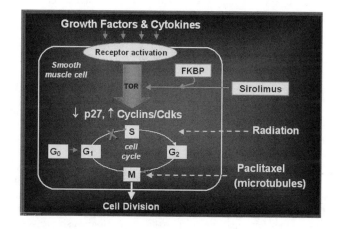

FIGURE 1. Therapeutic mechanism of action of paclitaxel.

7. How can drugs become embedded on a stent?

Several coatings, have shown adequate biocompatibility and low thrombogenicity. These coatings did not shown any intrinsic effect on ISR, (e.g., inert polymer, heparin, and phosforilcholine) but they have been considered as vehicles for an efficient antirestenotic drug. Drug release must be predictable and in controllable concentration and time spent. The delivery vehicle must be suitable for sterilization, must follow the geometric configuration change during stent expansion, and must resist mechanical injury caused by the inflation of the balloon. Today these problems are controlled, guaranteeing intact coating during clinical applications.

8. How long does it take for the drug to be totally released from the stent?

It depends on the amount of polymers layers used as a vehicle for drug delivery. The drug could be released slowly ($\leq$ 30 days), moderately ($\leq$ 2–3 weeks), or fast ($<$ 2 weeks).

9. Could drug-eluting stents have side effects?

Yes, but it depends on the amount of drug released. For example, paclitaxel has a very narrow therapeutic window. At toxic levels of paclitaxel, apoptosis can occur and lead to vessel closure. Local delivery doses of sirolimus are about less than 3% of systemic dose used in patients with renal transplantation, therefore, side effects do not occur in these patients.

10. Has ISR decreased in the era of drug-eluting stent?

Drug-eluting stents have dramatically reduced intimal hyperplasia more than 90% (Sirius, Ravel, Taxus). All large, randomized trials comparing drug-eluted stents (sirolimus or paclitaxel) with bare stents have shown an impressive reduction of ISR (from about 25% to $<$ 5%). Those results are shown in the table.

In-Stent Restenosis in the Drug-Eluting Stent Trials

TRIAL	PATIENTS, N	DRUG-ELUTING STENT, %	BARE STENT, %
FIM	30	0	–
RAVEL (sirolimus)	238	0	26
SIRIUS (sirolimus)	1058	3.2	35.4
TAXUS II (paclitaxel)	534	2.3	17.9

11. What are the indications for drug-eluting stents?

Patients with symptoms of myocardial ischemia and obstructive coronary artery disease suitable for percutaneous revascularization could be good candidates for drug-eluting stents. Patients with some of the classic villains of PCI (e.g., multivessel disease, diabetes, left main stenosis, small diameter vessels, long lesions, saphenous vein grafts, bifurcations) may well benefit from stents implantation of drug-eluting.

12. Which medications are used before, during and after a procedure of drug-eluting stents?

Acetol-salicylic acid (aspirin) should be administrated at a dose of at least 100 mg/day 12 hours before the procedure and continued indefinitely. Regarding the adjunctive use of a thienopiridine drug, a loading dose of 300 mg of clopidrogel must be administrated 24 hours before the procedure and followed with a 75 mg daily dose for 8 weeks. Alternatively, ticlopidine could be given at a dose of 250 mg twice a day, which should be started at least 1 day before the procedure and continued for a total of 8 weeks.

13. How could intimal hyperplasia be evaluated after drug-eluting stent placement?

Intimal hyperplasia is the scar tissue that develops in response to vessel wall injury and is the most important surrogate of ISR. There are several ways to identify the amount of intimal hyperplasia that develops after stent implantation. Noninvasive tests such as an exercise stress test and nuclear medicine are able to detect myocardial ischemia, which suggests that intrastent neointimal formation limits coronary blood flow.

Invasively, coronary angiography can quantify intimal hyperplasia by measuring late lumen loss (minimum lumen diameter at follow up minus minimum lumen diameter immediately after stent deployment). Several reports from bare stent trials revealed late lumen loss values from 0.8 to 1.0 mm. Recently, a 70% to 90% reduction of those late loss values have been observed with the placement of sirolimus-eluting stents. The assessment by intravascular ultrasound (IVUS) allows us a more accurate and detailed description of the amount and pattern of neointimal formation. Moreover, IVUS analysis conveys data not only of a single cross-sectional area but also of the entire treated segment such as stent, lumen, and neointimal volumes. Neointimal volume after bare stent implantation ranges from 35 to 40 mm^3 in a 15- to 20-mm stent. However, with sirolimus-eluting stent implantation, neointimal volume has been decreased to 1 to 10 mm^3 (> 75% reduction).

14. What are some tips for implanting a drug-eluting stent in order to set a good long-term result?

Based on the vast experience provided by the FIM, RAVEL, and SIRIUS trials, we have learned that restenosis and late loss were much higher in-lesion segments (stented + injured references segments) compared with the stented segments alone. The latter is essentially caused by some injury triggered by stent deployment and postdilatation compromise of proximal and distal margins. Certainly, the presence of significant plaque burden at edges of the stent carries a risk for the development of edge restenosis and calls for a much longer lesion segment covered with stent. Moreover, it is also advisable to avoid aggressive pre- and postdilatation with balloon longer than the stents.

Interestingly, several reports have showed that whenever a gap is left between two deployed drug-eluted stents, a significant amount of intimal hyperplasia develops. Therefore, it is strongly recommended to overlap whenever two or more stents are to be implanted.

15. What are the long-term results sustained after drug-eluting stents?

A drug-eluting stent is a rather complex device composed of a triad: the drug, the coating, and the stent. The long-term outcome after placement of drug-eluting stents depends on the intricate interaction between these three components and the patient's vascular response. Nevertheless, there were no clinical events reported between 24 to 36 months follow-up in patients who received sirolimus-eluting stents as part of the FIM trial.

BIBLIOGRAPHY

1. Leon MB, Moses JW, Popma JJ, et al: A multicenter randomized clinical study of the sirolimus-eluting stent in native coronary lesions. Available at http://www.tctmd.com.
2. Marx SO, Marks AR: The development of rapamycin and its application to stent restenosis. Circulation 104:852–855, 2001.
3. Morice M-C, Serruys PW, Sousa JE, et al: A randomized comparison of a Sirolimus-eluting stent with a standard stent for coronary revascularization. N Engl J Med 346:1773–1780, 2002.
4. Sousa E, Costa M, Abizaid A, et al: Lack of neointimal proliferation after implantation of sirolimus-coated stents in human coronary arteries. Circulation 103:192–195, 2001.
5. Sousa JE, Costa MA, Abizaid AC, et al: Sustained suppression of neointimal proliferation by sirolimus-eluting stents: one-year angiographic and intravascular ultrasound follow-up. Circulation 104:2007–2011, 2001.
6. Sousa JE, Costa MA, Sousa AGMR: What is "the matter" with restenosis in 2002? Circulation 105: 2932–2933, 2002.
7. TAXUS II: Final 6-month results. Available at http://www.tctmd.com.
8. Teirstein PS: Living the dream of no restenosis. Circulation 104:1996–1998, 2001.
9. Teirstein PS, Kuntz RE: New frontiers in interventional cardiology: intravascular radiation to prevent restenosis. Circulation 104:2620–2626, 2001.
10. Waksman R, White RL, Chan RC, et al: Intracoronary radiation therapy after angioplasty inhibits recurrence in patients with in-stent restenosis. Circulation 101:2165–2171, 2000.

X. Balloon Valvuloplasty and Septal Closure

47. MITRAL VALVULOPLASTY AND AORTIC VALVULOPLASTY

Farouc A. Jaffer, M.D., Ph.D., and Igor F. Palacios, M.D.

1. What are the indications for percutaneous mitral vaulvuoplasty (PMV)?

PMV is an effective alternative to surgical mitral commisurotomy in the treatment of patients with mitral stenosis. Candidates for PMV include those with symptomatic mitral stenosis (mitral valve area < 1.5 cm^2 measured on echocardiography and by hemodynamics) with a favorable valve morphology (noncalcified, pliable), without evidence of severe mitral regurgitation. Asymptomatic candidates who are likely benefit from PMV include those with at least moderate mitral stenosis (MS) (MVA < 1.5 cm^2) and pulmonary hypertension (pulmonary artery systolic pressure > 50 mmHg at rest or > 60 mmHg with exercise). Another possible indication for PMV is patients with new-onset atrial fibrillation.

2. What are the contraindications to PMV?

Moderate or severe mitral regurgitation (MR) on angiography or left atrial thrombus is a contraindication to PMV. Transesophageal echocardiography is, therefore, required in all patients before PMV. Thrombus in the left atrial appendage is not an absolute contraindication, although care must be taken to avoid clot dislodgment. From an anatomical standpoint, severe calcification of the mitral valve and commissures is a relative contraindication because PMV is likely to be unsuccessful.

3. What is the mitral valve echo score? What are its components?

The mitral valve echo score (Echo-Sc) described by Wilkins et al. is useful for stratifying patients likely to benefit from PMV. The four components of the Echo-Sc are mitral valve leaflet mobility, valvular thickening, subvalvular thickening, and valvular calcification. Each component receives a score of 1 (favorable) to 4 (unfavorable), and the Echo-Sc is calculated by summing the four components. An Echo-Sc of ≤ 8 predicts a favorable outcome for PMV. Recent data show that PMV patients with an Echo-Sc of ≤ 8 had greater increases in MVA, less repeat PMVs or mitral valve surgery, and a substantially improved 12-year survival (82% vs. 57%).

4. How is mitral regurgitation graded on angiography?

MR is based on Seller's classification, which evaluates left atrial opacification, clearance of left atrial contrast dye within 1 beat, and whether the contrast dye in the left atrium (LA) is equal to or greater than that of the left ventricle (LV):

GRADE	FULL LA CONTRAST	CLEARS < 1 BEAT	LA ≥ LV CONTRAST
1+ (mild)	No	Yes	No
2+ (moderate)	Usually	No	No
3+ (moderately severe)	Yes	No	Yes
4+ (severe)	Yes	No	Yes, within 1 beat

5. What are the two basic techniques used to perform PMV?

The two most common are the Inoue (single) balloon system and the double balloon system, both of which are antegrade techniques from the LA to LV, where the balloon is centered across the mitral valve. Retrograde methods are more technically demanding and require larger balloon sizes The Inoue single balloon technique is technically faster than the double balloon technique but has a steeper learning curve.

6. What is the mechanism of mitral valve area increase by PMV?

Several echocardiographic studies have shown the PMV increases the mitral valve area by opening of fused mitral commissures.

7. What is the initial critical step for both the Inoue and double balloon methods? What are its main complications?

After hemodynamic confirmation of significant MS, transseptal puncture of the atrial septum is performed. A sheath can then be guided from the right atrium into the LA to allow for delivery of either the Inoue balloon or double balloon across the mitral valve.

The main complications of transseptal puncture stem from accidentally perforating the aortic root (superior and anterior to the fossa ovalis), coronary sinus (posterior wall of the left atrium), or posterior wall of the right atrium. Such complications may lead to severe bleeding and cardiac tamponade. Inadvertent aortic puncture can be reduced by placement of a pigtail catheter in the noncoronary aortic cusp to serve as an anatomic landmark.

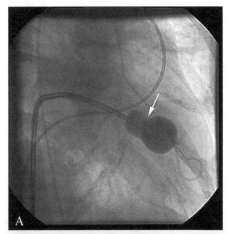

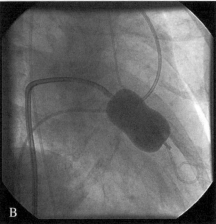

FIGURE 1. Percutaneous mitral valvuloplasty in a woman with rheumatic mitral stenosis using the Inoue balloon method. *A,* The Inoue balloon straddles the mitral valve (denoted by the asterisk). The distal end of the balloon inflates first followed by the proximal end. *B,* Complete inflation of the proximal and distal end results in mitral valve dilatation and commisural splitting.

8. What are the other complications that may occur with PMV?

Death ($<$ 2%; usually from complications of transseptal pucncture or guidewire perforation of the LV), severe mitral regurgitation ($<$ 10%), and stroke or systemic embolization ($<$ 2%) may occur.

9. How is the Inoue balloon size determined?

The size of the Inoue balloon ranges from 24 to 30 mm. The size is calculated using the following formula: [patient height in centimeters/10] + 10 mm.

10. How is PMV success determined?

A successful PMV is defined by a post-PMV mitral valve area greater than 1.5 cm^2 and post-PMV mitral regurgitation less than Seller's grade 3. Repeated balloon inflation may be necessary to achieve a satisfactory MVA. An alternative definition of success is if one of the fused mitral commissures opens during PMV.

11. What are the indications for percutaneous aortic valvuloplasty (PAV)? Why is its use much more limited compared with PMV?

PAV may be an option for patients with severe aortic stenosis. Indications are based on whether the aortic valve is noncalcified (e.g., congenital aortic stenosis [AS] or rheumatic non-calcified AS), or calcified (the typical elderly patient with AS). For noncalcifed AS, PAV may be a reasonable option to aortic valve surgery.

In calcific AS, PAV has a very limited role because of a very high rate of restenosis, relative high complication rate compared with surgery, and the inability to greatly increase the aortic valve area (AVA) beyond 1 cm^2. PAV is not an acceptable alternative to routine aortic valve replacement (AVR). Appropriate indications include patients with severe AS who are hemodynamically unstable and require a "bridge" to AVR, patients who are not AVR surgical candidates, and possibly patients with critical AS who require emergency noncardiac surgery. PAV can be used diagnostically in patients with low-output, low-gradient AS, but the risks of the procedure outweigh the alternative of dobutamine infusion.

12. What are possible contraindications to PAV?

Contraindications include significant aortic insufficiency, aortic valve endocarditis, and LV thrombus.

13. How is PAV performed?

The most commonly used method is a retrograde passage of a single balloon across the aortic valve. A double balloon retrograde technique may also be used in cases in which single balloon method provides a suboptimal result. First, to measure hemodynamics, a pulmonary artery catheter is placed and a 5-Fr pigtail is placed in the ascending aorta via the left femoral artery. In the right femoral artery, an 8-Fr sheath is placed, and the aortic valve is crossed using a straight-tip wire inside a second pigtail catheter. The transaortic gradient is determined from simultaneous aortic and LV pressure measurements. The cardiac output is then measured, and the AVA is determined by the Gorlin equation.

The straight-tip wire is then exchanged for a double curve exchange-length 0.038-inch guidewire. The second pigtail is removed with the 8-Fr sheath and exchanged for a 12-Fr sheath containing the PAV balloon. The balloon is 20-mm in diameter and 5.5 cm long. The balloon is filled with dilute contrast dye and then slowly inflated. Particular care must be taken to avoid dislodgment of the balloon from the valve, which may cause the stiff guidewire to perforate the left ventricle.

During balloon inflation for roughly 10 to 15 seconds, the arterial pressure is monitored. It is not uncommon to see patients lose consciousness during balloon inflation, and cardiac arrest may transiently occur. After inflation, the transaortic gradient and cardiac output are measured, and the post-PAV AVA is determined.

Antegrade PAV using a transseptal approach is a useful technique in patients with severe peripheral vascular disease.

14. What are the possible acute complications from PAV?

In a large National Institutes of Health study, roughly 25% of patients had a significant complication within 24 hours, including death (3%), stroke (3%), embolus (2%), vascular surgery (7%), or emergency AVR (1%). As stated previously, PAV is only indicated when surgical AVR is not an option.

15. How is a successful PAV defined?

Success is defined as either a doubling of the AVA or increase of the AVA greater than 1 cm^2. If success is not obtained after dilatation with a 20-mm balloon, a 23-mm balloon or a double balloon method (each 15–18-mm) can be used.

16. What is the typical duration of benefit for a successful PAV?

In a study of PAV patients who required subsequent AVR, the average duration of PAV benefit was only 9 months because of aggressive aortic valve restenosis.

BIBLIOGRAPHY

1. Bonow R, Carabello B, de Leon AC Jr, et al: Guidelines for the management of patients with valvular heart disease: executive summary: a report of the American College of Cardiology/American Heart Association Task Force on Practice Guidelines (Committee on Management of Patients with Valvular Heart Disease). Circulation 98:1949–1984, 1998.
2. Palacios IF, Sanchez PL, Harrell LC, et al: Which patients benefit from percutaneous mitral balloon valvuloplasty? Prevalvuloplasty and postvalvuloplasty variables that predict long-term outcome. Circulation 105:1465–1471, 2002.
3. Percutaneous balloon aortic valvuloplasty: acute and 30-day follow-up results in 674 patients from the NHLBI Balloon Valvuloplasty Registry. Circulation 84:2383–2397, 1991.
4. Ports TA, Grossman W: Balloon valvuloplasty. In Baim DS, Grossman W (eds): Grossman's Cardiac Catheterization, Angiography, and Intervention, 6th edition. Philadelphia, Lippincott Williams and Wilkins, 2001, pp 667–684.
5. Sellers RF, Levy MJ, Amplatz K, et al: Left retrograde cardioangiography in acquired heart disease. Am J Cardiol 14:437–447, 1964.
6. Soyer R, Bouchart F, Bessou JP, et al: Aortic valve replacement after aortic valvuloplasty for calcified aortic stenosis. Eur J Cardiothorac Surg 10:977–982, 1996.
7. Wilkins GT, Weyman AE, Abascal VM, et al: Percutaneous balloon dilatation of the mitral valve: an analysis of echocardiographic variables related to outcome and the mechanism of dilatation. Br Heart J 60:299–308, 1988.

48. PULMONIC VALVULOPLASTY

Alvaro Galindo, M.D.

1. What are the different types of right ventricular (RV) outflow obstruction?

For the purpose of this discussion, the RV outflow tract (RVOT) anatomically consists of the infundibular or *subvalvar* region, the pulmonary annulus and *valvar* apparatus, and the *supravalvar* region of the main pulmonary artery. Obstruction to the RVOT can occur at any one or a combination of these levels. Additionally, patients with congenital heart defects may have had surgery to establish a *conduit or homograft* between the RV and the pulmonary artery. These prosthetic communications often develop areas of obstruction and are occasionally amenable to catheter-based interventional procedures.

2. Is subvalvar pulmonic stenosis amenable to balloon dilation?

Infundibular or subinfundibular stenosis consists of a muscular obstruction. More often than not, it entails a dynamic narrowing of the RVOT. As such, subvalvar pulmonic stenosis is not amenable to balloon dilation. In some situations, however, it may respond to stent placement. It is important to note that subvalvar stenosis may result from RV hypertrophy in association with valvar pulmonic stenosis. In these cases, relief of the valvar stenosis leads to eventual relief of the subvalvar component.

3. Is supravalvar pulmonic stenosis amenable to balloon dilation or stent placement?

Supravalvar pulmonary stenosis can be either congenital or acquired. Congenital supravalvar pulmonary stenosis, in turn, can be isolated, as may be the case with rubella or Williams syndrome, or it can be associated with other cardiac defects such as in tetralogy of Fallot. Balloon dilation of congenital supravalvar stenosis is effective only in the setting of discrete membranous stenosis.

Supravalvar pulmonary stenosis may occur as an acquired lesion after surgery such as banding or patch augmentation of the main pulmonary artery, surgical pulmonary valvotomy, or arterial switch procedure for transposition of the great arteries. The mechanism of this obstruction relates to postoperative scar formation, which may respond to balloon angioplasty. In some situations, the use of an intravascular stent may be advantageous.

4. What is the procedure of choice for isolated pulmonary valve stenosis?

The procedure of choice for isolated valvar pulmonary stenosis in all age groups is percutaneous balloon valvuloplasty.

5. What is the incidence of valvar pulmonic stenosis?

The incidence of valvar pulmonary stenosis is approximately 12% of all moderate to severe forms of congenital heart defects or 0.73 per 1000 live births.

6. What is the natural history of valvar pulmonic stenosis?

Data from the Second Natural History Study of Congenital Heart Defects indicate that valvar pulmonic stenosis is rarely progressive. Patients with peak gradients less than 25 mmHg do not have increased morbidity or mortality. Individuals may remain virtually asymptomatic even with moderate (gradients between 50 and 79 mmHg) to severe (> 80 mmHg) pulmonary valve stenosis. Mortality usually occurs after the fourth decade of life and is associated with RV hypertrophy.

7. What are the indications for intervention for isolated valvar pulmonic stenosis?

The indications for balloon pulmonary valvuloplasty are the same as those for surgical intervention. Balloon valvuloplasty is of little or no benefit for patients with trivial or mild stenosis (gradients < 25 or 25–49 mmHg, respectively). Valvuloplasty is indicated for moderate (50–79 mmHg) or severe (> 80 mmHg) valvar pulmonic stenosis. Doppler-derived gradients of pulmonary stenosis are reasonably accurate and can be used as the basis for decisions to intervene.

8. What vascular approach can be used for balloon pulmonary valvuloplasty?

The femoral veins are the most common vascular access for balloon pulmonary valvuloplasty. The procedure, however, can be performed via the subclavian or internal jugular veins.

9. What diagnostic data is required for balloon pulmonary valvuloplasty?

Decisions for pulmonary balloon valvuloplasty are based on the gradient across the pulmonary valve, the diameter of the pulmonary valve annulus, and the nature of the obstruction (i.e., subvalvar, valvar, or supravalvar). For practical purposes, there is no need to calculate pulmonary valve area. An RV cineangiocardiogram in the left anterior oblique (LAO) 90-degree projection provides the best perspective of the right ventricular outflow tract and main pulmonary artery (see Figure 2).

10. How is the diameter of the balloon used for pulmonary valvuloplasty determined?

When using a single balloon, the recommended balloon diameter should be 1.2 to 1.4 times the diameter of the pulmonary annulus. Balloons that are smaller are ineffective in reducing the gradient across the valve. Balloon-to-annulus ratio in excess of 1.5 can result in hemorrhage into the RV myocardium.

11. When should you use two balloons for pulmonary valvuloplasty, and how do you determine the diameter of each balloon?

Two balloons should be used if the pulmonary annulus is too large for a single balloon. When using two balloons of equal size, each balloon should have a diameter of approximately 0.86 times the diameter of the pulmonary annulus. Otherwise, the combined diameters of the two balloons should be 1.35 times the ideal diameter of a single balloon.

12. What is the recommended technique for balloon pulmonary valvuloplasty?

Pulmonary balloon valvuloplasty is performed from an antegrade approach via the femoral, internal jugular, or subclavian vein. Saturation data are recorded in the superior vena cava, right atrium, RV, and pulmonary artery in order to evaluate for any possible sources of left-to-right shunting that may exaggerate the gradient across the RVOT. An atrial septal defect, for example, may have a 2.5:1 shunt and may cause a mild pulmonary valvar stenosis to manifest a gradient in excess of 50 mmHg. The appropriate management in that setting would involve either percutaneous or surgical closure of the atrial septal defect and reevaluation of the gradient across the RVOT.

Pressure data should be recorded in the RV and pulmonary artery. If there is any doubt as to the level of obstruction, a careful pullback tracing over a wire using an end-hole catheter will define the gradients along the course of the RVOT (Fig. 1).

An RV cineangiocardiogram should be recorded in the LAO 90-degree projection. This view provides images from which to estimate the diameter of the pulmonary valve annulus measured from hinge point to hinge point of the doming pulmonic valve. This perspective also provides anatomic detail of the RVOT (Fig. 2).

A determination is then made regarding the number and diameter (or diameters) of the balloon or balloons that will be required. Whether using one or two balloons, balloon length should be 3 to 5 cm in adults. The longer balloons facilitate stabilization of the balloon across the pulmonary annulus. Inflation pressures in excess of 5 atm should be avoided. After the balloon catheters are positioned straddling the pulmonary valve, they are simultaneously inflated using dilute contrast dye (1:4 contrast in saline). A waist should be evident at the level of the pulmonary valve, but will disappear upon full inflation (see Figure 2). Pressures are then recorded in the RV and pulmonary artery to assess the results of the intervention.

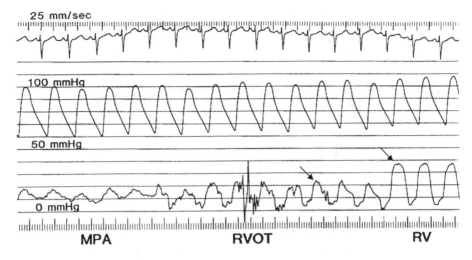

FIGURE 1. Pressure tracings representing aortic pressure and simultaneous pullback tracing over a wire from the main pulmonary artery (MPA) to the right ventricular outflow tract (RVOT) and then to the right ventricle (RV) following balloon pulmonary valvuloplasty. Note the absence of residual gradient from the MPA to RVOT. The gradient occurs within the RVOT representing dynamic obstruction associated with right ventricular hypertrophy.

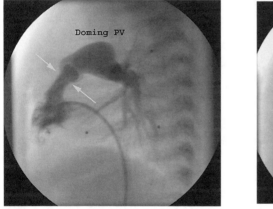
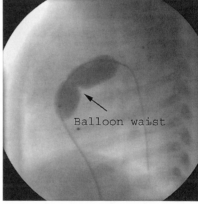

FIGURE 2. *A,* Lateral right ventricular cineangiocardiogram showing a thickened, doming pulmonary valve. The pulmonary valve annulus is measured at the valve hinge points *(arrows). B,* Pulmonary balloon valvuloplasty performed with single balloon. Note balloon waist at level of pulmonary valve annulus.

13. What should you consider if the gradient across the RVOT remains high after balloon pulmonary valvuloplasty?

If the gradient remains elevated (> 36 mmHg), a careful pullback pressure tracing should be recorded across the RVOT as described previously. It is common to find a dynamic infundibular stenosis after successful valvuloplasty because of ventricular hypertrophy. The contribution from this level of obstruction resolves spontaneously with time (Fig. 3).

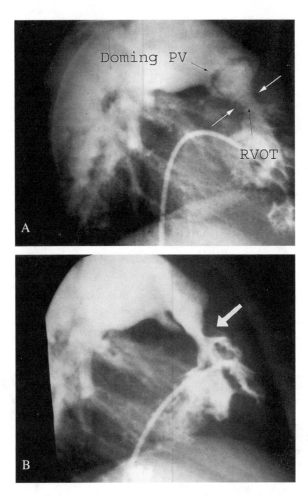

FIGURE 3. *A,* Lateral right ventricular cineangiocardiogram demonstrating valvar pulmonic stenosis as well as subvalvar stenosis due to right ventricular hypertrophy (*white arrows*). PV = pulmonary valve. RVOT = right ventricular outflow tract. *B,* Following successful balloon pulmonary valvuloplasty, the gradient from right ventricle to pulmonary artery was decreased from 95 to 65 mmHg. Note increased dynamic stenosis at the subvalvar region (*white arrow*). At 1-year follow-up, the gradient was 16 mmHg by echo.

14. What are the results of balloon pulmonary valvuloplasty?

Successful pulmonary valvuloplasty is defined as a residual valvar gradient of 36 mmHg or less. By this criterion, a successful outcome can be expected in 80% of patients. As noted, long-term follow-up indicates that residual gradients either remain stable or gradually decrease with time. Predictors of failure include hypoplasia of the pulmonary annulus, low balloon-to-annulus ratios (< 1.2:1), and markedly dysplastic valves.

15. Will residual gradients progress?

Residual RVOT gradients immediately after pulmonary balloon valvuloplasty may represent a combination of valvar stenosis and of dynamic infundibular stenosis related to underlying ventricular hypertrophy. As the RV hypertrophy resolves over a period of weeks to months, the dynamic subvalvar stenosis contribution to the overall gradient disappears. After this initial improvement, residual gradients tend to remain static thereafter.

16. When should balloon pulmonary valvuloplasty be considered during pregnancy?

Mild to moderate degrees of pulmonary stenosis are well tolerated during pregnancy. Severe pulmonary stenosis (gradients in > 80 mmHg) may pose a problem because of the associated gestational volume overload on an already pressure-loaded RV. Pulmonary balloon valvuloplasty may be indicated in the third trimester in the setting of severe pulmonary valvar stenosis. Regardless of the degree of stenosis, infective endocarditis prophylaxis is recommended during delivery.

BIBLIOGRAPHY

1. Butto F, Amplatz K, Bass JL: Geometry of the proximal trunk during dilation with two balloons. Am. J. Cardiol. 58:380, 1986.
2. Fawzy ME, Gala O, Dunn B, et al: Regression of infundibular pulmonary stenosis after successful balloon pulmonary valvuloplasty in adults. Cathet Cardiovasc Diag 21:77, 1990.
3. Galindo A, Perloff JK: Cardiac catheterization as a therapeutic intervention. In Perloff JK, Child JS (eds): Congenital Heart Disease in Adults, 2nd ed. Philadelphia, W.B. Saunders, 1998, pp 271–290.
4. Hayes CJ, Gersony WM, Driscoll DJ, et al: Second natural history study of congenital heart defects: results of treatment of patients with pulmonary valve stenosis. Circulation 87(suppl I):28, 1993.
5. Hoffman JIE, Kaplan S: The incidence of congenital heart disease. J Am Coll Cardiol 39:1890, 2002.
6. Kaul UA, Singh B, Tyagi S, et al: Long-term results after pulmonary valvuloplasty in adults. Am Heart J 126:1152, 1993.
7. McCrindle BW: Independent predictors of long-term results after balloon pulmonary valvuloplasty. Circulation 89:1751, 1994.
8. McFaul PB, Dornan JC, Lamkihboyle D: Pregnancy complicated by maternal heart disease: a review of 519 women. Br J Obstet Gynaecol 95:861, 1988.
9. Perry SB, Lock JE: Intracardiac stent placement to relieve muscular and non-muscular obstruction. J Am Coll Cardiol 21:(suppl A):261, 1993.
10. Rao PS: How big a balloon and how many balloons for pulmonary valvuloplasty [editorial]? Am Heart J 116:577, 1986.
11. Rao PS: Transcatheter treatment of pulmonary outflow tract obstruction: a review. Prog Cardiovasc Dis 35:119, 1992

49. SEPTAL CLOSURE DEVICES AND CONGENITAL HEART DISEASE

Alvaro Galindo, M.D.

1. Which atrial septal defects (ASDs) are amenable to device closure?

There are a variety of defects of the atrial septum; however, only patent foramen ovale (PFO) and secundum ASDs are candidates for device occlusion. The term *foramen ovale* refers to an oblique anatomic communication between the right atrium (RA) and the left atrium (LA) consisting of two offset openings known as the fossa ovalis in the septum secundum and the ostium secundum in the septum primum. This results in a natural shunt that allows blood (primarily from the inferior vena cava) to flow from right to left during fetal circulation. After birth, this communication begins to close as LA pressure increases and the cleft between the two septae is obliterated. In some people, it remains patent and represents a potential site for systemic venous thrombi to gain access to the left heart and thus the systemic arterial circulation.

ASDs of the sinus venosus and primum type cannot be closed by the transcatheter approach. These defects are characterized by deficient rims and by proximity to cardiac structures such as the atrioventricular valves, coronary sinus, vena cavae, or pulmonary veins. A device used to close these defects would affect the function of these adjacent structures or would become dislodged and embolize.

2. What is the incidence of PFO?

The true incidence of PFOs is not known because most patients remain asymptomatic. It is estimated, however, that the incidence in the general population may be 20%.

3. Describe diagnostic modalities and maneuvers used in establishing the diagnosis of a PFO.

The diagnosis of a PFO is most often made by careful interrogation of the atrial septum by echocardiography (Fig. 1). It is necessary to perform a saline contrast injection through a peripheral intravenous line with simultaneous Valsalva maneuver. The yield is further enhanced by transesophageal echocardiogram (TEE).

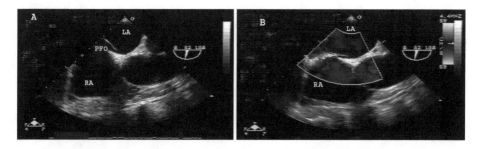

FIGURE 1. *A*, Transesophageal image of patent foramen ovale (PFO). *B*, Doppler interrogation of atrial septum depicting left to right flow across PFO.

4. What are cryptogenic strokes, and what is their association with PFO?

It is estimated that approximately 700,000 patients experience a cerebral stroke yearly in the United States. In 40% of these cases, no cause can be defined, thus, they are referred to as *cryp-*

togenic strokes. Using contrast echocardiograms, several investigators have found the incidence of PFO in patients who have experienced a cryptogenic stroke to be as high as 40% to 50% compared with the incidence of PFO in control groups of 4% to 10%.

5. What are the indications for closure a PFO?

The risk of recurrence of cryptogenic stroke in patients with PFOs is extremely high (50%). Current treatment strategies to prevent recurrence include anticoagulation therapy, surgical closure, or device occlusion of the PFO.

Indications for closure of PFO include history of stroke, transient ischemic attacks, or peripheral embolization in the absence of identifiable causes such as atrial fibrillation, hypercoagulable state, or cerebral artery disease.

6. Is anticoagulation therapy just as effective as surgical or device closure of PFO in reducing the incidence of recurrent strokes?

There is a high incidence of recurrent cryptogenic strokes in patients with PFO treated with warfarin. The recurrence rate may be as high as 50% in this population. Furthermore, anticoagulation therapy has an inherent risk of bleeding complications. The incidence of major bleeding events ranges between 1.5% and 11% per year.

Surgical closures have been shown to be effective in the prevention of recurrent strokes, as have device closures. These reports, however, have involved relatively small patient series. Large randomized trials of device closure compared with anticoagulation therapy are currently ongoing.

7. Describe the devices currently available for the occlusion of PFOs.

Several devices have been used for transcatheter occlusion of PFOs. These have included the Clamshell, Sideris Button, Das Angel Wings, Cardioseal, and Amplatzer PFO Occluder devices. Although several of these devices have undergone revisions and are still in use on an investigational basis in the United States, only the Cardioseal and Amplatzer devices have received Humanitarian Device Exemption designations by the Food and Drug Administration (FDA) and are in widespread use internationally.

The Cardioseal device consists of a double umbrella with four radial coil spring arms made of MPn35 (a nickel alloy). The fabric material is polyester. The Amplatzer PFO Occluder consists of a self-expandable, double disk device made of a nitinol wire mesh. Each disc has a thin polyester fabric. The connecting portion consists of a short flexible waist, which allows free motion of each disk (Fig. 2).

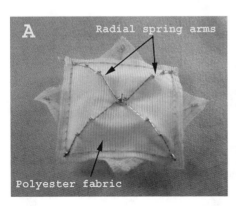
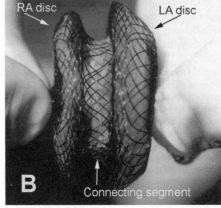

FIGURE 2. *A,* Cardioseal device. *B,* Amplatzer Septal Occluder and delivery calbe. LA = left atrial, RA = right atrial.

8. What are the results of device closure of PFOs?

Successful occlusion of the PFO can be defined as no bubbles crossing the atrial septum during saline-enhanced TEE Valsalva release. Early follow-up results indicate successful PFO occlusion can be achieved in more than 95% of cases. Because of the continued process of device endothelialization, this rate should approach 100% on late follow-up.

9. What is the incidence of secundum ASDs?

The overall incidence is approximately 0.94 per 1000 live births.

10. What are the indications and contraindications for device closure of an ASD?

Indications for device closure include echocardiographic documentation of a secundum ASD and clinical evidence of right ventricular (RV) volume overload. Evidence of the latter can consist of RV enlargement or a 1.5:1 left-to-right shunt.

Contraindications for device closure of a secundum ASD include presence of other cardiac defects that require surgical intervention, partial anomalous pulmonary venous return, pulmonary hypertension, intracardiac thrombi, sepsis, defects with margins of less than 5 mm, or defects with stretched diameters greater than 38 mm.

11. Describe the devices currently available for occlusion of ASDs.

A number of devices have been used for transcatheter occlusion of secundum ASDs. These have included the Clamshell, Sideris Button, Das Angel Wings, Cardioseal, Starflex, Helex, and Amplatzer Septal Occluder devices. Although several of these devices have undergone revisions and are still in use on an investigational basis in the United States, only the Amplatzer Septal Occluder is approved by the U.S. FDA.

The Amplatzer Septal Occluder consists of a self-expandable, double-disk device made of a nitinol wire mesh. The disks are joined together by a short, cylindrical connecting segment whose diameter corresponds to the stretched diameter of the defect to be occluded. Each disk and the center segment have a thin polyester fabric. Available device sizes range from 4 to 38 mm corresponding to the diameter of the center segment.

12. What are the current techniques for determining the size of the device to be used for ASD occlusion?

Device closure of an ASD should only be attempted with both fluoroscopic and echocardiographic guidance. The latter can be achieved with either TEE or intracardiac (ICE) echocardiography (Fig. 3). This allows for a more detailed evaluation of the number of defects and their location, distance from adjacent cardiac structures (mitral and tricuspid valves, coronary sinus, right pulmonary veins, and superior vena cava), and rim size.

It is imperative to determine the stretched diameter of the ASD. The stretched diameter can be calculated by pulling a round, compliant balloon across the defect and measuring the diameter of the largest balloon that can be pulled through. Otherwise, a large sizing balloon (24 or 34 mm diameter) can be inflated straddling the atrial septum. The waist on the balloon represents the atrial septum. The diameter of the balloon at the waist is, therefore, the stretched diameter (Fig. 4). The appropriate Amplatzer device is one whose middle segment diameter is the same size or slightly larger (1 mm) than the stretched diameter of the ASD.

13. What are the results of device closure of secundum ASDs?

The Amplatzer Septal Occluder could be placed successfully in 95.7% of attempted interventions. Successful occlusion as defined as residual shunt of less than 2 mm was achieved in 96.7% at 24 hours and 98.5% at 12-month follow-up.

14. Name the risks of ASD or PFO device occlusion.

As with most cardiac catheterization interventional procedures, the risks include air embolization, reaction to contrast material, exposure to x-rays, blood loss requiring transfusion, and

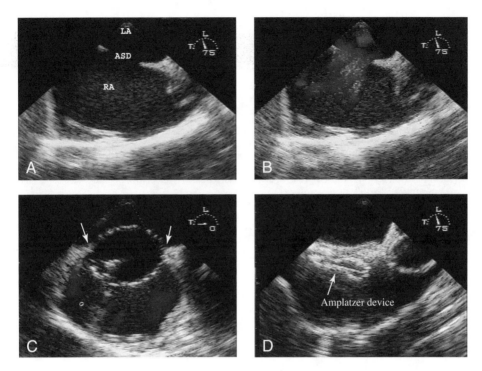

FIGURE 3. TEE of atrial septal defect (*A*), left to right shunt (*B*), balloon sizing of ASD (*C*), and Amplatzer device occlusion of ASD (*D*).

trauma to blood vessels or heart chambers. Risks more specifically related to device closure of ASDs or PFOs include device embolization, perforation of atrial wall, arrhythmias, infection, headaches or migraines, stroke, or transient ischemic attack.

15. What other septal defects can be closed using these occlusion devices?

In addition to occlusion of secundum ASDs and PFO, occlusion devices have been used in a variety of other settings. These include Fontan fenestrations, congenital ventricular septal defects, and postinfarction ventricular septal defects.

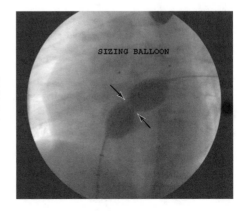

FIGURE 4. Cranial long axial oblique projection of sizing balloon across atrial septum. The diameter of the waist that forms on the balloon (*arrows*) represents the stretched diameter of the atrial septal defect.

BIBLIOGRAPHY

1. Beitzke A, Schuchlenz H, Gamillscheg A, et al: Catheter closure of the persistent foramen ovale: mid-term results in 162 patients. J Intervent Cardiol 14:223–230, 2001.
2. Cao QL, Du ZD, Joseph A, et al: Immediate and six-month results of the profile of the Amplatzer Septal Occluder as assessed by transesophageal echocardiography. A J Cardiol 88:754–759, 2001.
3. DiTullio M, Sacco RL, Gopal A, et al: Patent foramen ovale as a risk factor for cryptogenic stroke. Ann Intern Med 117:461–465, 1992.
4. Latson LA: Per-catheter ASD closure. Pediatr Cardiol 19:86–93, 1998.
5. Omeish A, Hijazi ZM: Transcatheter closure of atrial septal defects in children and adults using the Amplatzer Septal Occluder. J Intervent Cardiol 14:37–44, 2001.
6. Perry SB, Van der Velde ME, Bridges ND, et al: Transcatheter closure of atrial and ventricular septal defects. Herz 18:135–142, 1993.
7. Sacco RL, Ellenberg JH, Mohr JP, et al: Infarcts of undetermined origin: NINCDS stroke data bank. Ann Neurol 25:382–390, 1989.
8. Windecker S, Wahl A, Becker U, et al: Percutaneous closure of patent foramen ovale in patients with paradoxical embolism: long-term risk of recurrent thromboembolic events. Circulation 101:893–898, 2000.

XI. Peripheral Vascular Disease

50. DIAGNOSIS AND EVALUATION OF PERIPHERAL ARTERIAL DISEASE

Darwin Eton, M.D.

1. What are the guiding principles in the management of patients with peripheral arterial disease?

Except for aneurysms, pseudoaneurysms, embolic lesions, and arteriovenous fistulas, most peripheral vascular diseases are primarily treated medically, with intervention reserved for failure of medical therapy.

2. With all the technology available today, what is the role of a medical history and physical examination?

A well-performed clinical evaluation is the basis of diagnosis and treatment. It provides the information needed to establish the relevance and clinical magnitude of the disease and to guide the clinician in selecting the most cost-effective method (if any) among the wide array of diagnostic tests available. The diagnostic tests generally provide additional hemodynamic, physiologic, or anatomic information needed to plan the most appropriate therapy. The decision to intervene should be made on the basis of the clinical assessment. Despite all the newer and increasingly sophisticated diagnostic tools, the basis of the modern approach to diagnosis in vascular patients remains the history and physical examination. Because medical therapy includes atherosclerotic risk factor modification, the history needs to encompass review of these risk factors in detail. These risk factors include age, hypertension, tobacco use, hyperlipidemia, hypertension, homocystinemia, coronary artery disease, stroke, renal failure, genetic predisposition, hypercoaguability, autoimmune disorders (vasculitis), and (in the case of aneurysms) emphysema.

3. What are absolute contraindications to limb revascularization?

- Flexion contracture of the knee or hip precluding ambulation
- Rigor mortis of the calf (see acute ischemia section)
- Hemiplegia or severe hemiparesis precluding ambulation
- Extensive tissue destruction precluding foot salvage proximal to the midfoot unless an intervention is needed to heal a more distal amputation
- Life-threatening limb infections such as necrotizing fasciitis or *Clostridium perfringens* that extend onto the proximal foot or calf unless an intervention is needed to heal a more distal amputation.
- Severe comorbidities precluding safe anesthesia
- Nonhemodynamically significant disease unless it is embolic or aneurysmal
- Projected inability to withstand the hyperkalemic acidotic washout from reperfusion of profoundly ischemic muscle (e.g., acute renal failure with hyperkalemia that cannot be corrected before or during the reperfusion phase or severe cardiomyopathy and uncorrectable shock before reperfusion)

4. What are the relative contraindications to limb revascularization?

- Severe hypercoaguability and a lack of compliance with anticoagulation
- Mild to moderate symptoms (e.g., nondisabling calf claudication)
- Severe comorbidities with short life expectancy
- Poor bypass options (e.g., small or absent conduit, unreconstructable pedal outflow occlusive disease)
- No hope for rehabilitation or ambulation based on comorbidities
- Calcaneal or midfoot osteomyelitis unless needed to heal a more proximal amputation
- Extensive plantar necrosis unless needed to heal a more proximal amputation
- Coexistent unresectable sarcoma or other tumor in the limb
- Severe comorbidities that could be complicated by the intervention

5. What is acute ischemia?

Acute ischemia is characterized by sudden onset of pain, followed by pallor, paresthesias, poikilothermia (coolness), and paresis (the five P's). Typically, the calf remains soft until rigor mortis sets in, at which point the calf is doughy and the joints stiffen. If this physical finding is present, revascularization is contraindicated because the muscle death is extensive and irreversible and the resultant hyperkalemia and acidosis from reperfusion are lethal. If the calf remains soft, expeditious revascularization is required. Although 6 hours is often quoted as the interval of opportunity, my experience is that the opportunity exists as long as the muscle remains soft. The first tissue to be **irreversibly** damaged by ischemia is muscle. Nerve is quickly but **reversibly** injured by ischemia, and peripheral neurologic ischemia alone is not a contraindication to revascularization.

6. What is chronic limb ischemia?

Chronic limb ischemia is manifested by claudication and, if it is severe, by ischemic rest pain of the forefoot, nonhealing ulcers, or gangrene. These warrant reconstructive efforts within the limits described previously.

Unlike claudication, ischemic rest pain is experienced *not* in a muscle group but rather in the foot, specifically the toes and metatarsal heads. It should not be confused with *night cramps,* which are common in patients with atherosclerosis and occur as painful cramps of the calf muscle that usually begin after the patient has fallen asleep and are relieved by massage of the muscle. In its earliest manifestations, rest pain may be experienced as dysesthesias in the foot after it has been elevated for some time. At this stage, the patient can usually relieve the pain by dangling the affected extremity over the side of the bed or, paradoxically, by getting up and walking around. Because this pain typically occurs at night, some clinicians call it *night pain* to distinguish it from the more severe rest pain that is constant and present even with dependency.

Ischemic rest pain implies a reduction of blood flow in the extremity to a level below that required for normal resting tissue metabolism. If left untreated, tissue necrosis results. The affected limb is relatively useless or incapacitated by the constant pain and paresthesias. Because patients with ischemic rest pain typically keep the limb dependent, there is often edema, which further compromises tissue perfusion. Angiography in such extremities invariably demonstrates at least two—and often three or more—serial obstructions of the arterial tree. By contrast, in claudicants, usually only one or, at most, two segments are involved.

7. What are the hemodynamic considerations in the ischemic leg?

Blood flow is directly proportional to arterial pressure and inversely related to peripheral resistance. *Arterial pressure* is determined by cardiac output, peripheral resistance, and circulating blood volume. *Peripheral resistance* in the normal limb is a function of the precapillary arterioles, blood viscosity, tissue pressure, and venous pressure. A hemodynamically significant stenosis results in a decrease in distal perfusion pressure and an increase in peripheral resistance, reducing blood flow.

The Poiseuille equation provides a relationship between fluid flow in a straight tube (Q) and the pressure gradient (ΔP), viscosity (μ), radius of the vessel (R), length of the stenosis (L), and mean flow velocity (V):

$$Q = \Delta P \, (\pi R^4) \, / \, 8L\mu = \Delta P \, r^2 \, / \, 8 \, VL\mu$$

The flow through a stenosis or through narrow collateral vessels is proportional to the radius to the fourth power and inversely to the length of the stenosis.

When a main limb artery is occluded, the total resistance to flow that results is the sum of the parallel resistances (r) imposed by the collateral vessels that bypass that segment and is expressed by the formula

$$\frac{1}{r} = \frac{1}{r_1} + \frac{1}{r_2} + \frac{1}{4_n}$$

As the vessels dilate over time, this resistance diminishes and flow improves. If a second segment of the same artery becomes occluded, adding a resistance *in series,* the total resistance is expressed by the formula:

$$r_{total} = r_1 + r_2 + \ldots r_n$$

The impact of resistance in series is additive and further diminishes the capacity of the arterial tree to meet the functional demands imposed by exercise, infection, or the dissipation of external heat. Finally, even the minimal flow needed to sustain viability is compromised, and tissue necrosis ensues.

8. What is the impact of the collateral circulation?

Collateral vessels are generally preexisting pathways that enlarge when a stenosis or an occlusion develops in the distributing branches of large and medium-sized arteries. In general, collaterals are not a result of neovascularization. Anatomically as well as functionally, the collateral bed is divided into:

- Stem arteries
- Mid-zone collaterals
- Reentry arteries

5. What is the effect of exercise on the collateral circulation?

The pressure differential that develops across the collateral bed after arterial occlusion causes a reversal of flow in the distal mid-zone collateral channels and increases the velocity of flow through them as they dilate in response to this stimulus. Exercise enhances this by producing relative tissue hypoxia and acidosis, which reduces peripheral resistance, thus magnifying the pressure gradient across the occlusion.

10. What is the relationship between collateral flow and symptoms?

Collateral channels that form in response to a chronic, unisegmental occlusion can usually provide adequate blood flow to meet the resting needs of the limb and sufficient additional flow to sustain moderate exercise. Sudden occlusion of a previously normal vessel, however, as might occur with an arterial embolus, may not allow sufficient time for the collateral circulation to compensate for the acute ischemia and may result in tissue necrosis or frank gangrene. If the collateral development around an arterial stenosis keeps pace with any progression of the disease, there may be little change in symptoms. The patient may experience a transient period of severe limb ischemia that gradually relents over the next few weeks as the collateral circulation expands to its ultimate potential.

Although atherosclerosis usually spares the mid-zone collaterals, progressive intimal disease or extension of the main vessel thrombosis may occlude the stem or reentry vessels, thus compromising the effectiveness of the entire collateral network. In the absence of occlusion, collateral blood flow may be reduced by decreased cardiac output, increased blood viscosity, hyper-fibrinogenemia, or dehydration.

11. What are the anatomic variations of the collaterals at different levels, and what are their clinical relevance?

Occlusion of the distal abdominal aorta recruits stem collaterals from the intercostal and lumbar arteries to connect with reentry collaterals of the iliolumbar, gluteal, deep circumflex iliac, and epigastric arteries. A secondary visceral pathway arises from the left colic branch of the superior mesenteric artery, continues through the meandering mesenteric artery, and finally reenters the hypogastric artery via the hemorrhoidal plexus. For external iliac or common femoral artery occlusions, collateral supply develops by way of the hypogastric artery and its gluteal branches with the femoral circumflex branches of the profunda femoris (deep femoral) artery; this important collateral pathway is known as the *cruciate anastomosis*. The relationship between the aortoiliac collateral vessels and the visceral circulation explains how occlusive disease involving both systems may predispose patients to bowel ischemia and necrosis if these channels are disrupted at surgery or if flow through them is altered after aortofemoral bypass.

The interconnection of the perforating branches of the profunda femoris artery and the genicular branches of the popliteal artery readily compensates for occlusion of the superficial femoral artery. This network in the upper leg depends largely on the profunda femoris artery as a critical link between the cruciate and genicular networks and emphasizes the importance of a patent popliteal artery that serves as the reentry vessel for this vital collateral pathway. In a similar fashion, the genicular arteries, via their tibial connections, bypass popliteal obstructions. Occlusion of the anterior and posterior tibial arteries is often compensated for by the peroneal artery, which sends large collateral branches to the patent distal segments of the tibial arteries at the ankle. The paucity of collaterals in the lower leg explains why even unisegmental occlusion of the distal popliteal and proximal tibial arteries may result in such severe ischemia of the distal lower extremity.

12. What is the role of the vascular laboratory?
- Confirmation of physical findings
- Objective documentation
- Establishment of a baseline
- Sequential follow-up

13. What arterial tests are commonly performed in the vascular laboratory?
- Ankle brachial index
- Segmental pressures
- Doppler-derived waveforms
- Pulse volume recording
- Transcutaneous oxygen tension
- Duplex imaging

14. What is continuous-wave Doppler?

This is the hand held or pencil Doppler used clinically at the patient's bedside. It is helpful in locating pulses that are not palpable and is used to calculate the ankle brachial index (ABI). The ABI is the ratio of the highest systolic pressure measured by Doppler in the dorsalis pedis or posterior tibial artery with the cuff at the distal calf compared with the highest systolic pressure measured by Doppler of the two brachial arteries, with the cuff placed on the upper arm. Normal ABI ranges from 0.95 to 1.2. Mild resting ischemia ranges from 0.70 to 0.94. Moderate resting ischemia ranges from 0.50 to 0.69. Severe ischemia at rest ranges from 0.00 to 0.49. The standard error of the measurement is 15%. A normal ABI at rest does not mean the patient has no vascular disease. Caveats include incompressible vessels that artificially elevate the ABI (diabetes, renal failure), and subcritical stenosis. In the latter case, exercise or stress testing on a treadmill will be abnormal. An ABI repeated after onset of claudication will show a decrease compared with at rest. This suggests subcritical stenosis uncovered by exercise.

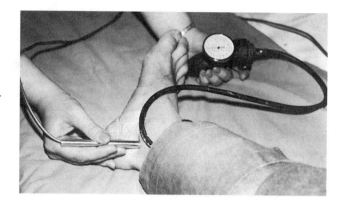

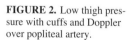

FIGURE 1. Ankle cuff for ABI calculation.

15. What are segmental pressures?

Segmental Doppler-derived pressures are measured with appropriate-sized blood pressure cuffs (Table 1). The Doppler is used to measure the systolic pressure below the cuff. Typically, high and low thigh cuff pressures are measured with the Doppler over the popliteal artery, but many laboratories select the dorsalis pedis (DP) or posterior tibial (PT) at the ankle for the entire exam. High and low calf cuff pressures are measured with the Doppler over the DP and PT (Fig. 2). Transmetatarsal pressures are measured typically with the cuff around the mid foot and a photoplethysmograph (PPG) probe over a digital artery distally (Fig. 3). Toe pressures are obtained with an even smaller cuff placed around the toe and the PPG probe is placed on the same toe (Fig. 4). Penile pressures can be measured similarly. Again, segmental pressures are subject to error based on the extent of medial calcification of the underlying artery below the cuff.

Table 1. Cuff Size for an Average Limb

CUFF LOCATION	ADULT CUFF SIZE (CM)
Upper thigh	11.0
Lower thigh	19.0
Thigh (contour type)	22.0
Ankle	12.0
Finger	2.0–2.5
Toe	2.5–3.0

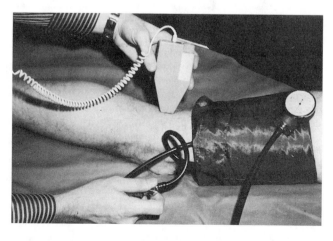

FIGURE 2. Low thigh pressure with cuffs and Doppler over popliteal artery.

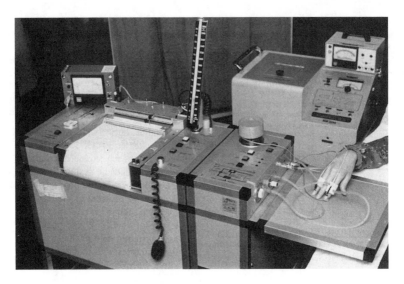

FIGURE 3. Digital PPG.

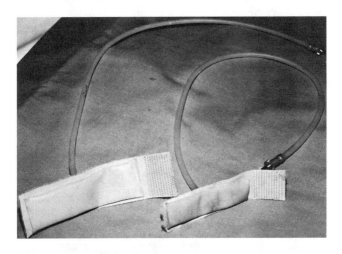

FIGURE 4. Toe pressure.

16. What are Doppler-derived waveforms?

These are the most helpful qualitative measure of flow over an artery. The test requires skill because the probe needs to be placed between 45 and 60 degrees of the axis of the artery and be pointed solely at the artery because any nearby venous signal will affect the tracing. The tracing is a representation of the Doppler shift frequencies obtained as sound is reflected back from the flowing blood particles (Fig. 5). A normal artery has a "triphasic" pattern throughout the cardiac cycle, with an immediate steep upsweep of the tracing followed by a downsweep below the baseline (flow reversal) and then another shorter upsweep. The tracing is sharp: there is little broadening of the tracing or "filling in" below the tracing. Spectral broadening and filling in of the window indicate turbulence. As the artery stiffens, the reversed flow disappears and the waveform looks "biphasic." As the stenosis worsens, the waveform becomes monophasic and the spectral window fills in and broadens. An occluded vessel has no flow. Distal to the occlusion, a patent vessel will likely show a monophasic flattened waveform. These are helpful guidelines in eval-

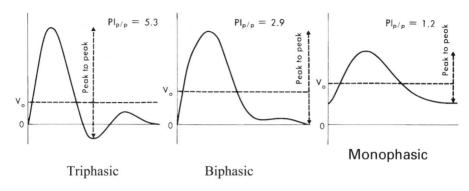

FIGURE 5. Doppler-derived waveforms. Pulsatility index = peak to peak amplitude divided by the mean amplitude (V_0) over the cardiac cycle. The Y axis is frequency shift; the X axis is time. Velocity is calculated from the frequency shift by the Doppler equation.

uating the hemodynamics in patients in whom calcified vessels give erroneous high systolic segmental pressures.

17. What is a pulse volume recording (PVR)?

This test is used to identify flow characteristics in an extremity (Fig. 6). Similar to the segmental pressure test, cuffs of different sizes are placed on the extremity at different levels. They are then inflated to 65 mmHg to give a snug fit. As the cardiac cycle unfolds, blood enters the leg, expanding its volume into the cuff. This raises the pressure within the cuff, which is then recorded at each cuff position (i.e., thigh, high calf, low calf, transmetatarsal, and toe) as the blood flows down the limb. The PVR is not influenced by leg edema.

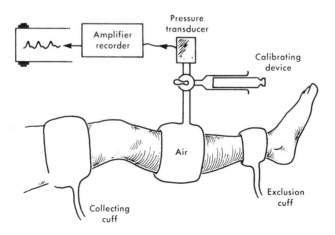

FIGURE 6. Pulse volume recorder cuffs at three positions.

Extremity occlusive disease is documented by PVR as a decrease in rise of the anacrotic limb, rounding and delay in the pulse crest, decreased rate of fall of the catacrotic limb, and absence of reflected diastolic wave (Table 2).

Table 2. Correlating PVR Chart Deflection in Millimeters and Presence of Reflected Wave with Wound Healing

CATEGORY	CHART DEFLECTION (MM)		REFLECTED WAVE	WOUND HEALING
	THIGH + ANKLE	CALF		
1.	> 15	> 20	Yes	Likley
2	> 15	> 20	No	Likely
3	5–15	5–20	No	Probable
4	< 5	< 5	No	Unlikely
5	Flat	Flat	No	Unlikely

18. What is transcutaneous oxygen measurement (TCpO2)?

This test is used to estimate amputation or ulcer healing ability in the extremity based on blood flow. It is especially useful in diabetic or renal failure patients whose vessels are calcified. The test is invalid in the presence of swelling, infection, or cellulitis. A probe is placed on the foot near the lesion. With the patient breathing room air, the normal $TCpO_2$ is 40 to 70 mmHg; if it is less than 20 mmHg, no healing will occur. Healing is likely if the $TCpO_2$ is greater than 30 mmHg (Table 3).

Table 3. Ankle and Toe Pressures Correlated to Healing Potential

PRESSURE (mmHg)	HEALING PROBABILITY (%)	
	NO DIABETES	DIABETES
Ankle Pressure		
< 55	0%	0%
55–90	85	45
> 90	100	85
Toe Pressure		
< 20	25	29
20–30	73	40
30–55	100	85
> 55	100	97

19. What is duplex imaging?

Similar to echocardiography, duplex imaging provides real time hemodynamic information throughout systole and diastole, along with two-dimensional images. The primary limitation is inability to insonnate through severe calcium. The test results are technician dependent, so validation of each laboratory is required.

Table 4. Duplex Sensitivity and Specificity in Predicting Disease Compared with Angiogram

ARTERY	N	SENSITIVITY	SPECIFICITY
Aorta	25	100%	100%
Iliac	110	89	90
CFA	50	67	98
SFA	123	84	93
Profunda	48	67	81
Popliteal	37	75	97
All	393	82	92
Grafts	10	67	100

20. What cerebrovascular diagnostics are offered in the vascular laboratory
- Indirect examinations:
  Oculopneumoplethysmography
  Periorbital Doppler study

- Direct examinations
  - Carotid and vertebral artery duplex ultrasound imaging
  - Transcranial Doppler examination

21. What is ocular pneumoplethysmography (OPG)?

Described by Gee in 1974, this is a technique by which the ophthalmic artery's systolic pressure (OSP) is indirectly measured via suction ophthalmodynomometry. Without being able to pinpoint stenosis location, OPG does detect the presence of a hemodynamically significant arterial stenosis (> 50–60% by diameter or > 75% by area) anywhere between the heart and the ophthalmic artery (Table 5). This includes disease in the cervical, thoracic, and intracranial (carotid siphon) portions of the carotid artery. The latter two areas are not visualized by conventional duplex ultrasonography.[1]

Table 5. Percent Diameter Stenosis versus Percent Area Stenosis Assuming Concentric Circles

% STENOSIS BY	
Diameter	Area
0	0
10	19
20	36
30	51
40	64
50	75
60	84
70	91
80	96
90	99
100	100

Percent diameter stenosis = $\% D_s = 100 \times [1 - (\text{inner diameter/outer diameter})]$
Percent area stenosis = $\% A_s = 100 \times [1 - (\text{inner area/outer area})]$
$\% A_s = 100 - 100 \times [1 - (\% D_s/100)]^2$

A less frequent use of OPG is the assessment of collateral ophthalmic artery pressure. For this assessment, common carotid artery (CCA) compression is used during OPG measurements (Table 6). This maneuver is purportedly useful in determining which patients may require intraoperative shunting during carotid endarterectomy, identifying patients who will tolerate carotid artery ligation, and predicting which asymptomatic patients with significant stenoses are at increased risk of stroke.

Table 6. Normal Carotid Artery Characteristics

VESSEL	WAVE SHAPE	SPECTRAL BROADENING	RESISTANCE	FLOW TURBULENCE
CCA	Biphasic	Absent	Mixed	Absent
ICA	Biphasic	Absent	Low	In bulb
ECA	Triphasic	Absent	High	Absent

Despite these potential applications, the use of OPG has been largely supplanted by direct duplex ultrasound imaging and transcranial Doppler.

22. What is a periorbital Doppler study?

Intracranial collateralization between the branches of the external (ECA) and internal carotid (ICA) arteries develops in the presence of a hemodynamically significant stenosis (> 75% area stenosis) in the ICA (Table 7). As an ICA stenosis progresses toward occlusion, the flow in the ophthalmic artery reverses as the ECA branches become the primary source of blood supply to the eye and to the intracranial ICA branches. With the use of a bidirectional Doppler system, this flow reversal may be detected.

Table 7. Classification of ICA Stenosis

DIAMETER STENOSIS	PEAK SYSTOLIC VELOCITY, CM/SEC	END-DIASTOLIC VELOCITY, CM/SEC	SPECTRAL BROADENING
0%	< 125		Mild to none during the deceleration phase of systole
1–15	< 125		Mild during the deceleration phase of systole
16–49	< 125		Mild during systole
50–79	> 125		Increased
80–99	> 125	> 100–140*	Marked
100	N/A	N/A	No flow

In the absence of a hemodynamically significant ICA stenosis, flow in the frontal and supra-orbital arteries should be antegrade (i.e., toward the probe). Flow should either augment or not change with compressions.

23. What does duplex ultrasonography add to the cerebrovascular examination?

Carotid duplex is a form of ultrasonography that combines two modalities: B-mode imaging and Doppler spectral waveform analysis. B-mode imaging, also referred to as the *brightness-mode,* provides a high-resolution grayscale anatomic image of both tissue and vessels on a monitor. The presence, contour, severity, and composition of atheromatous plaque is ascertainable. Doppler spectral analysis provides information concerning blood flow hemodynamics. With the color-flow imaging modality, speed and direction of flow are represented as different intensities of color.

In addition to screening for the presence of carotid atherosclerosis, the carotid duplex has become an essential factor in the management of the patient after carotid endarterectomy. Follow-up carotid duplex scans are done 1 and 6 months postoperatively, and every 6 months to 1 year thereafter.

The reported EDV used as the predictor for 80% to 99% disease classification varies among authors.

24. What is transcranial Doppler (TCD)?

Aaslid developed TCD in the early 1980s. It enables a focused ultrasonic beam to penetrate through selective windows in the head, including parts of the skull, in order to insonate the basal cerebral blood vessels. Information about blood flow, including velocity (cm/sec), direction, and relative downstream resistance, is ascertained. TCD measures flow velocity and *not* regional cerebral blood flow (rCBF). Arteries commonly insonated are the ophthalmic, internal carotid (ICA), (siphon and distal portion), proximal middle cerebral (MCA), proximal anterior cerebral (ACA), distal vertebral artery (VA), and proximal basilar artery (BA).

25. What are summary statistics?

Every vascular laboratory needs to correlate its observations with clinical and anatomic data obtained by other techniques. Statistics are vital to this comparison. t = true, f = false, p = positive, n = negative.

Sensitivity: Ability to recognize disease: tp/(tp+fn)

Specificity: Ability to recognize absence of disease: tn/(tn+fp)

Positive predictive value: Probability that a positive test result implies disease is present: tp/(tp+fp)

Negative predictive value: Probability that a negative test result implies disease is absent: tn/(tn+fn)

Overall accuracy: (tp+tn)/(tp+tn+fp+fn)

Prevalence: (tp+fn)/(tp+tn+fp+fn)

BIBLIOGRAPHY

1. Baker JD, Barker WF, Machleder HI: Ocular pneumoplethysmography in the evaluation of carotid stenosis. Circulation 62(suppl I):1–3, 1980.
2. Barnes RW, Garret WV, Slaymaker EE, et al: Doppler ultrasound and supraorbital photoplethysmography screening of carotid occlusive disease. Am J Surg 134:183, 1977.
3. Barnes RW, Russell HE, et al: Doppler cerebrovascular examination: Improved results with refinements in technique. Stroke 8:468, 1977.
4. Bluth EI, Wetzner SM, Stavros AT, et al: Carotid duplex sonography: a multicenter recommendation for standardized imaging and carotid Doppler criteria. RadioGraphics, 8:487–506, 1988.
5. Brockenbbroug EC: Screening for prevention of stroke: use of a Doppler flowmeter [brochure]. Washington/Alaska Regional Medical Programme, 1970.
6. Daigle RJ, et al: Velocity criteria for differentiation of 60–79% carotid stenoses from 80% or greater stenoses. J Vasc Technol 7:177–183, 1988.
7. Eikelboom BC: Evaluation of carotid artery disease and potential collateral circulation by ocular pneumoplethysmography [thesis]. Utrecht, The Netherlands, 1981.
8. Executive Committee for the Asymptomatic Carotid Atherosclerosis Study Endarterectomy for Asymptomatic Carotid Artery Stenosis. JAMA 273:1421–1428, 1995.
9. Faught WE, Mattos MA, van Bemmeler PS, et al: Colorflow duplex scanning of carotid arteries: new velocity criteria based on receiver operator characteristic analysis for threshold stenoses used in the symptomatic and asymptomatic carotid trials. J Vasc Surg 19:818–827, 1994.
10. Gee W, Oller DW, Wylie EJ: Noninvasive diagnosis of carotid occlusion by ocular pneumoplethysmography. Stroke 7:18, 1976.
11. Hood DB, Mattos MA, Mansour A, et al: Prospective evaluation of new duplex criteria to identify 70% internal carotid artery stenosis. J Vasc Surg 23:254–262, 1996.
12. Machleder HI, Barker WF: Noninvasive methods for evaluation of extracranial cerebrovascular disease. Arch Surg 112:944, 1977.
13. Moneta GL, Edwards JM, Chitwood RW, et al: Correlation of North American symptomatic carotid endarterectomy trial (NASCET) angiographic definition of 70% to 99% internal carotid artery stenosis with duplex scanning. J Vasc Surg 17:152–157, 1993.
14. Roederer GO, Langlois YE, Chan AW, et al: Ultrasonic duplex screening of extracranial arteries: improved accuracy using new features from the common carotid artery. J Cardiovasc Ultrasonogr, I, 1982.
15. Roederer GO, Strandness DE, et al: A simple spectral parameter for accurate classification of severe carotid diseease. Bruit 8:174–178, 1984.

51. ILIAC ARTERY INTERVENTION

Alex Powell, M.D., Barry T. Katzen, M.D., James F. Benenati, M.D.,
Gerald Zemel, M.D., Gary J. Becker, M.D., and Margaret Kovacs, Ed.D., M.S.N.

1. Should the symptomatic (ipsilateral) or asymptomatic (contralateral) leg be punctured for a diagnostic angiogram of the extremities?

In general, the contralateral limb should be accessed when performing a diagnostic angiogram. The reasons for this are multiple. If puncture and catheter placement were to be made through a critical stenosis on the ipsilateral limb, the presence of a catheter or vascular sheath could occlude the vessel. Furthermore, symptoms of claudication may be caused by infrainguinal disease. A retrograde puncture central to this disease would rule out any treatment options through this approach. However, lesions of the superior femoral artery (SFA) and tibial vessels can be treated from a contralateral approach or the patient could be brought back for an antegrade puncture through the affected groin. Although it is true that an antegrade puncture can be performed after an ipsilateral puncture, the frequent small hematomas encountered postangiogram and the increase in patient discomfort make this a secondary rather than a preferred method of treatment.

The one exception may be in cases in which a high-quality diagnostic magnetic resonance angiogram has been performed and an isolated iliac artery stenosis has been identified in the affected limb. If it is believed that this lesion alone is responsible for the patient's symptoms, then puncture of the ipsilateral groin may be indicated. The one possible pitfall to avoid in this scenario is a critical stenosis in which placement of the diagnostic catheter or sheath results in occlusion of flow. With flow occluded, it is difficult to assess the true extent of the disease adequately. Moreover, if the artery remains occluded for any significant length of time, thrombus could develop, which would obviously significantly complicate treatment.

2. Should an ipsilateral or contralateral approach be used in iliac interventions?

The answer to this depends on a number of issues. It is certainly possible to perform an angioplasty or stent procedure for either the ipsilateral or contralateral groin in many iliac interventions. However, in some situations, the ipsilateral approach has definite advantages. When stenting a lesion at the origin of the common iliac artery, precision is needed so that the stent covers the lesion but does not overlap into the aorta and possibly disrupt flow to the contralateral iliac artery. In such a case, an ipsilateral approach is far more precise and should be favored.

To treat a lesion from the contralateral groin, it is first necessary to place a sheath over the aortic bifurcation. This allows for adequate imaging of the region of interest during balloon dilation or stent placement. Furthermore, this sheath allows for easy postintervention imaging without giving up guidewire access.

3. Is angioplasty or primary stenting the treatment method of choice for focal iliac artery lesions?

The Dutch iliac stent trial showed that there was no significant difference in patient outcomes when patients had a good angioplasty result compared with patients who had a primary stent. However, what this data fail to show is that achieving a good angioplasty outcome can often be time consuming and require repeated inflations. For these reasons, many operators choose to place a stent primarily.

4. When performing iliac artery angioplasty or stenting, what criteria should be used to determine the endpoint of the procedure?

The endpoint of iliac artery interventions is both the angiographic and hemodynamic result. After intervention, a completion angiogram should be performed in at least two views. Certainly, a poor angiographic result will be associated with a poor hemodynamic result. However, the converse is not necessarily true. Despite a good angiographic appearance postintervention, it is still important to obtain hemodynamic measurements above and below the lesion. This is best accomplished through the use of a vascular sheath and smaller angiographic catheter through the sheath. This allow for simultaneous pressure measurements. Moreover, access across the lesion does not need to be abandoned as would happen with pullback pressure measurements.

Hemodynamic recordings should be obtained with and without the administration of a vasodilator into the affected limb. Frequently, these measurements can uncover a radiographically occult residual lesion. Operators should strive for a final gradient of zero at rest and less than 10 mmHg after vasodilator dosing.

5. If a patient has disease of the distal aorta extending into the iliac arteries, what is the preferred method of treatment?

The answer to this depends on the extent of the aortic disease. If 1 cm or less of the terminal aorta is involved, the aortic bifurcation is typically raised by placing parallel "kissing" iliac stents (Fig. 1). In cases in which the distal aorta is extensively diseased, an "inverted Y" technique is used. With this, a single stent is placed into the aorta. Kissing iliac stents are then placed into the aortic stent.

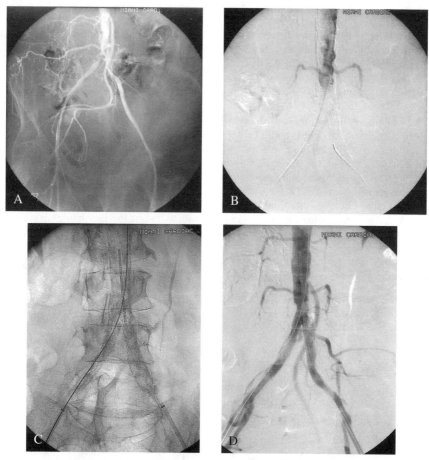

FIGURE 1. Kissing iliac stents. *A,* The initial diagnostic angiogram shows bilateral short segment common iliac artery occlusions. However, there is only minimal involvement of the distal aorta. *B,* Initial attempts at traversing the left-sided occlusion resulted in a subintimal dissection as evidenced by the guidewire lying clearly outside the vessel lumen. *C,* The guidewire was then repositioned with subsequent placement of kissing stents. The level of the aortic bifurcation was raised slightly to treat the distal aortic disease. *D,* The final angiogram shows now normal flow through the stented segments.

6. What is the most important patient sign or symptom to watch during iliac interventions?

Although it is obviously important to monitor all of the patient's vital signs, careful attention to any pain that a patient is having is probably the single most important factor to monitor. Mild or even moderate pain is not unusual during angioplasty or stenting. However, it is critically important to determine if the pain resolves after balloon deflation. If pain persists, an angiogram should be performed without delay to assess for possible rupture. Tachycardia and hypotension can also be signs of an iliac rupture; however, they occur after significant blood loss. Ideally, a rupture is detected and treated before signs of hemodynamic shock develop.

In addition to signifying potential rupture, patients' complaints of pain are also useful to gauge proper balloon size during interventions. If a patient complains of severe pain during balloon inflation, it is probably not wise to redilate with a larger balloon.

7. What type of artery is most prone to rupture during an iliac intervention?

Heavily calcified iliac arteries are the most likely to rupture during intervention. In particular, a heavily calcified external iliac artery is the most likely to rupture. Although the common iliac artery may rupture as well, care should be exercised when treating a patient with a calcified external iliac artery. If any debate exists as to the proper balloon size, a smaller balloon should be used first. A larger balloon can then be used if further dilation is needed and no problems were encountered with the first dilation. However, caution should be used and great care should be taken to avoid significant overdilation of a heavily calcified artery.

Although relatively rare, arteries that have been previously exposed to therapeutic radiation are also prone to rupture.

8. If, when performing an iliac intervention from a contralateral approach, an arterial rupture is encountered, what should be done?

The first maneuver that must be performed after an iliac rupture is immediate tamponade of the bleeding site. If this is not accomplished with alacrity, the patient may exsanguinate. If an iliac artery rupture is suspected, the initial postintervention angiogram should be performed through the bifurcation sheath, leaving the balloon within the sheath. If a rupture is confirmed, the balloon should then rapidly be readvanced and inflated over the site of the rupture (Fig. 2). After this is accomplished, it is important to perform another angiogram to confirm that the rupture has been temporarily sealed with the balloon; a larger balloon may be necessary if the bleeding persists.

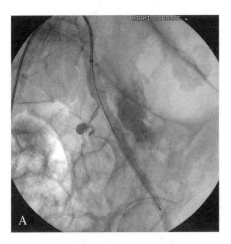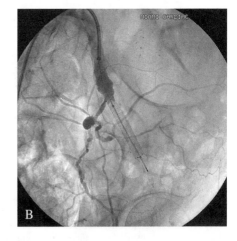

FIGURE 2. Iliac rupture. After stent placement and subsequent balloon dilation of a calcified external iliac artery lesion (*A*), significant contrast extravasation is observed. The angioplasty balloon (inflated with saline) was then immediately placed across the site of rupture. Injection through the up and over sheath (*B*) demonstrates successful temporary occlusion of the external iliac artery.

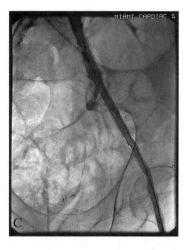

FIGURE 2. (*continued*) An ipsilateral (*left*) access was then made and a covered stent was placed across the site of rupture (*C*).

The next step is somewhat controversial. Some authors have reported successful repair of the injured vessel using a prolonged inflation across the site. However, delayed ruptures after this treatment have also been seen. Therefore, it is the opinion of the authors that the injury needs definitive repair. This can be accomplished with either surgical repair or placement of a covered stent. Although it is an off-label use, both Wallgrafts (Boston Scientific) and ViaBahns (Gore) make placement of a covered stent our procedure of choice.

If a covered stent is to be placed, the next step after temporary hemostasis is arterial access into the ipsilateral common femoral artery. After this is accomplished, the occlusion balloon must be temporarily deflated to allow guidewire passage. After the guidewire has been placed centrally, the covered stent can then be positioned. The occlusion balloon should then be deflated and withdrawn in rapid order as the covered stent is deployed.

9. What if the rupture occurs with an ipsilateral approach?

Typically, it is difficult to deliver a covered stent from the contralateral groin. Therefore, the first step in placing an ipsilateral covered stent is the placement of a new occlusion balloon from the contralateral groin. After this is accomplished, the procedure can proceed as described previously.

10. Can stents be placed across the origin of the internal iliac artery?

Because the proximal external iliac artery is a common site of disease, it is often necessary to angioplasty or stent across the origin of the internal iliac artery. Although a stent across the origin of the internal iliac artery does not usually lead to occlusion, operators must realize that the internal iliac artery can sometimes occlude after stent placement. Therefore, it is critically important to analyze the potential collateral pathways that can be lost if the internal iliac artery is occluded. Sometimes the internal iliac artery can be the only source of collateral flow to the opposite leg, as can be seen in Figure 3. In this case, the right internal iliac artery provided collateral blood flow to the left leg. The patient had a palpable pulse in the left leg via this collateral pathway.

11. How should acute iliac artery occlusions be treated?

Before definitive treatment, the thrombus burden needs to be removed. Although some operators use mechanical thrombectomy devices, the most widely accepted method to remove thrombus is pharmacologic thrombolysis. Typically, the lesion is approached from the contralateral groin. After the origin of the contralateral common iliac artery is engaged, a guidewire is passed through the thrombus. A multi side-hole infusion catheter is then placed so that the side holes cover the length of the thrombus. The lesion is typically infused overnight. If the procedure is successful, the patient then undergoes angioplasty or stenting of any underlying lesions that are uncovered during the thrombolysis procedure.

In cases in which there has been a previous aortic bypass or endovascular stent placement, the

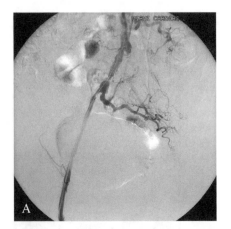

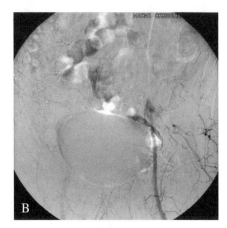

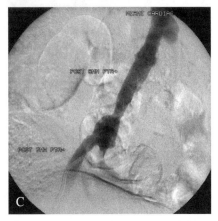

FIGURE 3. Cross-pelvic collateral flow. Early (A) and late (B) images from the initial diagnostic angiogram show a well-developed right internal iliac artery providing flow to the left leg in this patient with a left common iliac artery occlusion. The patient had previously undergone stenting of the right common and external iliac arteries; however, care was taken not to stent across, and possibly occlude, the origin of the right internal iliac artery. The patient now presents with recurrent left leg claudication. After balloon angioplasty of the right iliac system (C), the patient regained a palpable pulse in the left foot (the image is taken early in the run, and contrast dye has not yet fully opacified the internal iliac artery).

newly created aortic bifurcation may be too steep to traverse with a catheter. In these cases, thrombolysis may be performed through the ipsilateral groin (Fig. 4). Although there is at least a theoretical concern that bathing the puncture site with thrombolytic drugs may increase the risk of puncture site bleeding, this procedure has not been associated with a higher bleeding rate in our practice.

12. Should chronic iliac artery occlusions be approached from an ipsilateral or contralateral approach?

In general, the favored method for traversing an iliac artery occlusion is an ipsilateral approach. The reasons for this are mutlifactorial. First, an ipsilateral approach typically allows for better catheter and guidewire purchase. This catheter and guidewire positioning then typically allows for easier traversal of the occlusion.

Because initial attempts at traversing an iliac occlusion may result in a guidewire dissection, another advantage of the ipsilateral approach is that it is opposite to the direction of blood flow. This typically means that the dissection will be self-limiting and that another approach to the occlusion can be made. Whereas if a dissection occurs from a contralateral (antegrade) approach, the flowing blood may extend the dissection and render the case a failure.

However, this is not to say that an antegrade approach is not without its merits. If the ipsilateral approach is unsuccessful, an antegrade flow may allow for successful traversal of the occlusion. In addition, in cases in which the occlusion extends to the common femoral artery, there may be insufficient length of patent artery to puncture and still maintain access while stenting if an ipsilateral approach is attempted

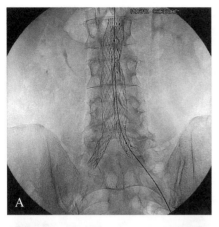
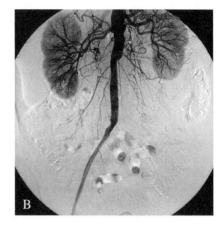
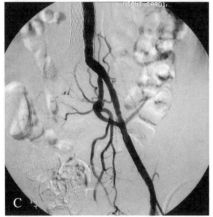

FIGURE 4. Retrograde lysis. Two weeks after endovascular stent placement, this patient complained of a cool, heavy-feeling left leg. A subsequent ultrasound (not shown) demonstrated a left iliac occlusion with a patent common femoral artery. Because the endovascular stent created a very steep aortic bifurcation, it was believed that it would not be possible to place an infusion catheter from the right. Therefore, a left-sided approach was undertaken (*A* and *B*). After uneventful overnight lysis, a repeat angiogram was performed. A left iliac stenosis was discovered and subsequently treated (*C*).

13. Should chronic iliac artery occlusions undergo lysis before further treatment is attempted?

The answer to this is controversial. Some operators believe that it is imperative that lysis should be attempted in all occlusions. Their rationale is that the lesion may be converted from a long-segment occlusion to a focal high-grade stenosis or occlusion that is more easily treated.

Other operators argue that the risk of performing thrombolysis in these patients is greater than the potential benefits. Therefore, they simply stent the entire length of the occlusion.

Still other operators have adopted a hybrid approach. Within this group, the tactile feel of the guidewire traversing the occlusion is of utmost importance. If the guidewire passes through the lesion "like butter," the lesion is assumed to contain a large amount of thrombus that will lyse. Thrombolysis is then initiated. If, however, the guidewire passage is difficult and the lesion feels hard and gritty, it is assumed that the lesion will be unchanged after lysis. Therefore, these lesions are stented primarily.

14. How should iliac artery aneurysms be treated?

Although surgery remains an option, most isolated iliac artery aneurysms can be repaired through endovascular methods. The first step in treatment planning is determining the extent of the aneurysm. The presence of a normal proximal and distal segment of artery ("landing zones") needs to be ascertained.

The lack of a suitable proximal neck leads to a very different treatment algorithm. Typically, it is necessary to place a bifurcated stent graft that extends into the aorta. Whereas this proximal extension is necessary to achieve an adequate seal, the contralateral, bifurcated segment is necessary to provide flow to the opposite leg. Another option in patients without a suitable proximal neck is coil exclusion of the aneurysm, thereby excluding it from flow. The patient would then need to undergo a femoral-to-femoral bypass to revascularize the affected leg.

The location of the distal landing zone has important implications. It is critical to determine the relationship of the landing zone to the origin of the internal iliac artery. If it is necessary to span the origin of the internal iliac artery, it is necessary to first occlude the internal iliac artery (Fig. 5). If the stent graft is placed across the origin of the internal iliac artery without first occluding the artery itself, it is possible for cross-pelvic collaterals to refill the internal iliac artery back to its origin. This results in an endoleak and nonexclusion of the aneurysm.

Although there are virtually no long term data, it is necessary to understand that placing a stent graft across the inguinal ligament may result in graft failure secondary to repetitive motion at the hip joint. Therefore, very careful consideration as to alternative therapies should be given before placing a stent graft across the inguinal ligament.

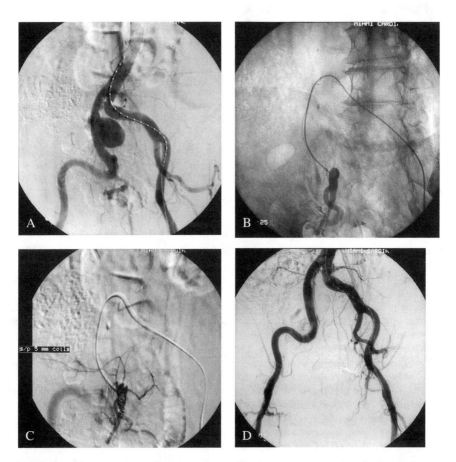

FIGURE 5. Iliac aneurysm. The initial diagnostic image (*A*) demonstrates a large aneurysm of the right common iliac artery. Because it was determined that there was insufficient distal landing space in the common iliac artery, it was decided to anchor the graft in the proximal external iliac artery. Before placing the graft, the right internal iliac artery first had to be catheterized (*B*) and subsequently coil embolized (*C*) to prevent a cross-pelvic endoleak. The completion angiogram (*D*) shows successful exclusion of the aneurysm without evidence for endoleak.

15. How should patients with isolated aneurysms of the internal iliac artery be treated?

The principle of cross-pelvic collateral circulation is of primary importance in the treatment of patients with isolated internal iliac artery aneurysms. These vessels can arise from the contralateral internal iliac artery or either profunda femoris artery. If all potential pathways are not occluded, it is possible for collateral vessels to refill the aneurysm. Therefore, it is necessary to determine the distal extent of the aneurysm. If the aneurysm ends before the internal iliac artery bifurcates, then it is only necessary to occlude the main artery distal to the aneurysm. Conceivably, even a short segment–covered stent could be placed into such an aneurysm.

However, most aneurysms extend at least as far as the bifurcation into the anterior and posterior divisions of the internal iliac artery. If this is the case, occlusion of each of the involved vessels distal to aneurysm is necessary.

If a suitable proximal neck exists, the internal iliac artery can be coil-occluded back to its origin to successfully complete exclusion of the aneurysm from the circulation. However, if no suitable proximal neck exists, it is then necessary to place a covered stent across the origin of the internal iliac artery from the common to the external iliac artery. The aneurysm would then be excluded from the circulation while maintaining flow to the affected leg.

16. Should incidentally discovered lesions of the internal iliac artery be treated?

Unlike coronary lesions, incidentally discovered stenoses of the iliac artery do not pose an imminent risk to the patient. Therefore, treatment of incidentally discovered lesions is generally not advised. Although rare, the risk of possible complications outweighs the benefits of treatment in these lesions. The one exception to this may be an incidental critical stenosis that poses an imminent risk of occlusion. Because treatment of iliac occlusions can be significantly more difficult and may even require surgery, it may be wise to treat an incidentally discovered critical stenosis. The other indication for treatment of incidentally discovered stenoses is occlusion of flow after placing a vascular sheath or balloon pump through the stenosis. If such a lesion is treated, great care should be exercised when recrossing the lesion so that the newly placed stent is not displaced.

17. How should iatrogenic dissections of the iliac artery be treated?

The first step in treatment is to determine the extent and severity of the dissection. Small non–flow-limiting dissections almost certainly heal on their own and no treatment is usually necessary. If, however, the lesion is flow-limiting, treatment is mandatory. Most flow-limiting dissections have a proximal reentry point. This reentry point allows for antegrade flow of blood into the false lumen. This pressurized flow within the false lumen then compromises flow within the true lumen. Therefore, treatment of iatrogenic dissections is based on closing off the reentry point.

If a significant flow limiting dissection is encountered (Fig. 6), the first step is to withdraw

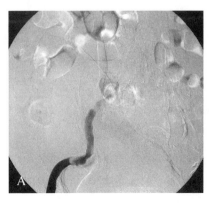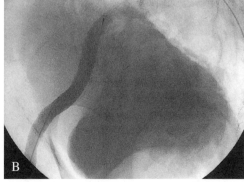

FIGURE 6. Iatrogenic guidewire dissection. *A,* After initial attempts at performing a routine diagnostic angiogram from the right groin, a flow limiting dissection was observed. *B,* After careful manipulation of the catheter through the true lumen, the site was successfully stented.

the diagnostic catheter or sheath to a point where it is clearly distal to the dissection. After this has been accomplished, great care should be made to locate and then traverse the true lumen. After the catheter has been placed in the true lumen above the level of the dissection, a detailed angiogram is necessary to confirm the location of the catheter within the true lumen as well as to delineate the proximal reentry point of the dissection. This reentry point can then be stented open. Additional stents are then placed as necessary to establish normal flow within the iliac artery.

BIBLIOGRAPHY

1. Blum U, Gabelmann A, Redecker M, et al: Percutaneous recanalization of iliac artery occlusions: results of a prospective study. Radiology 189:536–540, 1993.
2. Dormandy JA, Rutherford RB: Management of peripheral arterial disese (PAD). TASC Working Group: TransAtlantic Inter-Society Consensus (TASC). J Vasc Surg 31(1 pt 2):2–296, 2000.
3. Dyet JF, Gaines PA, Nicholson AA, et al: Treatment of chronic iliac artery occlusions by means of percutaneous endovascular stent placement. J Vasc Interv Radiol 8:349–353, 1997.
4. Rees CR, Palmaz JC, Garcia O, et al: Angioplasty and stenting of completely occluded iliac arteries. Radiology 172(3 pt 2):953–959, 1989.
5. Reyes R, Maynar M, Lopera J, et al: Treatment of chronic iliac artery occlusions with guide wire recanalization and primary stent placement. J Vasc Interv Radiol 8:1049–1055, 1997.
6. Sapoval MR, Chatellier G, Long AL, et al: Self-expandable stents for the treatment of iliac artery obstructive lesions: long-term success and prognostic factors. Am J Roentgenol 166:1173–1179, 1996.
7. Verwerk D, Guenther RW, Schurmann K, et al: Primary stent placement for chronic iliac artery occlusions: follow-up results in 103 patients. Radiology 194:745–749, 1995.

52. RENAL ARTERY STENOSIS

Christopher J. White, M.D.

1. What is the incidence of renovascular hypertension?

The incidence of renovascular hypertension (RVH) is less than 0.1% in the general population. RVH occurs in about 4.0% of in patients with hypertension. However, in patients with atherosclerotic vascular disease of the heart or peripheral vessels, the incidence of RVH is much higher. In patients with suspected coronary artery disease (CAD) the risk is 10% to 20%; in patients with malignant hypertension, the risk is 20% to 30%; and in those with malignant hypertension and renal insufficiency, the incidence of RVH is 30% to 40%.

Therefore, patients with known or suspected atherosclerosis of the heart or cerebral or peripheral vessels are at markedly increased risk of atherosclerotic renal artery stenosis. These patients often present with difficult-to-control blood pressure (BP), loss of renal function, and acute cardiac decompensation such as flash pulmonary edema or unstable angina.

2. What is the natural history of renal artery stenosis?

The natural history of atherosclerotic renal artery lesions is to progress in severity over time. Progression to occlusion is more common with more severe stenoses. The risk of progression to occlusion for greater than 50% diameter stenoses is about 15% over the first year.

Even when BP is controlled with medical therapy, lesions progress in severity and there is evidence of progressive loss of renal function. In patients with normal renal arteries, the development of renal artery stenosis at follow-up is associated with loss of renal function. The presence of critical renal artery stenosis is associated with a decreased 4-year survival. Patients with bilateral renal artery stenosis have a worse survival rate than those with unilateral disease.

3. What is the pathophysiology of RVH?

Unilateral renal artery stenosis, with a normally functioning contralateral kidney, results in vasoconstrictor-mediated hypertension. Renin release is stimulated by the renal artery stenosis, causing release of angiotensin and aldosterone. The normal kidney prevents salt and water retention, but there is sustained vasoconstriction caused by angiotensin II production.

Bilateral renal artery stenosis or renal artery stenosis of a solitary kidney results in volume overload–dependent hypertension (Fig. 1). The lack of the normal kidney prevents natriuresis and results in volume overload. The volume overload suppresses further angiotensin II production. These are the patients that present with "flash" pulmonary edema.

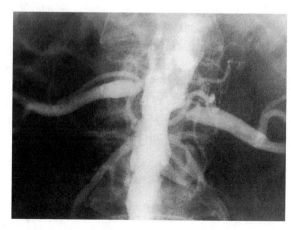

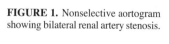

FIGURE 1. Nonselective aortogram showing bilateral renal artery stenosis.

4. What are the causes of renovascular hypertension?
- Atherosclerosis is the most common (60% to 70%)
- Fibrous dysplasias (or fibromuscular dysplasia [FMD]) (20% to 30%) (Fig. 2)
- Renal artery aneurysm
- Renal artery fistula
- Renal artery thrombosis or embolism

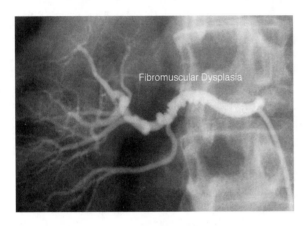

FIGURE 2. Selective renal angiography of FMD.

5. What are the clinical reasons to suspect renal artery stenosis?
- Onset of hypertension ≤ 30 years or ≥ 55 years
- Previously well-controlled BP that is now uncontrolled
- Malignant hypertension
- Hypertension resistant to medical therapy
- Presence of an abdominal or flank bruit
- Discrepancy of renal sizes on non-invasive imaging
- Azotemia with an angiotensin-converting enzyme (ACE) inhibitor
- Azotemia in elderly patients with other atherosclerotic disease

6. What is the best test to screen patients for renal artery stenosis?
There is no single best noninvasive test. The accuracy of the tests depends on the institution and experience of the physician.

1. **Renal duplex** is an excellent test to screen individuals for renal artery stenosis. It is very technician dependent and can be difficult in obese patients. It detects renal size and is useful for bilateral disease. Accessory renal arteries may be missed.

2. **Magnetic resonance angiography (MRA)** and **computed tomographic angiography (CTA)** are becoming more attractive as screening tools for renal artery stenosis. CTA can screen arteries for in-stent restenosis.

3. **Radionuclide renography** is limited as a screening tool because it compares kidneys with each other and 30% of patients have bilateral disease. It is a time-consuming test and is expensive. Its main use is in conjunction with an ACE inhibitor to determine the clinical significance of a unilateral borderline stenosis (i.e., 50–70%).

7. Should every patient with a history of hypertension undergoing cardiac catheterization be screened for renal artery stenosis?
Not all patients with a history of hypertension should undergo renal angiography at the time of catheterization. The pejorative term "drive-by angiography" should not be used because it connotes lack of planning and lack of forethought regarding patients in whom renal angiography is performed. Screening for renal artery stenosis at the time of cardiac catheterization is re-

served for patients who are clinically suspected of having renal artery stenosis. Not every stenosis requires intervention. Identifying patients with renal artery stenosis allows them to be followed closely and treated appropriately. This author often screens patients with noninvasive testing before elective catheterization and then performs angiography in patients who are likely to have renal artery stenosis.

8. Are selective renal angiograms or nonselective aortograms better for screening patients for renal artery stenosis?

There are reasons to favor both approaches. **Selective angiography** has the advantage of better quality imaging and providing angulated views of the proximal or ostial portion of the renal artery. Some lesions can be very difficult to detect without selective angiography. Pressure gradients across lesions can be measured with small-diameter diagnostic catheters at the time of selective angiography.

Nonselective aortography visualizes the aorta and its branches, including accessory renal arteries, which can be missed if only selective angiography is performed. Some believe that this approach is less likely to generate atheroemboli because the selective catheter scrapes the wall of the aorta or causes trauma to the ostia of the renal arteries during selective intubation. However, no single approach is always correct, and operators can make individual decisions for each patient. Sometimes I perform selective angiography after having performed nonselective aortography to visualize more clearly a suspicious ostial narrowing.

9. Is there a role for provisional stenting in the renal arteries?

Yes. In general, non-ostial renal artery stenoses should be dilated with an appropriately sized (1:1) balloon. If less than a 20% residual stenosis is the result and there are no flow-limiting dissections, then balloon dilation alone is sufficient.

Renal artery aorto-ostial lesions located within 1 cm of the origin of the vessel, percutaneous transluminal angiography (PTA) restenosis lesions and failed PTA lesions should receive stents.

10. What is the strongest predictor of renal artery patency after stent placement?

The single strongest predictor of long-term patency is post-stent deployment minimal luminal diameter. The larger the stent, the better the patency (Figs. 3 and 4). However, oversizing of stents can lead to severe complications. It is recommended that some objective measure of the reference be obtained. This can be either quantitative angiography or intravascular ultrasound. We attempt to achieve a 1:1 diameter stent placement compared with the reference vessel.

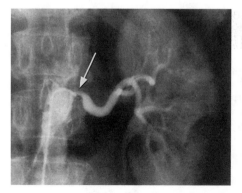 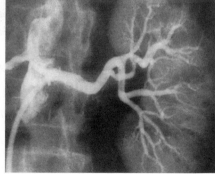

FIGURE 3. Left renal ostial stenosis with an optimally deployed stent.

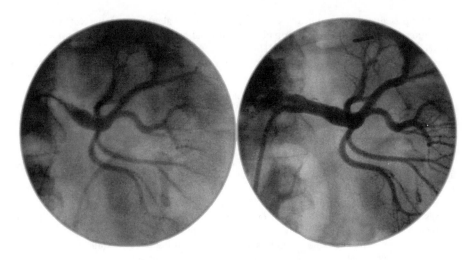

FIGURE 4. Left renal ostial stenosis with a suboptimal stent result.

11. What percentage of patients with uncontrolled hypertension are improved with percutaneous coronary intervention for renal artery stenosis?

In several large trials, it appears that overall improvement occurs in about 75% of patients. However, only a minority (< 20%) of patients are actually cured of their hypertension.

12. Do renal stents preserve the patency of stenotic renal arteries?

The answer to this question is not known. It is clinically accepted that critically narrowed arteries (> 90%) benefit from stent placement, but this has never been tested in any controlled trial.

13. Are the results of renal stents superior to balloon dilation for FMD lesions?

Although this has never been subjected to a comparative trial, the results of balloon angioplasty alone for FMD lesions has been so good as to not require stent placement unless a PTA failure occurs.

14. Does successful renal stent placement preserve renal function?

Two published trials have demonstrated that, in patients with impaired renal function at baseline and renal artery stenosis, the successful placement of a stent improves or stabilizes renal function.

15. Is renal stent restenosis dependent on reference vessel size?

Although not a linear relationship, it does appear that larger renal stent sizes have lower restenosis rates. The largest diameter stent that can safely placed should be used.

16. Is atherosclerotic renal artery stenosis a common cause of renal failure?

Yes, the incidence of atherosclerotic renovascular disease is about 15% in patients beginning dialysis. Renal failure is usually multifaceted. Traditionally, unilateral renal artery disease should not impair global renal functon as long as the contralateral kidney is unaffected. However, in elderly patients with systemic atherosclerotic disease, hypertension, or diabetes mellitus, a unilateral tight renal artery stenosis may contribute to renal insufficiency; an attempt to relieve this stenosis is usually warranted.

17. Is atheroembolism a significant problem during renal stent placement?

With the introduction of emboli protection devices, such as the PercuSurge balloon catheter and various filter devices, investigators are reporting the retrieval of significant amounts of embolic debris in association with renal intervention. The bulky atheroma in continuity with the aortic wall plaque may contribute to atheroemboli. Determining whether pharmacologic or device strategies are preferable to reduce the impact of atheroemboli will require clinical trials.

18. Is there a role for interventional cardiologists in treating renal artery stenosis?
The diagnosis and treatment of RVH is within the scope of practice of cardiologists. The technical skills required to treat renal artery lesions are very similar to those used for large ostial saphenous vein graft lesions. The impact of poorly controlled hypertension on stroke, heart failure, and coronary ischemia is devastating. It is cost effective to bundle renal artery angiography with a cardiac catheterization.

19. What are the indications for renal artery intervention?
1. A significant renal artery stenosis is present.
   - $\geq 70\%$ diameter stenosis
   - ≥ 15 mmHg pressure gradient across the lesion
2. Refractory hypertension is present.
   - $\geq$ two antihypertensive medications
   - Flash pulmonary edema
3. Renal insufficiency is present.
   - Dialysis dependent $\geq 75\%$ renal mass in jeopardy
   - Chronic with $\geq 75\%$ renal mass in jeopardy
4. Congestive heart failure is present.
   - Difficult-to-manage BP (vasoconstrictor-mediated renovascular hypertension)
   - Volume overload
5. Refractory coronary ischemia is present.
   - Difficult-to-manage BP (vasoconstrictor-mediated RVM)
   - Volume overload

BIBLIOGRAPHY

1. Dorros G, Jaff M, Jain A, et al: Follow-up of primary Palmaz-Schatz stent placement for atherosclerotic renal artery stenosis. Am J Card 75:1051–1055, 1995.
2. Dorros G, Prince C, Mathiak L: Stenting of a renal artery stenosis achieves better relief of the obstructive lesion than balloon angioplasty. Cathet Cardiovasc Diagn 29:191–198, 1993.
3. Greco BA, Breyer JA: The natural history of renal artery stenosis: who should be evaluated for suspected ischemic nephropathy? Semin Neph 16:2–11, 1996.
4. Harden PN, MacLeod MJ, Rodger RSC, et al: Effect of renal artery stenting on progression of renovascular renal failure. Lancet 349:1133–1136, 1997.
5. Harding MB, Smith LR, Himmelstein SI, et al: Renal artery stenosis: prevalence and associated risk factors in patients undergoing routine cardiac catheterization. J Am Soc Nephrol 2:1608–1616, 1992.
6. Jean WJ, Al-Bittar I, Xwicke DL, et al: High incidence of renal artery stenosis in patients with coronary artery disease. Cathet Cardiovasc Diagn 32:8–10, 1994.
7. Meany TF, Dustan HP, Novick AC: Natural history of renal arterial disease. Radiology 9:877–887, 1968.
8. Olin JW, Melia M, Young JR, et al: Prevalence of atherosclerosis renal artery stenosis in patients with atherosclerosis elsewhere. Am J Med 88(suppl N):46–51, 1990.
9. Schreiber MJ, Pohl MA, Novick AC: The natural history of atherosclerotic and fibrous renal artery disease. Urol Clin N Am 11:383–392, 1984.
10. Watson PS, Hadjipetrou P, Cox, SV, et al: Effect of renal artery stenting on renal function and size in patients with atherosclerotic renovascular disease. Circulation 102:1671–1677, 2000.
11. White CJ, Ramee SR, Collins TJ, et al: Renal artery stent placement: utility in difficult lesions for balloon angioplasty. J Am Coll Cardiol 30:1445–1450, 1997.

53. INFRAINGUINAL PERCUTANEOUS INTERVENTION

Juan A. Pastor-Cervantes, M.D., Craig M. Walker, M.D., and David E. Allie, M.D.

1. What is the most common symptom of lower extremity arterial disease?

Atherosclerotic vascular disease affecting the lower extremities is the most common form of peripheral vascular disease and can lead to clinical conditions ranging from intermittent claudication or pain at rest to ulceration and gangrene. Intermittent claudication is the most common symptom of peripheral arterial disease, resulting from a flow-limiting lesion that causes exercise-induced muscle ischemia.

2. What is the incidence and prevalence of lower extremity arterial disease?

Data from The Framingham Study have reported an annual age-adjusted incidence of intermittent claudication of 0.3% in men and 0.1% in women. The prevalence of symptomatic peripheral arterial disease among the general population is highly age related and has been estimated to be between 10% and 20% for patients older than age 55 years. The prevalence of asymptomatic peripheral arterial disease is as high as 25% to 35%, as shown in the Systolic Hypertension in the Elderly Study and the Women's Health and Aging Study, respectively.

3. What is the ankle-brachial index (ABI)?

The ABI is the ratio of the highest systolic blood pressure (BP) at the arm to the systolic BP at the ankle. This simple test is performed similarly to taking a standard blood pressure with more complete information obtained when Doppler systems are used.

These systems allow recording of Doppler waveforms that can be correlated with clinical findings. An ABI is a quick, cost-effective, simple test used to screen for upper and lower extremity arterial disease.

An ABI examination is recommended for any patient who has signs and symptoms of peripheral arterial disease. The American Diabetes Association in collaboration with the American Heart Association have recommended that ABI studies be performed in insulin-dependent diabetic patients older than age 35 years and in patients with more than 20 years' duration of diabetes.

4. How is the ABI performed and calculated?

Begin by taking a BP reading at the arm:
1. Place a BP cuff around the patient's arm.
2. Palpate for the radial or brachial artery.
3. Place gel on the skin for Doppler systems.
4. Apply the Doppler probe at a 45- or 60-degree angle for Doppler systems.
5. Take the systolic BP by inflating the cuff to 20 mmHg over pressure cessation.
6. Deflate the cuff at a slow rate of 3 mmHg until you hear the first Doppler sound or, conventionally, if regular BP measurement is obtained.
7. Record the systolic BP when you hear the first sound or again; if the conventional method is used, record the systolic BP.
8. Repeat the test on the other arm.
9. For ABI measurement, use the highest systolic BP.

Take the systolic BP at the ankle.
1. Place the BP cuff above the ankle.
2. Apply gel to the skin at the posterior tibialis artery or dorsalis pedis.
3. Hold the probe at 45- or 60-degree angle against the posterior tibialis or dorsalis pedis

artery and listen for Doppler sound. If the conventional method is used, the respective pulses must be palpated.

4. Inflate the cuff to 20 mmHg over pressure cessation.

5. Deflate the cuff at a slow rate of 3 mmHg until the first Doppler sound is heard. If the conventional method is used, do this until palpable pulses are felt again.

6. Record the systolic BP.

7. Repeat the test at the posterior tibialis or dorsalis pedis artery of the other ankle.

To calculate the ABI, divide the highest ankle pressure by the highest arm pressure.

$$\text{ABI} = \frac{\text{Ankle systolic pressure}}{\text{Arm systolic pressure}}$$

The systolic BP in the arterial system increases from the central aorta to the periphery. This is because of the fact that the arteries toward the periphery have increased resistance and become stiffer; therefore in normal individuals the ankle-to-arm ratio should be greater than 1.0.

5. What is the relationship between ABIs and the degree of obstruction?

Interpretation of ABI Results

ABI	INTERPRETATION
> 0.91	Normal
0.71–0.90	Mild obstruction
0.40–0.70	Moderate obstruction
< 0.39	Severe obstruction

6. Which conditions can cause a false-negative ABI measurement?

It is important to understand that lower extremity and ankle systolic pressures may be falsely elevated in patients with:

- Calcified or noncompressible arteries (e.g., diabetes mellitus), for which a toe/brachial index or Doppler waveform analysis should be evaluated
- Smaller than required BP cuff usage
- Upper extremity peripheral arterial disease

7. Which treatment options are currently available for lower extremity arterial disease?

Treatment options are categorized and divided according to the severity of the initial presentation. For patients with intermittent claudication, initial therapy should begin with aggressive risk factor modification (e.g., appropriate treatment of hyperlipidemia, hypertension, and diabetes), the institution of exercise programs, and smoking cessation clinics, followed by adequate medical therapy. An antiplatelet agent should be administered, usually aspirin. Although the CAPRIE study showed clinical benefit with clopidogrel over aspirin, with an 8.7% relative risk reduction in the occurrence of stroke, myocardial infarction (MI), or vascular death, the use of this agent has been limited by a large cost disadvantage when compared with aspirin. Cilostazol has demonstrated to increase walking distance significantly in patients with intermittent claudication; however, it is contraindicated in patients with abnormal left ventricular systolic function, limiting its use to a very select population. Other modalities of treatment include gene therapy, although results of initial studies need to be corroborated before widespread use can be recommended.

Treatment options for patients with pending tissue loss include all of the above measures plus limb salvage strategies that need to be performed urgently. In general, we perform an initial ultrasonographic and angiographic evaluation of the limb at risk to assess the characteristics and extension of the disease; after performing such a stepwise approach, we then proceed with either percutaneous or surgical revascularization strategies. Our preference in most cases is to begin with percutaneous intervention, always leaving surgical alternatives open for adjunctive therapy. After access to the lesion is obtained, several key factors must be kept in mind, including the ability to cross the blockage, open the blockage, and maintain vessel patency.

8. What are the indications for the percutaneous treatment of infrainguinal arteries, and why should endovascular therapy be the first line of intervention over surgery?

The indications for treatment of the femoropopliteal arteries are similar to those for the iliac vessels. Claudication that limits lifestyle, rest pain, ischemic ulceration, and acute limb ischemia are indications for percutaneous intervention. Peripheral interventions are associated with less pain, cost, and risk of infection, as well as less trauma to patients and the ability to treat multiple segments of disease at one setting with a very low complication rate and an average length of hospital stay of 1.4 days. Angioplasty also offers the advantage of saphenous vein preservation and may be used repetitively to treat arterial lesions, maintain blood flow, and improve secondary patency rates.

9. What is the patency rate of infrainguinal percutaneous intervention?

More than any other vascular segment, technical success and patency in the infrainguinal region depend on the characteristics of the lesion treated. The primary patency rate (i.e., uninterrupted patency with no procedures performed on or at the margins of the treated segment) for lesions smaller than 3 cm in length fluctuates between 75% and 85% at 1 year, gradually declining to less than 60% at 3 years and less than 40% at 5 years. There are much worse outcomes when stenosis of more than 3 cm or occlusions are included, demonstrating that the patency rate of such lesions at 1 year are less than 60%, with an abrupt decline to less than 40% at 3 years and less than 30% at 5 years.

10. What is the anatomic and functional relationship of the infrainguinal vessels above the knee?

The common femoral artery is an extension of the external Iliac artery, which originates at the inguinal ligament and then bifurcates (usually at the lower portion of the femoral head) into the superficial femoral artery (SFA) anteromedially and the deep femoral artery (DFA), or profunda, posterolaterally. The DFA has two major branches, the lateral circumflex and medial circumflex femoral arteries. The DFA provides circulation to the majority of the muscles of the thigh as well as the feeding arteries to the femur. The SFA proceeds down the anteromedial thigh and dives deep at the adductor (Hunter's) canal, where it becomes the popliteal artery running posterior to the femur. Major popliteal branches include the sural artery, which provides flow to the calf muscles and geniculate (superior, middle, and inferior) arteries around the knee.

11. What is the anatomic and functional relationship of the infrainguinal vessels below the knee?

Below the knee, at the border of the popliteus muscle, the popliteal artery divides, with the anterior tibial (AT) artery that brings circulation to the adjacent muscles in the anterior aspect of the leg proceeding laterally and anterior to the tibia toward the foot. As it passes over the ankle onto the dorsum of the foot, it continues as the dorsalis pedis (DP) artery. After the takeoff of the AT, the popliteal continues as the tibioperoneal trunk (TPT), which subsequently bifurcates into the posterior tibial (PT) and peroneal arteries. The PT courses posteromedially in the calf and gives circulation to the adjacent muscles in the posterior aspect of the leg as well as feeding arteries to the tibia. The peroneal artery runs near the fibula between the AT and PT arteries. The peroneal artery then rejoins the PT above the ankle via its posterior division and the AT via its anterior division. On the dorsum of the foot, the DP artery has lateral and medial tarsal branches. After the PT artery passes behind the medial malleolus, it divides into the medial and lateral plantar arteries. The lateral plantar and distal DP arteries join to form the plantar arch.

12. How should a lesion be approached from the technical aspect?

Before the onset of any intervention, a thorough understanding of the anatomy, lesion morphology, lesion location, patient's history, contraindications to anticoagulation, and thrombolytic therapy must be obtained. In most cases, our preference is to initiate diagnostic procedures from a site remote from the ischemic extremity. Thus, if the left leg is ischemic, the right leg or left arm is used for diagnostic angiographies. In this regard, one will not worsen the involved limb or mask more proximal lesions by the placement of catheters or sheaths. Careful attention to the inflow (aorto-iliac) and a complete assessment of the outflow are mandatory to help plan therapy and define a baseline.

Inflow lesions should be corrected early in the course of treatment. Our general approach in the lower extremity is to use a preformed sheath, such as a Balkin sheath (Cook Incorporated) or a metal flex sheath (Arrow International, Inc.), positioned in the external iliac from the contra lateral groin.

This provides the interventionalist with two benefits. The relative stiff system provides support and an easy exchange mechanism for catheter and guidewire manipulations. In addition, contrast dye administered through the side port of the sheath allows frequent visualization of the distal arterial tree without removal of any of the interventional devices being used to treat the lesion.

13. What anticoagulation therapy is used for peripheral intervention?

After a decision to intervene percutaneously has been made, anticoagulation therapy is advised. An initial bolus of heparin 60 to 100 U/kg with frequent monitoring of the activated clotting time (ACT) to maintain a level of more than 200 seconds in combination with glycoprotein (GP) IIb/IIIa is recommended. For patients in whom a previous diagnosis of heparin-induced thrombocytopenia have been made, another alternative to the use of heparin includes the use of direct thrombin inhibitors, alone and in combination with GP IIb/IIIa inhibitors. These agents may completely replace the use of heparins during the performance of percutaneous interventions because of intrinsic drug characteristics, which make them more effective, predictable, and reliable.

14. What technique is used to cross an occlusion?

Our preference is to use a 5-Fr glide catheter with a 0.035 in-angled glidewire, with initial attempts to cross the lesion done with the glide catheter alone, followed by the use of a glidewire if initially unsuccessful. If both initial strategies fail to cross the lesion, then a straight glidewire can be used with caution after a successful crossage has been performed advancement of the glide catheter beyond the lesion is undertaken with subsequent confirmatory angiograms. This is done to ensure an intraluminal position distal to the thrombosis or occlusion.

Then the wire is advanced into the distal arterial circulation and therapeutic options are considered, including the use of percutaneous transluminal angioplasty (PTA) or stenting.

15. After lesion is crossed and dilated, should it always be stented?

It is well known that traditional approach with balloon or stenting to infrainguinal interventions has lacked similar long-term results compared with results from iliac interventions. (However, this is a very active and evolving field, with multiple ongoing trials that use laser intervention, newer stent designs, and ultimately the use of pharmacologic coated stents, with the goal of improving current outcomes.) Recently, the Food and Drug Administration approved the first stent to be used in the superficial femoral artery and popliteal artery. The Intracoil stent (Sulzer Intratherapeutics, Inc.) (Fig.1) has a coil design that allows deployment at flexure points (Fig. 2), preservation of side branches (Fig. 3), and comparable long-term results to standard percutaneous angioplasty, with improved acute (30 days) results, including angiographic and procedural success (Fig. 4). Other important findings included lower in-hospital MACE (major adverse cardiac events) and lesser major complications (decreased abrupt closure, subacute closure, distal embolization, and renal failure) when compared with conventional balloon angioplasty.

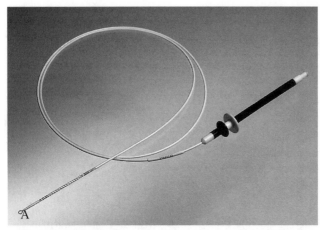

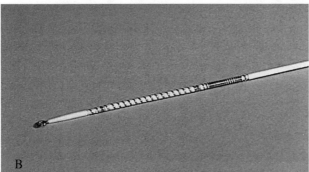

FIGURE 1. The IntraCoil self-expanding peripheral stent consists of a 40-mm nitinol coil stent with evenly placed coils in the open configuration, an over-the-wire delivery catheter with radiopaque proximal, and distal marker bands that aid in placement of the stent.

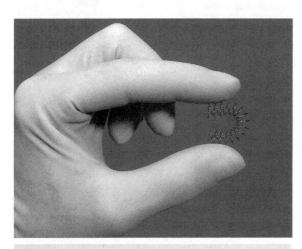

FIGURE 2. The IntraCoil self-expanding peripheral stent. This stent is indicated for improving peripheral luminal diameter in patients with symptomatic atherosclerotic disease caused by stenotic lesions (length < 15 cm) or occlusive lesions (length < 12 cm) in femoropopliteal arteries, to the bifurcation of the tibial artery, with a reference vessel diameter of 3.0 to 7.8 mm.

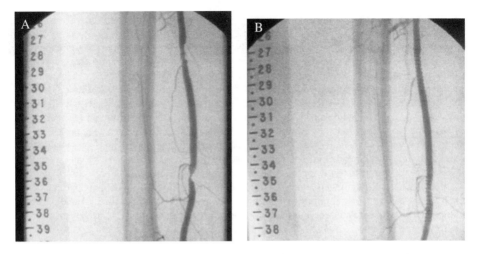

FIGURE 3. *A,* Diagnostic angiogram from the left CFA demonstrates a significant mid-right SFA stenosis, followed by a critical distal right SFA stenosis at the adductor canal. *B,* Subsequent percutaneous angioplasty of the stenotic segments and IntraCoil stent deployments revealed optimal results, with preservation of side branches and adequate stent uniformity.

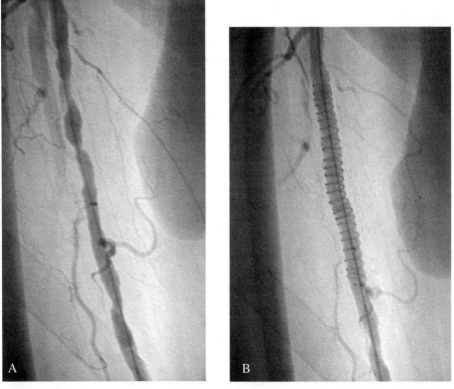

FIGURE 4. *A,* Diagnostic angiogram from the left CFA demonstrates a proximal right SFA with significant sequential eccentric lesions. *B,* Subsequent percutaneous angioplasty of the stenotic segments and IntraCoil stent deployment demonstrate that there is no longer evidence of residual stenosis and adequate results.

16. What other access technique is useful in the management of distal SFA or infrapopliteal percutaneous intervention?

An antegrade puncture to the common femoral artery (CFA) has been used with enormous success for the treatment of distal SFA or infrapopliteal disease; however, this access modality can be technically challenging. First of all, one must be careful to enter the CFA, under fluoroscopic guidance at the midfemoral head, below the inguinal ligament and above its bifurcation. The guidewire must then be selectively advanced into the SFA. Several techniques have been developed to redirect the guidewire that preferentially advances into the profunda femoral artery (PFA). After documenting that the entry point is into the CFA, the needle can be redirected to the contralateral wall and the guidewire readvanced; alternatively, the floppy tip of a moveable core wire can be advanced into the profunda and allowed to protrude into the SFA. Another method is to exchange the needle for the 4- or 5-Fr dilator and redirect the guidewire into the SFA under fluoroscopic guidance; finally, a dilator with a side hole proximal to the end hole (Cope-Saddekni SFA Access dilator, Cook Group, Bloomington, IN) can be advanced into the PFA and retracted until a guidewire can be advanced through the side hole and into the SFA. After the guidewire is in place in the SFA, a vascular sheath is introduced.

17. Have other techniques been used with success aside from percutaneous balloon angioplasty and stenting in the management of infrainguinal intervention?

Laser application may be well suited for infrainguinal percutaneous intervention because the diffuse nature of the disease. In addition, occlusions outnumber stenosis three to one. SFA occlusions are five times more common than iliac occlusive disease. Difficulty in crossing occlusions greater than 5 cm has led to alternative techniques of recanalisation, including laser angioplasty. Debulking the atheromatous material with laser techniques may theoretically lower the high restenosis rate in SFA stenosis with PTA alone. Long-term patency is negatively influenced by longer lesion length, occlusion, poor distal runoff, and diabetes. Case selection for femoropopliteal laser intervention include visible proximal stump, reconstitution at the popliteal artery, minimal to no calcification and at least one vessel runoff.

Percutaneous peripheral revascularization with excimer laser has been used extensively for the treatment of infrainguinal lesions (Figs. 5 and 6). The recent advances in catheter technology

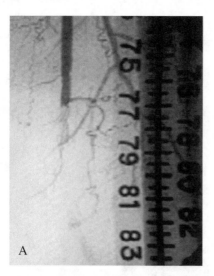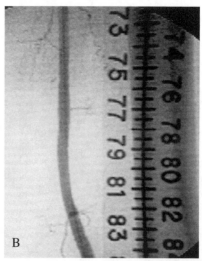

FIGURE 5. *A,* Diagnostic angiogram from the right CFA demonstrates a long total occlusion of the left SFA. *B,* Subsequent percutaneous intervention assisted with the excimer laser catheter activated at 45 mJ/mm^2 and 25 pulses/s permits further advancement of the guidewire across the lesion and performance of angioplasty with complete revascularization of the treated segment.

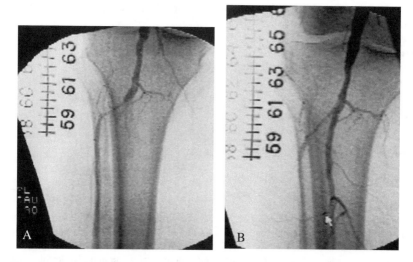

FIGURE 6. *A,* Diagnostic angiogram demonstrates a long total occlusion of the right tibioperoneal trunk. *B,* Post-excimer laser and percutaneous transluminal angioplasty, the angiogram reveals complete revascularization of the right tibioperoneal trunk without significant residual stenosis and preservation of side branches.

have allowed much better outcomes compared with previous laser delivery systems. These modifications have included optimally spaced fibers, athermic 308-nm wavelength spectrum catheters, and saline infusion techniques, which have greatly reduced the previously concerning problems of vessel injury, dissections, and perforation. Biamino et al. reported a secondary patency rate of 75.1% at 12 months, with the use of excimer laser for the treatment of long chronic total occlusions; the mean length lesion in this study was 19.4 ± 6 cm. More results should become available from the ongoing PELA (Peripheral Excimer laser vs. Angioplasty) trial comparing laser to balloon angioplasty in 10 cm or longer SFA occlusions.

18. Why is antiplatelet therapy essential in the treatment of patients undergoing peripheral interventions?

Thromboembolic and ischemic complications are frequently encountered during and after endovascular procedures. Because the use of adjunctive therapy with GP IIb/IIIa receptor blockade in noncoronary interventions is new, the reported data of controlled randomized and prospective studies are limited mainly to coronary use. Platelet adhesion, activation, and aggregation occurring at the site of arterial injury are mediated by local factors, after balloon angioplasty subendothelial structures are exposed, and subsequent platelet activation is accompanied by activation of the coagulation cascade. Whereas reendothelialization of the injured arterial wall occurs from areas of the intact endothelium and is almost complete 2 weeks after arterial injury, the functional capacity of the endothelial cells is impaired for almost 4 weeks after intervention. *In vitro* studies have revealed that platelets rapidly accumulate on the stent surface after stent placement. GP IIb/IIIa receptor blockade has been used successfully both alone and in combination with fibrinolysis in noncoronary interventions. Recently, the PROMPT (Platelet Receptor antibodies in Order to Manage Peripheral Arterial Thrombosis) trial was completed and showed that the time to thrombolysis could be reduced by approximately 40% with adjunctive abciximab therapy. In summary, the data on the clinical use of GP IIb/IIIa receptor antagonist support the role of a highly potent antiplatelet therapy in the early course of injury to the vessel wall from percutaneous intervention.

19. What are the rate and type of complications seen during the performance of infrainguinal percutaneous interventions?

Major complications:	Minor complications:
Death in hospital: 0%	Hematoma: 2.2%
Q-wave myocardial infarction: 0%	Contrast dye reaction: 1.1%
Non–Q-wave myocardial infarction: 0%	
Amputation: 0.8%	
Abrupt closure: 2.3%	
Subacute closure: 1.5%	
Distal embolization: 0.8%	
Major bleeding complications: 0.8%	
Access site surgery: 0.5%	
Renal failure: 0.5%	

20. What is reperfusion syndrome?

Reperfusion syndrome is the damage done by reestablishment of blood flow to an ischemic extremity. This cycle of events can lead to limb loss after otherwise successful revascularization. Through various pathways, leukocyte adhesion molecules, procoagulant factors, and vasoconstrictive agents are released, leading to edema, neutrophil activation and platelet plugging, microthrombosis, and vasoconstriction. Endothelial integrity is disrupted, leading to loss of fluid into the interstitial space, release of toxins, and massive swelling. Two models have been used to describe the microcirculatory changes after revascularization of ischemic skeletal muscle. The no-reflow model states that damage is caused by persistent ischemia at the tissue level caused by edema and capillary plugging despite restoration of blood flow. The reflow model shows that damage is more active, demonstrating that oxygen release to ischemic cells damage organic molecules through the generation of free radicals. In addition, intracellular calcium overload and altered arachidonic acid metabolism occur.

21. How is reperfusion syndrome treated?

After appropriate diagnostic information is obtained and the degree of ischemia is sufficient to affect a potentially salvageable limb, efforts should be made to reestablish reperfusion as rapidly as possible. Immediate anticoagulation at therapeutic levels should be achieved essentially in all cases to keep important collateral pathways open; thereafter, either percutaneous or surgical revascularization are needed.

Percutaneous intervention or surgical revascularization offer numerous strategies that result in complete reperfusion of the threatened limb. These interventions can include combination therapy with GP IIb/IIIa, thrombolysis, or the use of mechanical thrombectomy devices. Adjunctive mannitol infusion as a scavenger for a free radical molecules have also been used successfully. Saline should be infused together with intravenous administration of a loop diuretic such as furosemide or bumetanide. Alkalinization of urine with sodium bicarbonate should be attempted only after careful assessment of the patient's volume and calcium status. The patient should be carefully monitored to avoid volume overload. When muscle compartmentalization is a problem, the situation should be promptly corrected by fasciotomy.

22. What are the do's and don'ts of infrainguinal percutaneous intervention?

Do:

1. Use appropriate anticoagulation with monitor ACT and adjunctive GP IIb/IIIa inhibitors for infrainguinal intervention.

2. Know the anatomofunctional relationships of the possible intervene vessels.

3. Use a glide catheter and a glidewire.

4. Perform angioplasty first, leaving stenting for bail-out situations.

5. Use self-expanding stents when necessary (IntraCoil stent), always sizing up to 1 mm in diameter.

6. Fix inflow before outflow.

7. Always keeps surgical options open.

Don't:

1. Intervene unless the anatomofunctional relationship of the affected area is well known.

2. Perform primary stenting of the infrainguinal vessel.

3. Stent across the CFA or the popliteal artery unless the patient is not a surgical candidate or under extenuating circumstances.

4. Lose the wire position.

5. Use closure device systems that have intravascular absorbable anchors because these devices can jeopardize flow to the intervene limb.

23. How is success defined in infrainguinal intervention?

There are several ways to assess success postintervention, including angiographic measures as well as clinical and noninvasive Doppler techniques. Angiographycally, less than 30% residual stenosis without embolic complication constitutes a successful result. However, all this analysis is meaningless without relief of or substantial improvement in symptoms; healing of ischemic ulcerations; increase in the ABI of at least 0.15; or normalization of the popliteal pulse, thigh/calf pulse volume recording, or Doppler waveforms.

24. Can closure devices be used after percutaneous infrainguinal interventions?

Infrainguinal percutaneous interventions are usually performed through the CFA. Hemostasis of the arteriotomy is usually achieved by manual compression followed by a prolonged period of bedrest. Thus, patient treatment after any interventional procedure is time consuming and affects the cost of revascularization. In view of these limitations, multiple arteriotomy closing devices have been used. The Angio-Seal and VasoSeal systems have collagen plugs that are intended to seal the artery entry site by applying pressure against the wall and forming a coagulum. The Angio-Seal has an additional intravascular absorbable anchor to facilitate collagen plug apposition.

However, leaving a potential obstructive anchor in an already diseased vascular territory can jeopardize flow to the treated segments and can have serious consequences, including total thrombosis of the lower extremity. Other systems have used a balloon-closed system assisted with thrombin infusion around and outside of the arteriotomy to promote clotting (Duett). A different approach has involved the development of a closing device that delivers needles and sutures (Perclose) through the arterial wall around the access site. A potential advantage of this device is the lack of delayed bleeding after the intervention because there are no collagen plugs that could become resorbed or dislodged. Sutured-mediated closure systems allow closure of the arterial access site without placement of any occlusive intraluminal or subcutaneous material, as mentioned previously.

25. What is the role of duplex ultrasonography in patients with peripheral arterial disease?

Native vessel arterial duplex ultrasonography is generally accepted and widely used as a method of defining arterial stenosis or occlusions. The sensitivity of duplex ultrasonography to detect occlusions and stenosis has been reported to be 95% and 92%, respectively, with specificities of 99% and 97%, respectively. Limitations have included tandem lesions, tibial vessel imaging, and difficulty imaging the inflow arteries. Using a 5.0- to 7.5-MHz transducer, imaging of the infrainguinal arteries is performed. The vessels are studied in the sagital plane, and Doppler velocities are obtained using a 60-degree angle. Vessels are classified into one of five categories: normal, or 1% to 19% stenosis; 20% to 49% stenosis; 50% to 99% stenosis; and occlusion. The categories are determined by alterations in the Doppler waveform and by increasing peak systolic velocities. For stenosis to be classified as 50% to 99%, for example, the peak systolic velocity must increase by 100% in comparison with the normal segment of artery proximal to the stenosis. Arterial duplex ultrasonography has been used to guide interventionalists toward appropriate access to a lesion potentially amenable to endovascular therapy. This technology has also been used after endovascular therapy to determine technical success and durability of the procedure.

26. What are the required credentialing criteria for the performance of peripheral interventions?

Noncardiac angiography (arterial and venous) and catheter-based interventional procedures are essential components of a modern clinical cardiology practice. Therefore, all interventional cardiologists should be knowledgeable in these techniques.

Current guidelines for competence indicate that trainees should perform at least 100 diagnostic peripheral angiograms, 50 peripheral angioplasties, and 10 peripheral thrombolytic infusions.

ACKNOWLEDGMENT

Chris Hebert, R.T., R.C.I.S., Cardiovascular Technician Director, Cardiovascular Institute of the South, Lafayette, LA; and Gary Chaisson, R.T., R.C.I.S., Cardiovascular Technician Director, Cardiovascular Institute of the South, Houma, LA.

BIBLIOGRAPHY

1. Creager MA, Cooke JP, Olin JW, White CJ: Training in vascular medicine and peripheral catheter-based interventions: Core Cardiology Training in Adult Cardiovascular Medicine (COCATS 2). J Am Coll Cardiol 39:1242–1246, 2002.
2. Das TS: Percutaneous peripheral revascularization with excimer laser: equipment, technique and results. Lasers Med Sci 16:101–107, 2001.
3. Duda SH, Wiskirchen J, Erb M, et al: Suture-mediated percutaneous closure. Radiology 210:47–52, 1999.
4. Gonze MD, Sternbergh WC, Salartash K, Money SR: Complications associated with percutaneous closure devices. Am J Surg 178:209–211, 1999.
5. Haji-Aghaii M, Fogarty TJ: Balloon angioplasty, stenting, and role of atherectomy in nonoperative management of lower-extremity arterial disease, part II. Surg Clin North Am 78:593–616, 1998.
6. Hoppenfeld BM: Vascular recanalization techniques. In Bakal CW, Silberzweig JE, Cynamon J, Sprayregen S (eds): Vascular and Interventional Radiology. New York, Thieme Medical Publishers, 2002, pp 71–88.
7. Lyden SP, Shortell CK, Illig KA: Reperfusion and compartment syndromes: strategies for prevention and treatment. Semin Vasc Surg 14:107–113, 2001.
8. Martin DR, Katz SG, Kohl RD, et al: Percutaneous transluminal angioplasty of infrainguinal vessels. Ann Vasc Surg 13:184–187, 1999.
9. Strandness DE: Noninvasive vascular laboratory and vascular imaging. In Young JR, Olin JW, Bartholomew JR (eds): Peripheral Vascular Diseases, 2nd ed. St. Louis, Mosby-Year Book Inc, 1996, pp 33–64, 1996.
10. Tepe G, Hahn U, Pusich B, et al: New strategies in platelet inhibition in noncoronary interventions. Semin Vasc Surg 14:143–149, 2001.
11. Weitz JI, Byrne J, Clagett P, et al: Diagnosis and treatment of chronic arterial insufficiency of the lower extremities: a critical review. Circulation 94:3026–3049, 1996.
12. Young JR: Clinical clues to peripheral vascular disease. In Young JR, et al (eds): Peripheral Vascular Diseases, 2nd ed. St. Louis, Mosby-Year Book, 1996, pp 3–17.

54. CLAUDICATION: A SURGEON'S PERSPECTIVE

Pranay T. Ramdev, M.D.

1. What is vascular claudication?

Tiredness and ache characterize vascular claudication. The disorder is always experienced in a functional muscle unit, is reproduced consistently, and is promptly relieved by rest.

2. What is the physiologic cause of vascular claudication?

Flow to the exercising muscle mass is unable to meet the requirements of increased metabolic activity or arterial occlusion or stenosis proximal to the affected muscle bed is responsible.

3. How does claudication impact on lifestyle?

- Maximal walking speed is 1 to 2 mph versus 3.3 mph for control subjects.
- Maximal walking distance is limited.
  - 30% have difficulty walking around the home.
  - 65% have difficulty walking 150 ft (~ half a block).
- Functional ability is similar to New York Heart Association class III congestive heart failure.
- Social, personal, and occupational activities may be limited by ischemic pain.

4. What is the prevalence of claudication?

Claudication increases with age. In Europe:

- < 1% in 30-year-old men
- 3% in 55- to 59-year-old men
- 3–7% in 60- to 69-year-old men
- > 7% in ≥ 70-year-old men
- **5–10 times** more prevalent than critical limb ischemia
- **20–30 times** more prevalent than acute limb ischemia per year

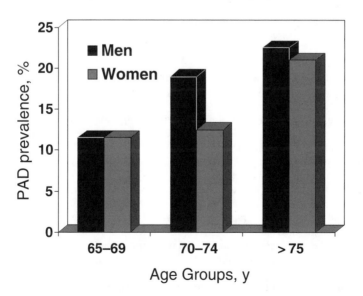

FIGURE 1. Age-related increase in peripheral vascular disease (PVD) prevalence by gender. (Adapted from Criqui MH, Fronek A, Barrett-Connor E, et al: The prevalence of peripheral arterial disease in a defined population. Circulation 71:510–515, 1985.

5. What is the true incidence of claudication?

The incidence is difficult to assess because many patients are older, and aging patients appear to accept increasing difficulty in walking as part of aging. Between 2010 and 2030 the number of elderly patients (age $\geq$ 65 years) will increase by 70%. An aging society means increasing incidence of the disorder.

6. Does arteriographically documented peripheral arterial occlusive disease (PAOD) correlate with clinical symptoms?

A total of 67% of patients with arteriographically proven leg arterial occlusions did not complain of claudication on an initial questionnaire. Additionally, 33% of patients steadfastly maintained that they were asymptomatic even after a detailed interview.

7. Because angiography does not always identify clinically relevant PAOD, what physiologic studies should be obtained?

The studies that identify physiologically relevant lesions include Doppler-derived waveforms, pulse-volume recordings (PVR), and transcutaneous oxygen levels (TcPO$_2$).

8. What are the indications for an angiogram?

An angiogram should only be obtained when a decision to intervene (either by open repair or catheter-based technology) has been reached based on the relevant physiologic testing. Intervention based solely on angiographic data is inappropriate.

9. How important is the pulse examination?

The pulse examination coupled with symptoms will identify the location of arterial lesions more than 80% of the time. An abnormal femoral pulse examination result is more than 95% accurate in predicting aortoiliac occlusive disease. Normal pedal pulses at rest do not rule out a vascular cause of claudication. Exercise the patient until symptoms develop (walk, tiptoe repetitions) and ascertain if the pedal pulses disappear. If so, a subcritical stenosis likely exists in the axial arterial flow stream. During clinic consultation, one can quickly measure the ankle-brachial index (ABI) at the end of exercise and time the return of pedal pulses from the onset of symptoms.

10. What is the risk of limb loss in patients with claudication?

In the Framingham Study, only 1.6% of patients with claudication observed for 8.3 years required amputation.

In the cardiology literature, a review of patients with claudication revealed the following:

- Seventy-five percent remain stable or improve 2–5 years after onset despite angiographic evidence of progression in the majority.
- Twenty-five percent worsen: 7–9% in first year, then 2–3% yearly.
- Five percent will undergo intervention within 5 years of diagnosis.
- **Only 2–4% of patients with claudication will require major amputation in their lifetime.**
- Smoking and diabetes predict rapid progression and higher intervention and amputation rates.
- ABI $<$ 0.5 is the most significant predictor of deterioration needing intervention.
- Men are at higher risk for progression.

11. What is the difference in the life expectancy of a patient with claudication versus an age-matched control subject?

The life expectancy for patients with claudication is 72% survival at 5 years and 50% at 10 years.

The life expectancy for control subjects is 90% expected 5-year survival rate (Fig. 2)

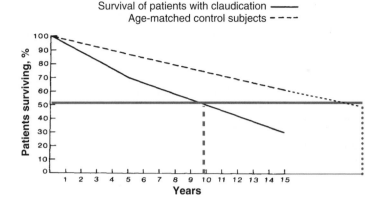

FIGURE 2. Kaplan-Meyer cumulative survival curves of patients with claudication compared with controls subjects. Data from Boyd, 1960; McAllister, 1979; Imparato, 1975; Peabody, 1974; Cronenwett, 1984; Rosenbloom, 1988; Jonason and Ringqvist, 1985; and Walsh, 1991.

12. What are the deaths in the patients with claudication secondary to?

- Atherosclerosis in other locations further reduced the survival of those patients
  - 61% 5-year survival with associated cerebrovascular disease
  - 59% 5-year survival with symptomatic coronary artery disease (CAD)
- 75% of deaths were caused by CAD.
- Hypertension had a slightly adverse effect on 5-year survival.
- Hypercholesterolemia had no significant effect on 5-year survival.

13. What is the incidence of CAD in patients with claudication?

In 1000 claudication patients undergoing elective surgery:
- CAD in 90% confirmed by angiogram
- CAD in 47% when only the clinical history and resting ECG were used for screening, emphasizing the asymptomatic nature of CAD
- Severe surgically correctable CAD: 14% of claudication patients with no history or ECG evidence of CAD

14. What are the risk factors for peripheral arterial disease (PAD)?

- Male gender
- Older age
- Hyperhomocysteinemia
- Ratio of total cholesterol to high-density lipoprotein
- Lipoprotein(a)
- Tobacco
- High triglyceride level
- Diabetes
- Hypertension

15. What are the noninterventional treatment goals for patients with claudication?

- Risk factor management:
  - Abstinence from all tobacco
  - Control of hypertension, diabetes mellitus, and hyperlipoproteinemia
  - Weight reduction
  - Treatment of CHF or azotemia

- Exercise, preferably a supervised program
- Meticulous foot care
- Platelet inhibition, which decreases the risk of ischemic stroke, myocardial infarction, and vascular mortality
- Agents directed at claudication

16. How does exercise help claudication patients clinically?
The greatest benefit comes from supervised programs, with a mean increase of 179% in initial claudication distance and a mean increase of 122% in maximal walking distance. A total of 34% of patients with claudication had a contraindication to exercise treatment (e.g., CAD). Neither ankle blood pressure nor calf muscle blood flow is better in claudication patients whose walking tolerance improves after an exercise program. Improved muscle performance results in part from adaptive changes in muscle enzymes, leading to a more efficient extraction of oxygen.

17. How does angioplasty compare with nonoperative treatment of claudication?
Initial improvement, as assessed by ABI, was greater in the angioplasty group. After 1 year, the patients in the exercise group could walk farther, both on the treadmill in the laboratory and as assessed by questionnaire, and there was no longer a significant difference between the ABI values of the two groups.

18. What are the indications for intervention for patients with claudication?
- Disability precluding gainful employment
- Unacceptable alteration in lifestyle

19. Trental was the original treatment of choice for nonoperative treatment of claudication. How was it thought to work?
- It was believed to act partly by a microrheologic mechanism. Whole blood viscosity would decrease by increasing whole blood filterability. This occurs presumably by the effect on white blood cells and, possibly, on plasma fibrinogen and platelet aggregation.
- Ehrly demonstrated an increase in muscle oxygen tension in patients with claudication, but these data have not been duplicated.
- It is not currently recommended as the drug of choice for medical treatment of claudication.

20. What is cilostazol (Pletal), and how does it work in patients with claudication?
- Significantly increases the pain-free and maximal walking distances
- Response may be seen as early as 2 to 4 weeks
- Beneficial effects may increase with time
- Well tolerated, with most adverse events of mild to moderate severity:
  Headache
  Loose or abnormal stools
  Palpitations
- Pletal inhibits phosphodiesterase III, which results in:
  Increased intracellular cyclic adenosine monophosphate (cAMP)
  Decreased intracellular calcium ion
- These effects result in:
  Inhibition of platelet aggregation
  Smooth muscle cell relaxation (vasodilation)

21. What is a contraindication of cilostazol (Pletal)?
CHF of any severity.

22. What is the current philosophy on the treatment of patients with claudication and peripheral vascular disease?

- Most nondiabetics can expect their claudication to remain stable, especially if they abstain from tobacco.
- Those with ischemic rest pain, ulcers, or gangrene are at high risk for both limb loss and premature death and merit limb salvage.
- Nevertheless, because every patient with symptomatic atherosclerosis is at greater risk for early death, the overall goals of therapy should be to relieve pain and preserve bipedal gait without further jeopardizing the patient's already limited life expectancy.
- Most patients with claudication improve symptomatically with conservative noninterventional or medical management.
- Claudication is a medically treated disease with intervention by either surgery or balloon angioplasty needed in a carefully selected handful of patients.

BIBLIOGRAPHY

1. Aquino R, et al: Natural history of claudication: long-term serial follow-up study of 1244 claudicants. J Vasc Surg 34:962–970, 2001.
2. Byrne J, et al: Infrainguinal arterial reconstruction for claudication: is it worth the risk? An analysis of 409 procedures. J Vasc Sur 29:259–269, 1999.
3. Current Therapy in Vascular Surgery, 4th ed. Ernst & Stanley. Vascular Surgery, 5th ed. Rutherford, NJ.
4. McDermott MM, Mehta S, Greenland P: Exertional leg symptoms other than intermittent claudication are common in peripheral arterial disease. Arch Intern Med 159:387–392, 1999.
5. Regensteiner JG, Steiner JF, Hiatt WR: Exercise training improves functional status in patients with peripheral arterial disease J Vasc Surg 23:104–115, 1996.
6. Salmasi AM, Nicolaides A, Al-Katoubi A, et al: Intermittent claudication as a manifestation of silent myocardial ischemia: a pilot study. J Vasc Surg 14:76–86, 1991.
7. Whyman MR, Fowkes FG, Kerracher EM, et al: Is intermittent claudication improved by percutaneous transluminal angioplasty? A randomized controlled trial. J Vasc Surg 26:551–557, 1997.

55. EVALUATION OF CAROTID DISEASE

Jose G. Romano, M.D., and Alejandro M. Forteza, M.D.

1. What is the impact of carotid disease on stroke and cardiac disease?

With 750,000 new strokes each year and 160,000 annual deaths, stroke is the third cause of death and leading cause of disability in the United States. Elderly individuals are particularly vulnerable because age is the most important risk factor for stroke. Cerebral ischemia accounts for 80% of all strokes, and 20% of these are caused by to carotid atherostenosis. Carotid disease is also a marker for coronary atherosclerosis and is associated with cardiovascular death: population studies have revealed that the presence of a carotid bruit doubles the mortality rate. Even in the absence of a defined carotid atherosclerotic plaque, the mere increase in the intima and media thickness is a predictor for greater risk of stroke and myocardial infarction (MI): the Cardiovascular Health Study showed an increase in stroke and MI from 5% to 25% at 7 years when comparing the lower and higher quintiles of intima and media thickness. In those with defined carotid plaques, the risk may even be higher.

2. How does carotid disease result in neurologic injury?

Atherosclerosis constitutes the main pathological process found at the origin of the internal carotid arteries. In response to common risk factors (e.g., as hypertension, diabetes, hyperlipidemia, tobacco use, hyperhomocystenemia), lipids, smooth muscle cells, fibroblasts, and calcium accumulate within the arterial wall. Initially, a fibrous cap covers these plaques, and at this stage they are unlikely to cause symptoms. The disruption of the fibrous cap is associated with plaque growth with higher degrees of stenosis, infection, and alterations in metalloproteins. The rupture of the fibrous cap leads to an ulcer on the endothelial surface. After blood is exposed to the thrombogenic influences of the plaque contents, thrombus formation on the plaque surface can occur. The thrombus, and occasionally plaque contents (e.g., cholesterol crystals and other debris), can embolize to the intracranial vessels and result in cerebral ischemia. Indeed, most strokes and transient ischemic attacks (TIAs) related to large vessel disease are caused by artery-to-artery embolism.

Although normal cerebral blood flow is about 50 cc of oxygenated blood per 100 grams of brain per minute, the brain can function with flow as low as 20 cc/100 g/min. Tissue exposed to flow of 10–20 cc/100 g/min is salvageable if flow is restored within minutes to hours, but blood flow under 10 cc/100 g/min results in cell death within a few minutes. Therefore, the onset of symptoms is directly related to the amount of flow reduction and the state of collateral flow to the affected area. Collateral flow usually arises from the external carotid artery through retrograde ophthalmic flow into the distal intracranial carotid artery; from the posterior circulation through the posterior communicating artery; or across the anterior communicating artery from the contralateral carotid artery. The anterior communicating artery is functionally the most important source of collateral flow. The source of collateral flow should be taken into account when deciding on carotid revascularization.

Different from myocardial ischemia in which plaque accidents result in total or near total vessel occlusion and distal hemodynamic insufficiency, carotid-related cerebral ischemia is caused most frequently by artery-to-artery embolism. If the embolus is promptly lysed, either therapeutically or spontaneously, symptoms resolve without deficits and the episode is characterized as a TIA. Hemodynamic symptoms related to poor blood flow through a narrowed carotid artery are associated with hypotensive or hypovolemic states. The border zone between the major cerebral branches are commonly affected with low flow states.

3. Describe the symptoms of carotid disease.

The carotid arteries carry 80% of cerebral blood flow; irrigate the territories of the middle cerebral, anterior cerebral, and anterior choroidal arteries; and provide blood flow to the eyes through the ophthalmic arteries. The symptoms of carotid embolism vary according to the recipient artery. Ophthalmic artery occlusion results in monocular visual loss (transient amaurosis fugax or permanent central or branch retinal artery occlusion), often described as blurring, graying, or curtaining of vision. Middle cerebral artery syndrome often includes contralateral weakness affecting the face and arm more than the leg, contralateral sensory loss, and aphasia if the dominant hemisphere is affected, or hemi-inattention or neglect with nondominant lesions. In addition, there may be gaze deviation toward the affected hemisphere. Anterior cerebral artery strokes affect the contralateral leg and shoulder more than face and arm and can have associated abulia and incontinence. The anterior choroidal stroke affects the basal ganglia and internal capsule, with contralateral hemiplegia, hemisensory loss, and hourglass-shaped homonymous visual field defects. Anterior choroidal infarcts may be difficult to differentiate from lacunar strokes because of occlusion of small penetrators.

4. Which clues found in the general examination point to carotid disease in stroke victims?

Clues for carotid disease include an audible bruit in the anterior neck, evidence of a cholesterol retinal embolus (i.e., Hollenhorst plaque), and a history of various spells of ischemia in the same arterial distribution. In addition, careful craniovascular examination may reveal asymmetric preauricular and orbital pulses that are stronger on the side of the stenosis and represent external carotid artery collateral flow. On occasions, dilatation of the extracranial vasculature may be noted.

5. What is the risk of stroke in patients with carotid stenosis?

Patients who have had symptoms of carotid disease (e.g., stroke, TIA, amaurosis fugax) are at a much higher risk of recurrent stroke. The seminal North American Symptomatic Carotid Endarterectomy Trial (NASCET) defined a 26% risk of ipsilateral stroke at 2 years in the presence of stenosis of 70% or more for those treated medically, with increasing risk at greater degree of stenosis. The risk of stroke after purely ocular symptoms (amaurosis fugax) is less than in those with cerebral symptoms. For stenosis of 50–69% in symptomatic patients, the risk of stroke was less impressive: at 5 years, the risk of ipsilateral stroke in those undergoing antiplatelet therapy was 22.2%. Stenosis under 50% is unlikely to result in stroke. The risk of stroke with asymptomatic carotid stenosis is clearly less than after a TIA or stroke. The Asymptomatic Carotid Atherosclerosis Study (ACAS) studied carotid stenosis of 60% or more; in the medically treated group, the risk of ipsilateral stroke was estimated at 11% at 5 years, suggesting an annual risk of 2.2%.

6. Is there a risk of stroke after carotid occlusion?

Yes. At the time of carotid occlusion, there is about 20% chance of distal embolism. In the first few weeks after occlusion, there is a small but significant risk of stroke. Because the internal carotid artery lacks cervical branches, there is stagnation of the distal blood column, with clot developing up to the first branch, the ophthalmic artery. Until the distal thrombus re-endothelizes, usually over 3 to 6 weeks, there is a risk of embolism from the top of the clot column, because the retrograde flow from the ophthalmic artery may "shave" off small emboli. This phenomenon is called *stump embolism* and may be prevented by anticoagulation for several of months after the occlusion. In the chronic stages of a carotid occlusion, hemodynamic factors determine the risk of ipsilateral stroke. Although the overall risk is about 1% per year, it may increase to 10% in those with poor collateral blood flow.

7. What is the best initial test to detect carotid disease?

Extracranial duplex ultrasonography is a reliable, noninvasive, and relatively inexpensive method to study the extracranial carotid system. It combines B-mode ultrasound and color-coded Doppler; whereas B-mode provides, in grayscale, an image of the common, internal, and external carotid arteries, Doppler techniques allow a physiologic evaluation of the blood flow characteristics. Whereas ultrasound allows direct imaging of the arterial wall and atherosclerotic plaque, conventional angiography depicts only the arterial lumen. Plaque characteristics provide information about stroke risk. Two findings are particularly important: (1) plaque ulceration provides a favorable milieu for the formation of thrombus that can secondarily embolize and (2) a hypoechoic plaque, representing either intraplaque hemorrhage or a lipid-rich plaque, is associated with the potential for plaque destabilization. Color-coded duplex ultrasonography is a color representation of the blood flow velocity; sampling at the level of the stenosis quantifies the acceleration of blood flow in this segment. Many ultrasonographic criteria have been established to estimate the degree of stenosis, and each ultrasound laboratory should validate its own criteria against angiographic standards. In general, a peak systolic flow velocity of 140 cm/sec correlates with about 50% stenosis, and velocities of 200 cm/sec or more suggest more than 70% stenosis. Carotid ultrasound has a sensitivity of 90–95% and specificity of 85% compared with catheter angiography. Ultrasound may be unable to detect high-grade stenosis and mistakenly diagnoses a carotid occlusion in 5% of cases. Although power Doppler and echocontrast agents may improve the odds of a correct diagnosis, for now it is standard practice to corroborate carotid occlusions with another imaging modality such as magnetic resonance angiography (MRA), computed tomographic angiography (CTA), or catheter angiography.

Both MRA and CTA adequately image the carotid system, with the advantage of visualizing the intracranial circulation. These techniques are more expensive and have accuracy that is similar to ultrasound for detecting extracranial carotid stenosis. The authors use them to confirm ultrasound findings.

8. Is it important to evaluate the intracranial circulation?

Yes. Evaluation of the intracranial circulation is important for various reasons. First, there may be tandem distal carotid stenosis that may increase the risk of cerebral ischemia and may tip the decision toward a certain method of carotid revascularization. Second, evaluation of the intracranial circulation allows the estimation of available collateral flow. This information is useful in estimating which asymptomatic patients are at a higher risk of stroke. Finally, the presence of asymptomatic microemboli detected by transcranial Doppler (TCD) over the ipsilateral middle cerebral artery suggests an unstable carotid plaque that increases the risk of stroke. Although MRA, CTA, and catheter angiography allow anatomic visualization of the intracranial vessels, TCD provides physiologic information. The anatomic modalities described above allow the detection of intracranial stenosis, vascular malformations, and aneurysms. On the other hand, TCD is an inexpensive and noninvasive technology based on the ability of low-frequency ultrasound waves to penetrate the skull and record echoes from the red blood cells in the large intracranial arteries. A segmental increase in blood flow velocity suggests a focal area of stenosis. Reversed direction of flow of the ophthalmic artery or anterior cerebral artery represents collateral flow through the external carotid or across the anterior communicating artery, respectively. The state of collaterals can be further evaluated by TCD vasodilatory CO_2 or acetazolamide challenge tests. Absence of autoregulatory capacity is seen in high-grade carotid stenosis without adequate collateral flow, because a maximally dilated distal vasculature cannot respond to further challenges. Finally, TCD allows the prolonged monitoring for microemboli.

9. Is carotid angiography needed to confirm carotid stenosis diagnosed by ultrasound?

Although ultrasound is usually the first diagnostic study, it is our belief that patients with significant stenosis in whom revascularization is being considered should have a confirmatory test. Establishing the degree of stenosis by ultrasound may be misleading in the presence of contralateral significant stenosis or occlusion, high carotid bifurcation, or severely calcified plaques, and in those with thick and short necks. Catheter angiography is the gold standard diagnostic test, but it carries a risk of clinical stroke of about 1%, although experienced centers have a lower rate of complications. With a reported sensitivity and specificity as high as 90%, MRA is playing an increasingly important role in the selection of surgical candidates and may replace catheter angiography in the future. Contrast-enhanced MRA holds particular promise. Most clinicians and surgeons are comfortable operating on asymptomatic carotid stenosis based on the information provided by the combination of ultrasound and MRA, particularly because the benefits of revascularization in asymptomatic patients are negated by combined angiographic and surgical risks in excess of 3%. However, for recently symptomatic patients, catheter angiography is commonly performed.

10. When is carotid revascularization indicated?

The risk of stroke after ischemic symptoms is significant, and carotid endarterectomy trials have unequivocally shown that those with **symptomatic** carotid stenosis should be revascularized. These data are strongest for stenosis of 70–99% and less robust for stenosis of 50–69%.

For patients with **asymptomatic** carotid stenosis, the decision to revascularize is more difficult; because the natural history of asymptomatic carotid stenosis is relatively benign (annual risk of stroke of about 2%), the decision to intervene should be weighed against the inherent risk of the procedure. To maintain the benefits of revascularization in asymptomatic individuals, the surgical morbidity and mortality should be kept under 3%. This concept should apply to both endarterectomy and endovascular procedures. In addition, endarterectomy trials have shown less benefit for women than men with asymptomatic carotid disease. Besides other traditional vascular risk factors, certain qualifiers increase the risk of stroke in patients with *asymptomatic* carotid stenosis and provide grounds to proceed with revascularization. These qualifiers include high-grade stenosis in otherwise healthy and relatively young patients; those with documented progression of carotid stenosis; individuals with poor collateral flow or vasomotor reactivity; and the presence of asymptomatic embolism detected by transcranial Doppler monitoring or by its sequelae, silent strokes on cerebral imaging.

Benefit of Carotid Endarterectomy

POPULATION	STENOSIS, %*	NONSURGICAL, %[†]	SURGICAL, %[†]	ABSOLUTE RISK REDUCTION, %	NNT[‡]
Symptomatic	50–69[¶]	22.2	15.7	6.5 at 5 years	20
Symptomatic	70–99[¶]	26	9	17 at 2 years	8
Asymptomatic	60–99[§]	11	5.1	5.9 at 5 years	83

*Measurement according to the NASCET method.
[†]Risk of ipsilateral stroke.
[‡]Numbers needed to treat to prevent one stroke at 2 years.
[¶]From NASCET.
[§]From ACAS.

11. When should endarterectomy be performed after symptoms of cerebral ischemia?

There is no reason to delay treatment after TIAs. However, after a stroke, the endothelium distal to the occlusion loses its tight junctions, which may result in extravasation of blood into the infarcted tissue upon restoration of blood flow, particularly in the presence of hypertension. This consideration should delay revascularization for a few weeks in large strokes. However, in small strokes, the risk of recurrent ischemia from a tight carotid stenosis outweighs the potential for hemorrhage; therefore; revascularization should not be delayed.

12. Should carotid occlusions be revascularized?

Revascularization of carotid occlusion is usually not indicated, because the occluded vessel promptly develops organization of the clot. Therefore, attempts to open the vessel are counterproductive, with a high risk of perioperative stroke. The exception is thrombectomy immediately after acute carotid occlusion, a risky procedure that is rarely performed. Another procedure is external carotid–to–internal carotid (EC-IC) bypass surgery, in which a branch of the external carotid artery, the superficial temporal artery, is anastomosed surgically to a middle cerebral artery branch through a craniotomy. This intervention was not proven to be effective in a large trial (the EC-IC Bypass Study), but the procedure may be used in selected patients with recurrent ischemia caused by carotid occlusion in whom collateral flow is clearly defective.

13. Is angioplasty and stenting equivalent to carotid endarterectomy?

Carotid angioplasty and stenting is now feasible and is increasingly performed. To date, the endovascular approach has not been proven to be as safe or more efficacious than endarterectomy. However, it is an evolving technique, and the development of new materials and distal protection devices, as well as stents coated with different vasoactive substances, may make it the procedure of choice in the future. In our opinion, endarterectomy, a time-proven and relatively safe procedure, should currently be the indicated approach for most individuals.

There are a number of situations in which endarterectomy is risky and in which angioplasty and stenting should be strongly considered for symptomatic patients:

- Cardiac or pulmonary contraindications to surgery such as unstable coronary disease and severe chronic obstructive pulmonary disease
- Patients with a contralateral high-grade stenosis or occlusion; these patients are at particular risk of perioperative stroke with endarterectomy, because the need to interrupt blood flow during the procedure may not be tolerated
- A high carotid bifurcation behind the mandible that is not surgically accessible
- Restenosis after endarterectomy
- Radiation-induced arteriopathy
- Contralateral vocal cord palsy; surgery may damage the remaining recurrent laryngeal nerve, resulting in bilateral vocal cord paralysis that necessitates tracheostomy

It is our belief that patients with asymptomatic carotid stenosis should not be treated with angioplasty and stenting until the risk–benefit profile is established in prospective randomized trials.

14. Should patients planned for carotid revascularization stop taking their antithrombotic agents before surgery?

No. Antiplatelet therapy should be continued; better outcomes are obtained after endarterectomy when patients remain on aspirin. Because endarterectomy denudes the endothelium, platelets promptly adhere to the exposed subendothelial matrix. Antiaggregant agents prevent the formation of platelet thrombi. In carotid angioplasty and stenting, after the coronary experience, the combination of aspirin and an adenosine diphosphate receptor platelet inhibitor (ticlopidine or clopidogrel) is prescribed before the procedure.

15. How should carotid stenosis be approached in the presence of known coronary disease?

When addressing carotid stenosis, it is important to evaluate for significant coronary disease because these often coexist. This evaluation is useful in assessing the risk and merits of the planned carotid revascularization. Those with stable coronary stenosis are probably safe undergoing endarterectomy with simple perioperative precautions such as beta-blockers and nitrates. Those with unstable coronary disease are at risk for MI and should be considered for coronary revascularization before endarterectomy. When severe coronary and carotid diseases coexist, a useful guideline is to first treat the symptomatic vascular bed. For those with unstable cardiac syndromes in whom coronary angioplasty and stenting is not feasible, carotid angioplasty and stenting (rather than carotid endarterectomy) should be considered.

16. What is the appropriate timing to revascularize carotid stenosis when coronary artery bypass graft (CABG) surgery is planned?

CABG is associated with a significant risk of stroke. Most perioperative strokes are embolic, either from an aortic arch plaque damaged by clamping or cannulation of the aorta or from fatty material recirculated in the cardiopulmonary pump machine. However, hemodynamic strokes distal to a significant carotid stenosis may occur and are caused by the significant hypotension achieved during surgery. The risk of intraoperative stroke can be estimated by the ability of the vasculature distal to the obstruction to autoregulate in the presence of vasodilatory challenges such as CO_2 inhalation during TCD monitoring. Controversy exists regarding the timing of carotid revascularization: should it be done before or during CABG? In our experience, a staged procedure of carotid revascularization followed by coronary surgery is most appropriate, but management decisions need to be individualized.

17. What other nonatherosclerotic conditions affect the carotid artery?

Carotid dissection is a common cause of stroke in young individuals. Contrary to general belief, its presenting symptom is frequently only an ipsilateral headache. In this condition, a tear in the endothelium leads to entry of blood into the arterial wall and formation of an intramural thrombus. Artery-to-artery embolism is usually the cause of cerebral ischemia, and it may occur because of a distal flap opening and exposing the thrombus to the carotid lumen; because of arterial occlusion as a consequence of significant expansion of the intramural thrombus, with a secondary thrombus forming in the distal segment of the occluded carotid; or in association to thrombus formation in a dissecting aneurysm. Carotid dissections often occur in the setting of trauma, but this trauma may be so minimal that many patients do not recall anything unusual. The vessel is damaged as it is compressed against the styloid process or cervical body with hyperextension of the neck or against the mandible with hyperflexion. There are clearly a number of individuals with minimal or no trauma who develop carotid dissections and who probably have defective collagen.

Fibromuscular dysplasia and Marfan's and Ehler-Danlos syndromes are often associated with arterial dissections, but more often no obvious collagenopathy is recognized. Carotid dissection often has associated ipsilateral neck and head pain, and Horner's syndrome (i.e., miosis and ptosis caused by interruption of sympathetic fibers traveling in the carotid sheath) may be found. On occasions, lower cranial neuropathy with tongue deviation and dysgeusia can be detected, resulting from compression of the nerve by a dissecting aneurysm, or to ischemic neuropathy by virtue of interruption of the vasa nervorum. As expected from the site of arterial injury, the distal extracranial internal carotid artery is most affected, and intracranial extension of the dissection is uncommon. Clinical suspicion should lead to appropriate corroborative diagnostic tests. Catheter angiography is the gold standard for diagnosis, and a flame-shaped stenosis or occlusion distal to the internal carotid artery origin is almost pathognomonic. Magnetic resonance imaging with fat saturation sequences has the advantage of detecting the arterial wall thrombus, seen as a bright halo around the lumen. Ultrasound techniques are less useful for diagnosis, but duplex ultrasonography can document a stenosis, and cerebral microemboli are found with TCD in most patients with recent carotid dissections. Anticoagulation for 6 to 12 weeks to prevent cerebral embolization is currently the preferred treatment of carotid dissection, but no prospective studies have studied alternatives to this. After the dissection heals, antiplatelet therapy can be initiated.

Giant cell arteritis (GCA), a disease that occurs almost exclusively in elderly individuals, deserves special mention because its complications can be prevented if they are recognized early. In this disease, mononuclear cells infiltrate the large and medium extradural vessel, and granulomas can be found in the media of the artery. Headache is the most consistent complaint of patients with GCA; it is usually temporal, may interfere with sleep, and can have associated scalp tenderness. Other common complaints include jaw claudication caused by masseter muscle ischemia and a palpable nodular or pulseless temporal artery. The symptoms of polymyalgia rheumatica often coexist and precede those of GCA. They include fever, weight loss, fatigue, malaise, and limb girdle myalgias; polymyalgia rheumatica appears to represent one end of the spectrum of the same disease. The most feared complication of GCA is vision loss. Anterior ischemic optic neuropathy caused by occlusion of the ciliary vessels is the most common mechanism of vision loss, but posterior ischemic optic neuropathy or central retinal artery occlusion can also occur. Stroke is less common, and if at all, the pathologic process may involve the posterior circulation. Diagnosis is based on clinical findings confirmed by an elevated sedimentation rate, usually greater than 50; elevated C-reactive protein level; and a confirmatory temporal artery biopsy. Prompt steroid therapy can prevent the ocular and cerebral complications.

CAROTID ATHEROSTENOSIS: ILLUSTRATIVE CASE

A 72-year-old woman with hypertension and diabetes is found to have a right anterior neck bruit. She denied symptoms suggestive of amaurosis fugax, stroke, or TIA, and the results of the neurologic examination were normal. An extracranial duplex ultrasonogram (Fig. 1) shows an irregular, heterogeneous plaque at the origin of the right internal carotid, with associated velocities across the stenosis of 350/140 cm/sec, resulting in an estimated luminal stenosis of 90%. This was confirmed by neck MRA (Fig. 2), in which there is segmental absence of time of flight enhancement at the origin of the right internal carotid artery (flow-gap) consistent with at least 70% stenosis. The hemodynamic impact of this stenosis is apparent on TCD: note the dampened flow velocity of the right middle cerebral artery (Fig. 3, *top panel*), ipsilateral to the carotid stenosis, compared to the contralateral left middle cerebral artery (Fig. 3, *bottom panel*). In addition, the direction of flow in the right ophthalmic artery is reversed (Fig. 4, *top panel*), but the contralateral one is antegrade (Fig. 4, *bottom panel*), indicating recruitment of collateral flow from the external carotid artery through the ophthalmic artery. A microembolic signal was found in the right middle cerebral artery (Fig. 5), as noted by the interruption of the normal Doppler flow pattern and coded as a red vertical line. Despite the patient's clinically asymptomatic status, carotid endarterectomy was recommended because of the significant stenosis and suggestion of plaque instability by the presence of microembolization.

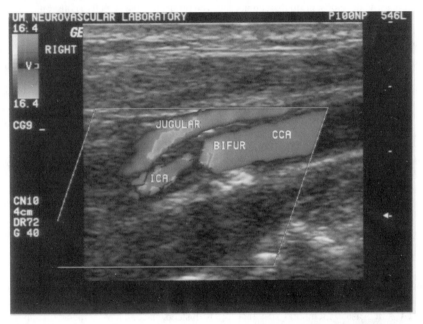

FIGURE 1. Color duplex ultrasonogram of the right internal carotid artery showing poststenotic turbulence.

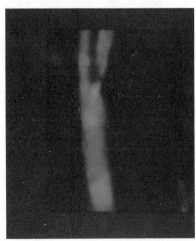

FIGURE 2. Right internal carotid MRA showing absence of flow-enhancement (flow-gap), suggesting stenosis of at least 70% (possibly more).

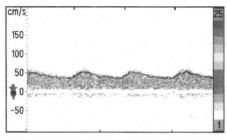

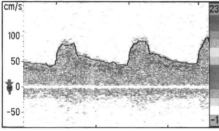

FIGURE 3. Transcranial Doppler flow patterns of the right (*top panel*) and left (*bottom panel*) middle cerebral arteries, with decreased or dampened flow velocity on the right, compatible with proximal high-grade carotid stenosis.

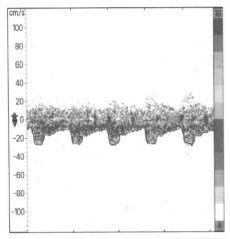

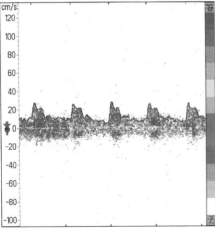

FIGURE 4. Transcranial Doppler flow patterns of the right (*top panel*) and left (*bottom panel*) ophthalmic arteries with reversed flow on the right, suggesting recruitment of the external carotid–ophthalmic collateral pathways.

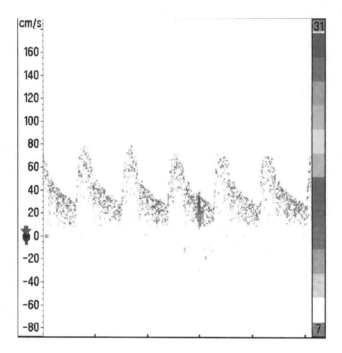

FIGURE 5. Transcranial Doppler flow pattern of the right middle cerebral artery interrupted by a high-intensity transient signal (in red), that represents a microembolic particle.

BIBLIOGRAPHY

1. Babikian VL, Feldmann E, Wechsler LR, et al: Transcranial Doppler ultrasonography: year 2000 update. J Neuroimaging 10:101–115, 2000.
2. Blakeley DD, Oddone EZ, Hasselblad V, et al: Non-invasive carotid artery testing: a meta-analytic review. Ann Intern Med 122:360–367, 1995.
3. De Bray JM, Glatt B, for the International Consensus Conference: Quantification of atheromatous stenosis of the extracranial carotid artery. Cerebrovasc Dis 5:414–426, 1995.
4. The EC/IC Bypass Study Group: Failure of extracranial-intracranial arterial bypass to reduce risk of ischemic stroke: results of an international randomized trial. N Engl J Med 313:1191–1200, 1985.
5. The European Carotid Surgery Trialists' Collaborative Group: Randomised trial of endarterectomy for recently symptomatic carotid stenosis: final results of the MRC European Carotid Surgery Trial (ECST). Lancet 351:1379–1387, 1998.
6. Executive Committee for the Asymptomatic Carotid Atherosclerosis Study: Endarterectomy for asymptomatic carotid artery stenosis. JAMA 273:1421–1428, 1995.
7. Filis KA, Arko FR, Johnson BL, et al: Duplex ultrasound criteria for defining the severity of carotid stenosis. Ann Vasc Surg 16:413–421, 2002.
8. Forteza AM, Koch S, Romano JG, Babikian VL: Detection of microembolus with transcranial Doppler. Rev Neurol 31:1046–1053, 2000.
9. Forteza AM, Rabinstein A: Angioplastía y stenting de la estenosis carotídea. Alternativa terapéutica o posibilidad técnica? Rev Neurol 32: 270–275, 2001.
10. Forteza AM, Romano JG, Latchaw RE: Non-invasive evaluation of extracranial and intracranial vascular disease. Rev Neurol 29:1321–1329, 1999.
11. Gomez CR: Carotid plaque morphology and risk for stroke. Stroke 21:148–151, 1990.
12. Heiserman JE, Zabramski JM, Drayer BP, Keller PJ: Clinical significance of the flow gap in carotid magnetic resonance angiography. J Neurosurg 85:384–387, 1996.
13. The North American Symptomatic Carotid Endarterectomy Trial Collaborators: Beneficial effect of carotid endarterectomy in symptomatic patients with high-grade stenosis. N Engl J Med 325:445–453, 1991.

14. The North American Symptomatic Carotid Endarterectomy Trial Collaborators: Beneficial effect of carotid endarterectomy in patients with symptomatic moderate or severe stenosis. N Engl J Med 339: 1415–1425, 1998.
15. O'Leary DH, Polak JF, Kronmal RA, et al, for the Cardiovascular Health Study Collaborative Research Group: Carotid artery intima and media thickness as a risk factor for myocardial infarction and stroke in older adults. N Engl J Med 340:14–22, 1999.
16. Polak JF, Shemanski L, O'Leary D, et al: Hypoechoic plaque at US of the carotid artery: an independent risk factor for incident stroke in adults aged 65 or older. Radiology 208:649–654, 1998.
17. Ringelstein EB, Zeumer H, Angelou D: The pathogenesis of strokes from internal carotid artery occlusion: diagnostic and therapeutical implications. Stroke 14:867–875, 1983.
18. Stary HC, Chandler AB, Dinsmore RE, et al: A definition of advanced types of atherosclerotic lesions and a histological classification of atherosclerosis: a report from the Committee on Vascular Lesions of the Council on Arteriosclerosis, American Heart Association. Circulation 92:1355–1374, 1995.

56. CAROTID STENTING AND ANGIOPLASTY

Johnny S. Sandhu, M.D., and Ajay K. Wakhloo, M.D., Ph.D.

1. How common is carotid stenosis? Who gets it, and why?

Although the precise prevalence of carotid artery stenosis is unknown, large studies have estimated that 0.5% of people in their sixties and 10% of people older than age 80 years have carotid artery stenosis. Atherosclerotic stenosis of the carotid artery has been estimated to be responsible for 20% to 30% of all strokes. More than 600,000 Americans suffer a stroke each year; more than one in four of them die. Currently, there are 4.6 million stroke survivors in the United States, where the disease is the third leading cause of death and the leading cause of major morbidity.

Age, race, gender, genetics, and family history are nonmodifiable factors that play a role in the development of carotid artery disease. Older age, African-American and Hispanic descent, male gender, and family history are all risk factors.

Modifiable risk factors include smoking, hyperlipidemia, sedentary lifestyle, increased body mass index, oral contraceptive use, alcohol and substance abuse, diabetes mellitus, hypertension, prior transient ischemic attack (TIA) or stroke, elevated homocysteine level, elevated anticardiolipin antibodies, presence of a carotid bruit, cardiac disease, increased fibrinogen, and low serum folate level.

2. How do these patients present?

Although many patients present with stroke, others present with a TIA that consists of ipsilateral amaurosis fugax, contralateral sensory or motor dysfunction limited to one side of the body, aphasia, contralateral homonymous hemianopia, or combinations thereof. The ocular symptoms are sudden, brief, painless, and last 1 to 5 minutes, rarely more than 30 minutes. Primary care physicians may also refer patients after auscultation of carotid bruits, although this is not a very sensitive sign.

3. What are the characteristics of carotid plaque?

Carotid plaques have a variety of characteristics that are distinguished as either homogenous or heterogenous plaques. *Arteriosclerosis* is a general term used for all structural changes that result in hardening of the arterial wall. Diffuse intimal thickening is growth of the intima through the migration of medial smooth muscle cells into the subendothelial space through the fenestrations of the internal elastic lamina, associated with increasing amounts of elastic fibers, collagen, and glycosaminoglycans (Fig. 1).

Homogenous plaques are stable, with deposition of fatty streaks and fibrous tissues. These plaques rarely have evidence of hemorrhage or ulcerations. On the other hand, heterogenous plaques are unstable, with histological characteristics of lipid-laden macrophages, monocytes, leukocytes, necrotic debris, cholesterol crystals, and calcifications. Plaques may be hard with calcium, lipid, and cholesterol accumulations within the vessel wall. The affected artery can be involved in a segmental or asymmetric manner.

The degree of carotid artery stenosis alone may not adequately predict which patients will suffer strokes. Extensive studies of plaque characteristics have revealed a correlation between the histologic features of a plaque and its susceptibility to cause thromboembolic events. These characteristics have been studied mainly to correlate ultrasonic findings, but research is ongoing to develop less invasive techniques, such as magnetic resonance imaging.

However, plaques that are more likely to be related to stroke have a low echogenicity on ultrasound. This corresponds with the weak reflection of ultrasound (i.e., echolucency) because of the lipid and hemorrhage content of the plaque. These plaques are soft and friable. Surface irregularities, or plaque ulceration, have also been shown to be a risk factor for thromboembolic events. These ulcerated plaques consist of soft, gelatinous clots that contain platelets, fibrin, white blood

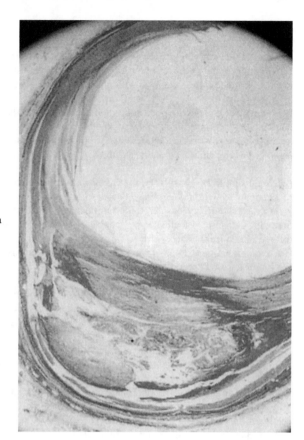

FIGURE 1. Tri-chrome staining of a carotid artery plaque.

cells, and red blood cells. Heterogenous plaques have been shown to be an independent risk factor for stroke regardless of the degree of stenosis.

The cholesterol-rich, slightly raised fatty streak becomes a fibrous plaque. The complicated plaque may undergo rupture, intraplaque hemorrhage, extensive necrosis, calcification, and subsequent thrombosis. Infiltration of the fibrous cap by foam cells may also contribute to the rupture.

4. Why do we treat patients with carotid artery atherosclerotic occlusive disease, and what is the standard of care?

We treat carotid artery disease to prevent embolic stroke and, on rare occasions, to improve hemodynamic-related neurologic symptoms caused by high-grade stenosis (e.g., radiation-induced stenosis). The North American Symptomatic Carotid Endarterectomy Trial (NASCET) was a randomized study that determined that carotid endarterectomy (CEA) reduced the risk of stroke in patients with ipsilateral carotid stenosis and a recent cerebrovascular event.

The study was published in 1991 and showed a statistically significant ipsilateral stroke reduction over a period of 24 follow-up months in symptomatic patients with high-grade carotid stenosis (> 70%) who underwent CEA (9%) versus patients who received medical therapy alone (26%). Patients in both groups received antiplatelet therapy (1300 mg) and antihypertensive, antilipid, and antidiabetic medications as indicated. The overall perioperative stroke and death rate for the 328 patients treated in the NASCET trial was 5.8%. However, other associated complications included cranial nerve injury (7.6%), myocardial infarction (0.9%), arrhythmia (1.2%), congestive heart failure (0.6%), wound infection (3.4%), wound hematoma (5.5%), and other cardiovascular problems (1.2%). Thus, CEA became the standard of care for carotid disease with high-grade stenosis (70% to 99%).

The annual stroke event rate for asymptomatic patients with hemodynamically significant carotid artery stenosis ranges from 2% to 5%. The 5-year stroke and death risk for an asymptomatic high-grade carotid stenosis with medical treatment was found to be 11%; the surgical arm had a stroke risk of 5.1%. The Asymptomatic Carotid Artery Stenosis (ACAS) trial justified CEA in asymptomatic men with 60% or greater stenosis only if the perioperative morbidity and mortality rate of the procedure is less than 3.0%. The acceptable perioperative morbidity and mortality rate for symptomatic patients is 6%. Although the findings were not as clear, women also experienced a reduction in stroke risk with CEA.

5. Who should be considered for carotid artery stenting or angioplasty?

Patients who are not good candidates for CEA and continue to have TIAs on optimal medical therapy should be considered for carotid stenting and angioplasty. Patients who fall into the following categories should also be considered for carotid artery stenting or angioplasty: lesions that are anatomically inaccessible to surgery, lesions with CEA restenosis, high-risk patients with severe comorbidities, lesions from radiation-induced stenosis, cases with associated dissections, and tumor-encased carotid arteries.

6. What are the current indications for carotid stenting and angioplasty?

Stenting is best used in a select group of patients. As seen in the NASCET study, a subgroup of patients is classified into a high-risk population. Patients were excluded from the NASCET study if they:

1. Were mentally incompetent or unwilling to give informed consent

2. Had inadequate angiographic visualization of both carotid arteries and their intracranial branches

3. Had an intracranial lesion that was more severe than the surgically accessible lesion

4. Had organ failure of the kidney, liver, or lung, or had cancer judged likely to cause death within 5 years

5. Had a cerebral infarction on either side that deprived the patient of all useful function in the affected territory

6. Had symptoms that could be attributed to non-atherosclerotic disease

7. Had a cardiac valvular or rhythm disorder likely to be associated with cardioembolic symptoms

8. Had previously undergone an ipsilateral carotid endarterectomy

9. Were older than age 79 years

10. Experienced angina or myocardial infarction (MI) in the previous 6 months

11. Had progressing neurologic signs

12. Had a contralateral CEA within 4 months

13. Underwent a major surgical procedure within 30 days

• Because stenting is still an investigational procedure that is currently being evaluated in randomized trials, it is best used in high-risk surgical patients such as the following:

Anatomic high-risk population:
- Surgically inaccessible lesion above C2 or below the clavicle
- Previous head or neck radiation therapy
- Surgery that included the area of stenosis or repair
- Ipsilateral neck dissection for cancer surgery
- Spinal immobility of the neck caused by cervical disorders
- Restenosis after previous or unsuccessful attempt
- Presence of laryngeal palsy
- Presence of tracheotomy
- Contralateral total occlusion of the carotid artery
- Tandem lesions

Medical high-risk population
- Congestive heart failure (New York Heart Association class III or IV)
- Unstable angina (Canadian Cardiovascular Society [CCS] class III/IV)
- Before coronary artery bypass graft surgery or valve replacement procedure
- Chronic obstructive pulmonary disease (forced expiratory volume < 30%)
- Left ventricular ejection fraction (LVEF) < 30%
- Age > 75 years
- Recent MI
- Two or more diseased coronary arteries > 70%

Inclusion criteria for stenting
- Symptomatic > 50%
- Asymptomatic > 80%

7. What are the exclusion criteria for stenting?
- Patients with bleeding disorders that preclude antiplatelet medication
- Allergy to antiplatelet medication
- Chronic carotid artery occlusion
- Positive blood culture results or sepsis
- Immunocompromised state
- Recent history of intracranial hemorrhage
- Acute large middle cerebral artery (MCA) stroke (infarct < 4–6 weeks' old)
- Fresh clot within stenosis
- Recent history of intracranial hemorrhage

8. What do we tell patients before stenting or angioplasty?
Patients should be informed that carotid stenting remains an investigational technique, even though it has been available for more than a decade and has proven to be effective. Case series have shown the benefit of stenting in subgroups as listed above. Periprocedural morbidity and mortality, including major and minor stroke, is less than 5% without the use of a distal protection device; the periprocedural risk of stroke is reduced by approximately 50% when a distal protection device is used. The restenosis risk is less than 5%; however, there is a need for follow-up studies that include Doppler ultrasound evaluations at 3, 6, and 12 months. Patients should also take clopidogrel (Plavix; 75 mg orally [PO] every day) and aspirin (325 mg PO every day) for 6 weeks and then low-dose aspirin only (81 mg/d) for life.

9. Are magnetic resonance imaging (MRI) studies safe after stenting?
With the use of current carotid stents, MRI studies can be immediately obtained without the risk of stent movement or deflection, which could potentially create thromboembolic complications. The use of magnetic resonance angiography (MRA) with gadolinium contrast may be used to study patency or in-stent stenosis, although some stents with metallic impurities may create artifacts in the region of interest.

10. Which stents are the most commonly used currently?
Precise S.M.A.R.T. Stent (Cordis, Johnson & Johnson, Miami Lakes, FL) (*see* Figure 2E), Wallstent (Boston Scientific Corp., Minneapolis, MN), and Acculink (Guidant, Indianapolis, IN) are the most commonly used stents.

11. What type of preprocedural testing is obtained from patients?
Before the procedure, all patients should undergo a thorough baseline physical assessment, a comprehensive neurologic examination, MRA or MRI, computed tomography (CT), electrocardiogram (EKG), and ultrasound. Blood work should include routine electrolytes, complete blood count, chemistry panel, blood urea nitrogen, creatinine, prothrombin time, partial throm-

boplastin time (PTT), international normalized ratio, red blood cell count, and platelet count. Also, women should undergo a urine pregnancy test before exposure to radiation.

12. What is the protocol followed for the actual procedure?

Patients should be NPO at least 6 hours before stenting. Beta-blockers should be ceased before the procedure because of the risk of exacerbating bradycardia associated with stenting carotid bulb lesions. Other medications such as insulin and Coumadin should also be closely monitored. Special attention should be paid to possible latex or contrast dye allergies.

Protocols may differ slightly based on the timing of the procedure, specifically if the procedure is elective or emergent. For elective procedures, patients are premedicated with clopidogrel (Plavix), 75 mg, and aspirin, 325 mg PO every day 2–4 days. In an acute procedure, a loading dose of Plavix, 450 mg, and aspirin, 650 mg PO, is given 3–4 hours before the procedure. Patients who cannot tolerate Plavix are provided with ticlopidine, 250 mg twice a day (total dose before the procedure of 500 mg), as an alternative. In the hyperacute setting, ketorolac (Toradol; cyclooxygenase A inhibitor), 30 mg IV, is provided, except in elderly patients and in patients with liver dysfunction. The dose is then reduced to 15 mg IV. Fentanyl, 50–150 mg IV, and midazolam (Versed), 1–2 mg, are used to initiate conscious sedation.

We perform carotid stenting with patients heparinized and maintain the activated clotting time (ACT) at 250 seconds. We keep patients fully heparinized for 24 hours with PTT values at 2 to 3 times normal. Based on the experiences with coronary artery stenting, glycoprotein (GP) IIb/IIIa receptor blockers are more aggressively used in carotid artery stenting. The ACT is maintained near 200 seconds if GP IIb/IIIa receptor blockers are used to avoid an increased risk of brain hemorrhage after revascularization. Options include an eptifibatide (Integrilin) 180 µg/kg bolus with a second 180-µg/kg bolus 10 minutes later. The other GP IIb/IIIa option is an abciximab 0.25 mg/kg bolus. In our practice, we do not maintain patients on continuous infusions after the initial bolus of GP IIb/IIIa receptor blockers. If GP IIb/IIIa receptor blockers are not used, the ACT is maintained between 250 and 300 seconds. However, an albumin 20% IV infusion over 20 minutes can be given every 4 to 6 hours as a volume expander in case the patient experiences significant periprocedural hypotension.

13. How is carotid stenting performed?

Primary stenting should be the goal to reduce periprocedural morbidity with angioplasty. This can be achieved in most patients, especially when using stents with minimal longitudinal shortening during deployment. Braided stents with significant shortening more frequently require PTA or otherwise tend to jump forward or backward proximally or distally to the stenosis ("watermelon seed effect").

Patient preparation includes the placement of an IV line with 0.9% normal saline infusion at 150 to 200 cc/h. Generally, we do not place an arterial line for continuous blood pressure monitoring.

The access point for the procedure is the femoral artery. Infrequently, the brachial, radial, or carotid artery might be directly accessed. A 5-Fr femoral sheath is then placed. An IV heparin bolus of 2000 to 2500 IU is provided. Angiography of both the iliac and femoral arteries is performed because many patients with carotid stenosis also have stenoses of the peripheral circulation, which might also require stenting.

A 5-Fr diagnostic catheter (Multipurpose, Sidewinder II) is used to perform four-vessel angiography of both the anterior and posterior circulation to evaluate the degree of stenosis (NASCET criteria) and other vascular abnormalities, such as tandem lesions or intracranial aneurysms. The diagnostic catheter is then parked into the common carotid artery (CCA) for acquisition of a road map. With the help of a 0.35-inch glidewire, the catheter is placed into the external carotid. The glidewire is then exchanged for a 0.038-inch, extra stiff 260-cm wire (Amplatz Wire, Cook, Inc., Bloomington, IN). The diagnostic catheter is then removed, and a guide catheter is inserted (6 or 7-Fr Shuttle) within the CCA, proximal to the target site. Angiograms are obtained to measure the arterial dimensions and the length of the lesion (Fig. 2A). At this point, a decision should be made for either primary stenting or preprocedural PTA.

For primary stenting, a 300-cm, 0.018-inch exchange wire (e.g., SV 5/8, Cordis, Johnson & Johnson) should be inserted into the stent delivery system. Either bony landmarks (vertebral body on lateral projection) or the road-mapping technique can be used for navigational reference. The plaque may help in localizing the area of stenosis for final stent placement. The wire is then navigated through the lesion, and the stiff part of the wire is placed across the stenosis (Fig. 2B). After stabilizing the wire, the stent is placed within the stenosis (Fig. 2D). The slack of the delivery system is taken out before deployment. The stent is then deployed, and the delivery system is subsequently removed. In tight lesions, the delivery system may need to be resheathed distal to the stented artery before removal to prevent the delivery system from being "caught" by the struts of the stent. A control angiography is then performed to visualize the stented segment (Fig. 2G) and the intracranial circulation. Depending on the remaining degree of stenosis, the stent is customized with a PTA balloon. We recommend slow inflation over several minutes; pressures of 6 to 8 atm (Fig. 2F) are generally adequate to open up the stent. In secondary stenting, the 0.018-inch exchange wire is navigated through the lesion with a PTA balloon (e.g., Savvy, 3. 0 to 3.5 mm × 20 mm, Cordis, Johnson & Johnson). The balloon is then placed within the stenosis and inflated very slowly (up to several minutes) at pressures ranging from 6 to 12 atm (Fig. 2C). Control angiography should be performed after the PTA and should include the intracranial circulation. Finally, stenting should proceed as discussed above.

One alternative is to perform primary stenting without the use of a guide catheter. This can be successfully accomplished in the right internal carotid artery (ICA) or a less tortuous left ICA, and it works for a stent mounted on a flexible 5-Fr delivery systems in conjunction with a stiff 0.018-inch wire. After completion of stenting, the introducer catheter (shuttle) is removed and the femoral access is percutaneously sutured (e.g., Perclose, Abbott Laboratories, Redwood City, CA; Angio-Seal, Sherwood Medical Company, St. Louis, MO; VasoSeal, Datascope Corp., Mahwah, NJ).

14. After stenting, are areas of flow stagnation within the plaque ulcer and carotid bulb thrombogenic?

No. Areas of contrast stagnation between the stent and the arterial wall are generally not present at 6- or 12-month follow-up angiography. Clotting of these areas with secondary endothelialization is most likely protective.

15. What are the common complications of stenting and how are they treated?

Common complications include bradycardia and hypotension that can be prevented by applying slow inflation and lower pressures during PTA. Atropine, 0.6–1.0 mg IV, and dopamine are very rarely necessary to treat these complications, but they are options if the need arises. Vasospasm during catheterization, PTA, or stenting generally does not require any treatment because of its spontaneous resolution, although papaverine, mannitol, or nipride may infrequently be used. Dissections during catheter manipulation, PTA, or stenting with an intimal flap may require extensive stenting to avoid vessel occlusion.

16. When are patients discharged, and what should they be told?

Patients are kept for 24 hours in a critical care or step-down unit before discharge. Special attention should be paid to hypo- and hypertension and new neurologic symptoms (National Institutes of Health stroke scale), including headaches that can be related to the hyperperfusion syndrome or cerebral hemorrhage.

Patients should ambulate the next day and resume normal activities. A carotid ultrasound of the stented artery can be obtained before patient discharge to rule out any larger clot burden on the endoluminal stent area.

Clinical follow-up visits are suggested at 1 month, 3 months, 6 months, and 1 year. Patients should watch for groin hematoma, fever, and neurologic symptoms (e.g., amaurosis fugax, headaches, aphasia, and sensory or fine motor impairment). Doppler ultrasound to monitor restenosis is recommended at 6 months and 1 year.

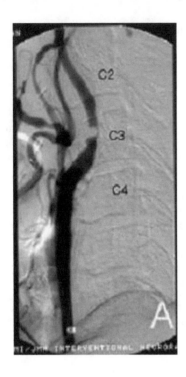

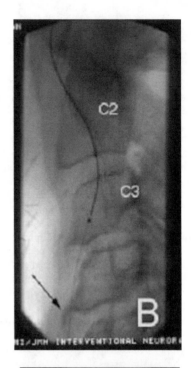

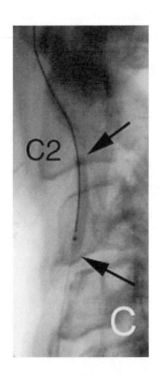

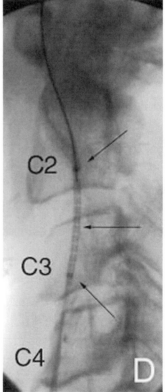

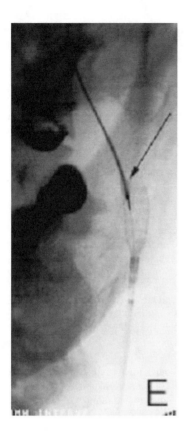

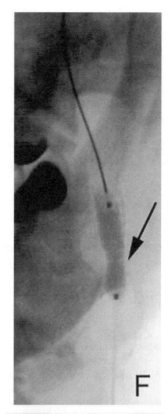

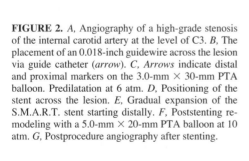

FIGURE 2. *A,* Angiography of a high-grade stenosis of the internal carotid artery at the level of C3. *B,* The placement of an 0.018-inch guidewire across the lesion via guide catheter *(arrow)*. *C, Arrows* indicate distal and proximal markers on the 3.0-mm × 30-mm PTA balloon. Predilatation at 6 atm. *D,* Positioning of the stent across the lesion. *E,* Gradual expansion of the S.M.A.R.T. stent starting distally. *F,* Poststenting remodeling with a 5.0-mm × 20-mm PTA balloon at 10 atm. *G,* Postprocedure angiography after stenting.

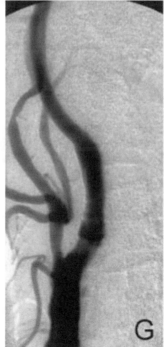

17. What are the long-term issues with anticoagulation, and how do we follow up patients?

Patients are put on clopidogrel, 75 mg PO every day, and aspirin, 325 mg PO, every year for 6 weeks after stenting. After 6 weeks, patients are instructed to take only aspirin 81 mg PO every day for life.

18. What are the long-term results of stenting?

In the largest review of more than 5000 carotid artery stenting procedures, 2.1% of patients were found to have restenosis of greater than 50% at 6 months. The restenosis rate after 12 months was found to be 3.5%. The major stroke and death rate at 1 year was 2.4%.

19. Are there any data available comparing CEA with stenting?

The Carotid and Vertebral Artery Transluminal Angioplasty Study (CAVATAS) was a randomized trial that sought to compare endovascular treatment with conventional carotid surgery. This multicenter trial in Europe, Australia, and Canada randomly selected 504 patients with carotid stenosis. Patients with stenosis of the common carotid artery, carotid bifurcation, or internal carotid artery that needed treatment were included only if both endovascular and surgical treatments were suitable. The CEA group included 253 patients, and the endovascular group included 251 patients. Stenting was used in 55 patients (26%), and angioplasty alone was used in 158 patients (74%).

The mean stenosis in the surgical group was 86.4%, and the 30-day stroke and death rate was 5.9%. In the endovascular group, the mean stenosis was 85.1% and the 30-day stroke or death risk was 6.4%. There was no significant difference between the two groups.

20. What is the value of distal protection devices?

Carotid plaques can be extremely friable, which has been known to create embolic problems. Any type of manipulation may cause distal embolization, fragmentation, or occlusion. More manipulation with guidewires, balloons, and stents may lead to increased number of fragments. Particle sizes range from 20 to 400 microns.

Although many distal protection devices have been developed to alleviate embolic complications, three main categories of devices exist. The most common type is the filter device, which is navigated distal to the stenosis and expanded to catch embolic particles. This device allows distal arterial perfusion through the holes of the filter, which is collapsed at the end of the procedure and retrieves the particulate matter after removal from the artery. However, it has been argued that the filter device allows the passage of tiny particulates that are less than 80 to 100 microns in size. Emboli smaller than 100 microns are thought to account for the majority of embolized debris, yet the clinical significance of such small emboli is not fully understood. This device is able to capture particles at prespecified filter sizes. The umbrella design of the filter is intuitively sensible and may be less traumatic to the vessel wall because of fewer external forces. Devices that are currently being used or tested include Accunet (Guidant Corp., Indianapolis, IN), FilterWire EX (Boston Scientific, Natick, MA), AngioGuard (Cordis Corp., Minneapolis, MN), and Med-Nova NeuroShield (MedNova Inc., Galway, Ireland).

The second type of device is the balloon occlusion device, which is expanded and completely prevents antegrade flow. The balloon is expanded as long as it takes to treat the vessel. Before deflation, the material is aspirated from the vessel through a special aspiration catheter. The most popular device on the market is the PercuSurge GuardWire Plus Temporary Occlusion and Aspiration System (PercuSurge, Inc., Sunnyvale, CA, a division of Medtronic, Inc., Minneapolis, MN). Also, The Guardian System (Rubicon Medical, Salt Lake City, UT) is a newer device that uses a similar balloon concept. The advantages include its ability to more completely capture both large and small particles; a technically easier to use design, with fewer potential mechanical problems because of the simple balloon inflation and deflation; and its ability to provide temporary and complete vessel occlusion during maximal times of embolization. However, temporary occlusion of the carotid may not be tolerated in all individuals, especially patients with significant bilateral carotid stenosis. It has been shown that fewer than 10% of individuals treated may not tolerate complete cessation of blood flow for greater than 5 to 15 minutes. Also, particles may be redirected into the external carotid artery during aspiration or pressure injection. The balloon may not completely deflate or could possibly get caught on the stent and subsequently tear.

The third type is a catheter occlusion device; the Parodi Anti-Emboli System (PAES; ArteriA Medical Science, Inc., San Francisco, CA) best exemplifies this type. It is a guiding catheter with an occlusion balloon at its distal end. It works by reversing the blood flow in the target artery. It is placed in the common carotid artery, and the balloon occlusion creates a negative pressure gradient distal to the balloon that causes retrograde flow into the internal carotid artery. The external carotid artery is also occluded to prevent flow and emboli from traveling in that vessel. The advantages include the ability to obtain complete protection before manipulation of the lesion. It is also able to capture particles of all sizes, and it facilitates treatment of tortuous and tight lesions because it does not have to be passed through the arterial lesion. It does, however, require a larger puncture site in the groin and interrupts flow during the protection time.

Currently, there are 10 carotid stent trials in the United States using distal protection devices, such as Cordis, Johnson & Johnson Nitinol SMART Stent Trial; BEACH (Wallstent + Filterwire, high-risk patients); Carotid Revascularization Endarterectomy Versus Stent Trial (CREST); and ARCHER Acculink with Umbrella as Distal Protection.

21. What are the restenosis rates for carotid stenting and angioplasty, and what can be done with restenosis?

Restenosis is not uncommon after CEA. Studies have reported incidences from 1.5% in symptomatic to 19% in asymptomatic patients. Furthermore, reoperation is frequently more difficult for restenosis after CEA, with higher rates of local and neurologic complications.

This may be compared with the coronary restenosis rates, which has been reported to be as high as 59%. Renal and femoropopliteal rates at 1 year after surgery have also been reported to exceed 30% and 40%, respectively. Several studies with follow-up of 1 year and less have reported in stent restenosis rates after carotid angioplasty and stenosis between 3.5% to 8%. Stenting of vessels has been shown to overcome previously high rates of restenosis with angioplasty alone.

22. When will a solid scientific randomized control trial begin to compare the advantages of PTA/S with CEA? What is the future of stenting?

The Carotid Revascularization Endarterectomy Versus Stent Trial (CREST) is currently enrolling patients for a multicenter clinical trial to compare the efficacy of CEA and carotid angioplasty-stenting in symptomatic patients with stenosis greater than or equal to 50%. SAPPHIRE (Stenting and Angioplasty with Protection in Patients at High-Risk for Endarterectomy) is the first randomized study to compare carotid stenting using a distal protection device with carotid endarterectomy (CEA) in high-risk patients. A total of 307 patients were entered in the randomized trial, with 156 patients enrolled in the stented arm and 151 entered in the CEA group. The composite endpoint of death, stroke, or MI was 5.8% for the stented patients and 12.6% for the surgical patients ($P = .047$).

The future use of carotid artery stenting will most likely growth safer, with less complications as biomedical technology advances with new materials and devices that accommodate current limitations. These include dedicated carotid stenting equipment with low profile stent delivery systems and a variety of stent designs and better access sheaths, specialty balloons, and guidewires. A variety of neuroprotective devices are likely to be optimized to decrease the incidence of embolic debris events. Drug-coated stents will also play a role in carotid stent development.

BIBLIOGRAPHY

1. AbuRahma AF, Wulu JT Jr, Crotty B: Carotid plaque ultrasonic heterogeneity and severity of stenosis. Stroke 33:1772–1775, 2002.
2. Association Heart Association: 2002 Heart and Stroke Statistical Update. Dallas, American Heart Association, 2001.

3. Biller J, Love BB: Vascular diseases of the nervous system—ischemic cerebrovascular disease. In Bradley WG, Daroff RB, Fenichel GM, Marsden CD (eds): Neurology in Clinical Practice, 3rd ed. Boston, Butterworth-Heinemann, 2000, pp 1125–1166.

4. CAVATAS Investigators: Endovascular versus surgical treatment in patients with carotid stenosis in the Carotid and Vertebral Artery Transluminal Angioplasty Study (CAVATAS): a randomised trial. Lancet 357:1729–1737, 2001.

5. Chakhtoura EY, Hobson RW, Goldstein J: In-stent restenosis after carotid angioplasty-stenting: Incidence and management. J Vasc Surg 33:220–226, 2001.

6. Executive Committee for the Asymptomatic Carotid Atherosclerosis Study: endarterectomy for asymptomatic carotid artery stenosis. JAMA 273:1421–1428, 1995.

7. Fasseas P, Orford JL, Denktas AE, et al: Distal protection devices during percutaneous coronary and carotid interventions. Curr Control Trials Cardiovasc Med 2:286–291, 2001.

8. Healy DA, Zierler RE, Michols SC, et al: Long-term follow-up and clinical outcome of carotid restenosis. J Vasc Surg 10:662–668, 1998.

9. Hobson RW: Update on the Carotid Revascularization Endarterectomy Versus Stent Trial (CREST) Protocol. J Am Coll Surg 194(Suppl 1):9–14, 2002.

10. Lal BK, Hobson RW II, Pappas PJ, et al: Pixel distribution analysis of B-mode ultrasound scan images predicts histologic features of atherosclerotic carotid plaques. J Vasc Surg 35:1210–1217, 2002.

11. Lanzino G, Mericle RA, Lopes DK, et al: Percutaneous transluminal angioplasty and stent placement for recurrent carotid artery stenosis. J Neurosurg 90:668–694, 1999.

12. Lopes DK, Mericle RA, Lanzino G, et al: Stent placement for the treatment of occlusive atherosclerotic carotid artery disease in patients with concomitant coronary artery disease. J Neurosurg 96:490–496, 2002.

13. Mericle RA, Kim SH, Lanzino G, et al: Carotid artery angioplasty and use of stents in high-risk patients with contralateral occlusions. J Neurosurg 90:1031–1036, 1999.

14. North American Symptomatic Carotid Endarterectomy Trial Collaborators: beneficial effect of carotid endarterectomy in symptomatic patients with high-grade carotid stenosis. N Engl J Med 325:445–453, 1991.

15. Ohki T, Veith FJ: Carotid artery stenting: utility of cerebral protection devices. J Invasive Cardiol 13:47–55, 2001.

16. Timsit SG, Sacco RL, Mohr JP, et al: Early clinical differentiation of cerebral infarction from severe atherosclerotic stenosis and cardioembolism. Stroke 23:486–491, 1992.

17. Wholey MH, Wholey M, Bergeron P, et al: Current global status of carotid artery stent placement. Cathet Cardiovasc Diagn 44:1–6, 1998.

18. Yadav JS: SAPPHIRE. In Proceedings of the 15th Annual International Symposium on Endovascular Therapy ISET, Miami, FL, January 19–23, 2003, p 111.

XII. Miscellaneous Interventional Topics

57. INTERVENTIONAL CARDIOLOGISTS AND THE CARDIAC SURGEON

Saqib Masroor, M.D., M.H.S., and Tomas Salerno, M.D.

1. What are the preoperative risk factors associated with increased postoperative mortality after coronary artery bypass graft (CABG) surgery?
- Age
- Left ventricular ejection fraction (LVEF)
- Number of vessels diseased or left main disease
- Emergency operation
- Gender
- Diabetes
- Congestive heart failure

2. What are the factors associated with surgical morbidity after coronary artery surgery?
- Previous stroke
- History of significant bleeding (dental or gastrointestinal)
- Hypertension
- Angina class
- History of previous myocardial infarction (MI)
- Concurrent remote-site infection (i.e., urinary tract infection)
- Significant chronic obstructive pulmonary disease
- Renal insufficiency or renal failure

3. What is the risk of perioperative stroke or neurologic deficits after CABG?
The risk is 1% to 3% for people of all ages. The risk is 3.8 times higher in those older than age 70 years. However, up to 61% of patients may experience new neurologic signs such as primitive reflexes, scotomata, areas of hypoesthesia, and temporary cognitive dysfunction at the time of discharge.

4. What are the proven benefits of off-pump (beating-heart) coronary artery surgery (OPCAB) versus conventional CABG?
Compared with conventional CABG, OPCAB has been shown to be associated with reduced myocardial injury, lower requirements for transfusions, and a shorter length of hospital stay.

There is no difference in survival, postcardiotomy dysfunction, requirement for intra-aortic balloon pump, degree of revascularization, need for subsequent revascularization, incidence of atrial fibrillation, perioperative MI, or stroke between OPCAB and CABG. No clinical study has clearly shown a reduced incidence of perioperative or late neurologic morbidity, partly because of the requirement of partial cross clamp for the proximal anastomosis in OPCAB. With the advent of new proximal connecting devices such as the St. Jude Aortic Connector System for anastomosis that obviate the need for partial cross clamping (Fig. 1), it will be interesting to see if there is a decrease in the incidence of neurologic deficits in patients undergoing OPCAB versus those undergoing CABG. It should be noted that transcranial Doppler (TCD) studies have shown

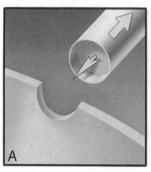 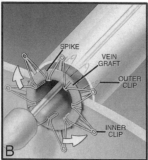 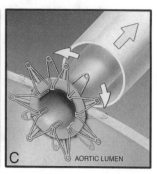

FIGURE 1. *A,* Circular hole in the aorta made with the punch followed by *B,* insertion of the vein graft mounted on spikes on the connector. *C,* Withdrawal of the delivery device deploys the inner clips, thus leaving the vein graft attached to the aorta. If the vein graft is not mounted properly on the spikes, the anastomosis can leak at that spot. (Courtesy St. Jude Medical, Minneapolis, MN.)

that clamping the aorta is either completely or partially responsible for most of the emboli to the brain associated with cardiac surgery.

5. What are the indications for surgical revascularization in patients with coronary artery disease (CAD)?

Surgery has been shown to provide survival advantage over medical therapy in the following situations.

- Left main coronary artery disease
- Three-vessel disease with left ventricular (LV) dysfunction
- Significant LV dysfunction

For patients with less severe disease and preserved LV function, no clear survival advantage has been demonstrated for medical or surgical therapy; however, patients initially treated with surgery experience the need for fewer revascularization procedures, antianginal medicines, or cardiac rehospitalizations than those on medical therapy or angioplasty.

In the Bypass Angioplasty Revascularization Investigation (BARI), *diabetics* (whether taking insulin or oral hypoglycemic agents) were the only class of patients in whom CABG was shown to provide survival advantage over percutaneous transluminal coronary angioplasty (PTCA).

6. What are the indications for emergency CABG?

- Unstable angina refractory to medical management and not amenable to PTCA
- Early postinfarction angina if not amenable to PTCA
- Failed PTCA with acute vessel closure
- Complications of PTCA such as dissection or perforation of the vessel wall
- Evolving acute MI
- Acute MI with mechanical complications such as ventricular septal defect or papillary muscle rupture
- Severe left main coronary artery stenosis

7. Which complications of MI warrant emergency CABG?

- Cardiogenic shock with surgically approachable coronary lesions
- Ventricular septal defect
- Papillary muscle rupture or dysfunction
- LV aneurysm
- Ventricular free wall rupture

In the absence of surgically approachable lesions and worsening cardiac function, consideration may be given to ventricular assist device placement as a bridge to cardiac transplantation.

8. What are the different approaches for surgical coronary revascularization?

The approaches include conventional CABG using cardiopulmonary bypass with either cardioplegia or intermittent aortic cross clamping and ventricular fibrillation with or without topical hypothermia.

Another approach is beating heart or OPCAB in which the heart is not arrested and the heart–lung machine is not used.

The surgical approach to the heart may be through median sternotomy, anterior thoracotomy (MIDCAB), posterolateral thoracotomy (in some reoperations), subxiphoid MIDCAB (in some obese patients), or totally endoscopic coronary artery bypass (TECAB) using robotic devices (still under investigation).

9. What are the different patterns of vein graft–coronary artery distal anastomoses?

There are three types of distal anastomoses:

1. Single graft, in which one vein graft is anastomosed in an end-to-side fashion to one target vessel

2. Multiple or sequential grafts in which one vein graft is anastomosed to more than one target vessels, in this case, the vein graft is anastomosed in a side-to-side fashion to the proximal vessel(s) although the last anastomosis is in an end-to-side fashion.

3. In Y-graft, a vein graft to one target vessel, instead of coming off the aorta, is sewed to another vein (arterial) graft at the proximal end, the distal anastomosis is an end-to-side one

10. What are the benefits of a sequential and Y-grafts?

There are two reasons for making sequential grafts: either the aorta has less available space for a suitable anastomosis or the length of the vein graft available is not enough for all separate anastomoses.

11. What are the disadvantages of a sequential graft?

Because more than one target vessel is being supplied by one graft, any technical problems at the proximal anastomosis can compromise flow to the entire heart.

Also, if the vein is small in diameter, side-to-side anastomosis is technically more difficult; therefore, there is a greater potential for a substandard anastomosis.

12. What are the causes of occlusion of vein grafts after coronary revascularization?

	ONSET AFTER SURGERY	INCIDENCE, %	REASON
Early	≤ 1 month	10–15	Technical
Delayed	1–12 months	5–10	Intimal hyperplasia
Intermediate	1–5 years	2–3 per year	Medial fibrosis
Late	> 5 years	5 per year	Atherosclerosis

13. What is the patency of the internal mammary artery (IMA) grafts?

The patency of the left IMA (LIMA) to the left anterior descending artery (LAD) graft is 92% to 97% at 1 year, 88% to 96% at 5 years, and 88% to 93% at 10 years. The 1-year patency of the right IMA is similar to the LIMA.

14. What is the incidence of significant cerebrovascular disease (CVD) in patients with CAD?

Hemodynamically significant (> 70%) carotid artery stenosis is present in between 3% to 12% percent of people requiring coronary revascularization.

15. What are the indications for screening duplex carotid studies in a patient with CAD?

- Symptomatic CVD
- Previous carotid endarterectomy (CEA)
- History of stroke or transient ischemic attack

- Presence of carotid bruits
- Left main disease

Relative indications include people older than age 65 years, with peripheral vascular disease and strong smoking history.

16. What are the indications for combined CEA/CABG?

1. Patients with less than 70% carotid stenosis should undergo CABG only.

2. Those with more than 70% carotid stenosis with a stable cardiac status should undergo staged CEA followed by CABG. This algorithm is used to prevent late neurologic deficits. There is no reported increase in the risk of perioperative stroke if only CABG is performed and the carotid disease is managed medically.

3. Those with more than 70% carotid stenosis and unstable angina, critical left main disease, or severe multivessel disease should undergo combined CEA/CABG, especially if there is a history of a recent TIA.

17. Who is a typical patient with postinfarction ventricular septal defect (VSD)?

In 60% of patients with postinfarction VSD, the defect is anteroapical in location after a full-thickness anterior wall infarction caused by occlusion of the LAD. In 20% to 40% of patients, it is in the posterior septum, after an inferoseptal infarction caused by occlusion of the dominant right coronary artery or dominant circumflex coronary artery.

A typical patient is a 65-year-old man with single vessel disease and no collaterals who presents 2 to 4 days after an acute MI.

18. How is a patient in cardiogenic shock and a postinfarction acute VSD managed?

Mortality of this patient's non-operative management is 80% to 90%. With aggressive management, including IABP/extracorporeal membrane oxygenation, inotropes, and diuresis, most of these patients can be stabilized to undergo cardiac catheterization followed by early or emergent repair or exclusion of VSD with revascularization. Using this management, current survival rates for these patients approach 75%. Percutaneous transcatheter closure of these VSDs has been reported but is not as effective as surgery because the tissue is too friable to seat the device adequately.

19. What is the role of coronary revascularization in patients with postinfarction VSD and cardiogenic shock?

People undergoing revascularization experience a longer survival compared with those who do not undergo revascularization. This difference was even more prominent in patients with anterior septal perforation. The main disadvantage of revascularization is the delay in getting cardiac catheterization; however, this is usually needed to stabilize the patient with IABP/ECMO and appropriate medical therapy before surgery.

20. What is the incidence of LV aneurysm formation after acute MI?

In people with VSD complicating an MI, the incidence of LV aneurysm formation is 35% to 68%. However, 12% of patients with an acute MI without VSD go on to develop an LV aneurysm.

21. What are the indications for repair of LV aneurysm?

- Drug-refractory angina with patent vessels
- Congestive heart failure refractory to medical therapy
- Ventricular tachycardia
- Arterial thromboembolism
- During surgical coronary revascularization in low-risk patients

22. What are the major physiologic effects of IABP?

IABP causes a reduction of LV afterload and an increase in aortic root and coronary perfusion pressures. This leads to a reduction in LV systolic wall tension and oxygen consumption and also the LV end-systolic and end-diastolic volumes. Cardiac output can increase by up to 10% to 20%.

23. What are the indications for the use of IABP?
- Cardiogenic shock
- Uncontrolled myocardial ischemic pain
- Postcardiotomy low cardiac output or failure to wean off cardiopulmonary bypass
- Failed or high-risk PTCA, atherectomy, or coronary stent placement
- Poorly controlled ventricular arrhythmias before or after the operation
- Postinfarction VSD or acute mitral insufficiency after MI
- Preoperatively in high-risk patients undergoing redo cardiac surgery: those with poor LV function and mitral regurgitation or low cardiac output caused by hibernating or stunned myocardium

24. What are the complications of IABP?
The incidence of complications is 13% to 29%. Leg ischemia is the most common complication (9% to 25%). Others include bleeding, false aneurysm formation, infection at the insertion site, septicemia, lymphocele, femoral neuropathy, balloon rupture, and thrombosis within the balloon.

25. What are the different routes of insertion of IABP?
- Transfemoral (most common)
- Transaxillary (in the presence of iliofemoral occlusive disease)
- Transaortic (for intraoperative use); always removed in the operating room

26. What are the indications for ECMO?
- Postcardiotomy cardiac support
- Postcardiotomy respiratory support
- Cardiac arrest or cardiogenic shock
- Posttransplantation or left ventricular assist device (LVAD) placement
- Support high-risk procedures in the cardiac catheterization unit
- Primary respiratory failure in children, neonates, and adults with or without trauma

27. What are the physiologic effects of ECMO?
ECMO unloads the right ventricle but does not unload the LV even though the LV preload is reduced. In a normal heart, the reduction in preload produced by the ECMO flow reduces the preload and end-diastolic volume of the LV. However, in a dilated failing heart, LV may not eject sufficient volume against the increased afterload to reduce the end-diastolic or end-systolic volume. Therefore, ECMO may increase LV wall stress and myocardial oxygen consumption unless an IABP is used to mechanically unload the LV.

28. What are the different modes of ECMO?
1. Veno-arterial mode for cardiac or cardiorespiratory support
2. Veno-venous mode for solely respiratory support

29. What are the complications of ECMO?
- Leg ischemia (most common)
- Renal dysfunction
- Bleeding and infection (now infrequent because of use of percutaneous catheters)
- Intracardiac clots, which are prevented by using heparin-coated circuits and heparin to keep the activated clotting time between 180 and 220 in veno-arterial ECMO; venovenous ECMO does not require anticoagulation when used with heparin-coated circuits
- Oxygenator failure caused by clots in the pump head

Patients on veno-venous ECMO usually have fewer and less serious complications.

BIBLIOGRAPHY

1. Baue AE, Geha AS, Hammond GL, et al (eds): Glenn's Thoracic and Cardiovascular Surgery, 6th ed. Stamford, CT, Appleton & Lange, 1996.
2. Bypass Angioplasty Revascularization Investigation (BARI) Investigators. Comparison of coronary by-pass and angioplasty in patients with multivessel disease. N Engl J Med 335:217–225, 1996.
3. Dijk DV, Nierich AP, Jansen EWL, et al: Early outcome after off-pump versus on-pump coronary bypass surgery: results from a randomized study. Circulation 104:1761–1766, 2001.
4. Edmunds HL Jr (ed): Cardiac Surgery in the Adult. New York, McGraw-Hill, 1997.
5. Goldstein DJ, Oz MC (eds): Cardiac Assist Devices. Armonk, NY, Futura Publishing Company, 2000.
6. Puskas JD, Williams WH, Duke PG, et al: Off-pump coronary artery bypass grafting provides compelte revascularization while reducing myoscardial injury, transfusion requirements and length of stay: prospective randomized comparison of 200 unselectd patients having OPCAB versus conventional CABG. Presented at the 82nd Annual Meeting of the American Association for Thoracic Surgery, Washington DC, May 5–8, 2002.
7. Salerno TA, Ricci M, Karamanoukian HL, et al (eds): Beating Heart Coronary Artery Surgery. Armonk, NY, Futura Publishing Company, 2001.

58. THE INTERVENTIONAL TRAINING PROGRAM

Alexandre C. Ferreira, M.D., and Eduardo de Marchena, M.D.

1. What are the goals of the interventional training program?

The cardiology training program prepares its interventional fellows for clinical performance in interventional cardiology. Trainees should develop an understanding of the clinical indications of angioplasty and the appropriate selection of patients for procedures. During training, they also develop the necessary catheter skills to perform percutaneous revascularization.

2. What are the components of the training in interventional cardiology?

The American College of Cardiology (ACC)/American Heart Association (AHA) guidelines for training in interventional cardiology establishes three phases for this training.

First, the trainees should learn the indications and limitations of coronary interventional procedures. In this phase of training, they also learn how to identify patients candidates for angioplasty and what types of devices are available for each intervention.

In a second phase of their training, interventional fellows develop cognitive and technical skills necessary to perform interventional cardiac procedures.

Finally, interventional trainees must develop the ability to incorporate new advances in interventional cardiology as they develop an attitude that accepts the need for continuous learning.

3. In which phases of patient care are trainees expected to be involved?

Trainees are involved in a preprocedural phase (or initial patient evaluation), a procedural phase (or actual intervention), an immediate postprocedural phase (or in-patient postprocedural care), and a late follow-up phase (or outpatient care).

4. What are the learning aspects of the preprocedural phase?

- Patient selection, which includes understanding the indication for the procedure in each particular patient
- Establishing a patient–physician relationship.
- Obtaining informed consent and understanding alternative treatments for each patient
- Reviewing preprocedural laboratory data and the noninvasive workup
- Developing awareness for possible relative contraindications for the procedure and identifying patient characteristic which could lead to higher risk (e.g., drug allergies and interactions, bleeding disorders, vascular anomalies)

5. What are the learning aspects of the procedural phase or intervention?

- Appropriate catheter, guidewire, and device selection
- Understanding lesion classification and procedural implications
- Identifying high-risk lesions and minimizing complications and risk
- Learning procedural pharmacotherapy, conscious sedation, and hemodynamic-guided therapy such as vasodilators and pressors
- Understanding intervention goals in stable angina, acute coronary syndromes, and acute myocardial infarction
- Dealing with life-threatening complication in the catheterization laboratory
- Understanding the role and limitations of cardiac surgeons
- Understand the interventional aphorism that "better is the enemy of good"

6. What are the learning aspects of the immediate postprocedural phase?
- Postprocedural vascular access care
- Postprocedure orders, including adjuvant pharmacotherapy
- Appropriate postprocedural and predischarge cardiac evaluation (physical, postprocedure electrocardiogram, and enzymes when indicated)
- Medical record documentation, procedure notes, and dictation
- Discharge and follow-up planning

7. What are the learning aspects of the late follow-up care of patients after intervention?
- Clinic follow-up care postprocedure, at least one clinic visit after the procedure, and appropriate referral for general cardiology follow-up
- Risk factor treatment
- Counseling for smoking cessation and risk factor modification
- Screening for restenosis, when appropriate, in high-risk patients

8. What are the academic relationships and faculty requirements for the interventional training program?

A training program in interventional cardiology should be affiliated with or be part of a comprehensive accredited cardiology training program.

There should be a minimum of three key faculty, with a key faculty-to-trainee ratio of 0.5 trainees per faculty member and with each key faculty member devoting at least 20 hours per week to the program, according to the ACC/AHA. The three members should consist of a program director and at least two associated faculty members. A larger number of associated faculty members allows trainees to be exposed to different approach and techniques in interventional cardiology.

9. What are the credential requirements for training program directors?

Program directors must be board-certified in interventional cardiology. The minimum number of procedures is a lifetime experience of 1000 coronary interventional procedures. The experience of at least 5 years after training is necessary.

10. What are the procedural requirements for the interventional faculty team?

Per year, at least 75 coronary interventional procedures should be performed by each faculty member. Although this activity level, recommended by the ACC/AHA, is a threshold level for maintenance of competence, it is a low activity level for individuals who have training responsibilities. Consequently, the ACC recommends that program faculty achieve a minimum clinical activity level of 125 procedures per year.

11. What is the procedural volume required for the training program?

A program must perform an absolute minimum of 400 coronary interventional procedures per year. The complexity of cases, clinical situations encountered, and types of devices used should allow trainees to be exposed to all aspects of coronary interventions. This exposure is done either directly through performing procedures or indirectly through conference reviews of cases.

12. What is the procedural volume required for trainees upon completion of training?

Trainees must perform at least 250 procedures during training. More is not necessarily better, and performing more than 600 procedures may jeopardize learning and quality of training, according to the ACC/AHA.

In order to benefit from a case, a trainee must play an active role in the entire process of patient selection and all technical and cognitive aspects of the case.

13. How do trainees document procedures performed during training?

Trainees are required to keep a log of all procedures performed during the training. Documentation required in each procedure includes the type of procedure performed, the interventional device used, and the type and number of vessels treated. We also recommend our fellows to annotate any complications arising from the procedure and the final result of each intervention. We expect them to have at least the absolute minimum of 250 cases per year evenly distributed in terms of complexity among the largest possible variety of pathology treated. We also expect them to work with different interventionists in our group in order to get exposure to more diverse interventional techniques.

14. How should each interventional case be counted when recording procedural volume?

A coronary interventional case is defined as all coronary interventional procedures performed during a single hospitalization. Staged procedures or emergent repeat procedures are counted as a single case if they are performed during the same hospitalization. Only one faculty member and one trainee can claim credit for each procedure.

15. How does the number of procedures performed by the operator correlate with patient outcome?

There is enough clinical evidence to indicate that although basic expertise may be maintained at 75 procedures per year, operators performing more procedures tend to have better outcomes.

16. What is the requisite knowledge base a program must ensure that its trainees acquire?

The program must establish a core curriculum to cover the basic science aspects of interventional cardiology, including cardiac and coronary anatomy, cardiac physiology, vascular biology and pathology, hemostasis, pathophysiology of ischemia, pharmacology, radiology imaging and radiation safety, intracoronary imaging and coronary flow physiology, interventional device design and performance, and clinical management strategies. This can done through the didactic seminars and conferences or study groups. Conferences should be performed at least once a week.

17. How are interventional fellows evaluated?

The number of procedures and the progress the trainee has made during the year are reviewed quarterly by the program director. Each faculty member of the training facility is expected to evaluate the trainee at least quarterly. General patient care, clinical evaluation, and improvement in catheter skills are all considered in the final evaluation of trainees.

18. What are the research requirements of the interventional program?

The interventional program should have an active clinical research program, and its trainees should be directly involved in research, according to the ACC/AHA. Fellows should be encouraged to write papers, case reports, and reviews. Participation in clinical research by trainees in extremely important because the field of interventional cardiology is constantly changing.

19. Is there a minimum number of publications absolutely required for graduating from a training program?

No. Although active involvement in research is required from trainees, there is no mandate for a specified number of publications in peer-reviewed journals or abstract presentations in national meetings.

20. Which are the training requirements for cardiologists willing to perform peripheral angioplasty?

A desired number of 100 diagnostic peripheral angiograms and 50 peripheral angioplasty procedures should have been performed under the supervision of an experienced peripheral interventionist (with > 50% performed as primary operator). The physician should also have had experiences in 10 cases of peripheral thrombolytic therapy and management.

The performance of peripheral angioplasty requires that the fellow take additional training. This includes understanding the natural history of peripheral vascular disease, noninvasive patient assessment, the indications for and risks and benefits of different therapeutic modalities (including conservative measures, angioplasty, surgical techniques, other interventional techniques and the indications for the use of and management of thrombolytic agents).

21. What number of procedures is recommended to maintain peripheral angioplasty skills?

The number of peripheral procedures required to maintain competence is estimated to be about one case per week. The ability to continue to perform peripheral procedures depends on the success and complication rates obtained by hospital quality assurance data and compared with expected standards.

Regular attendance at postgraduate seminars and continuing education through meetings in new endovascular techniques and equipment are also necessary.

22. Who should perform peripheral interventions?

The performance of peripheral interventions is not specialty specific. Physicians with the knowledge and skills according to the requirements of their institutions should be able to perform the procedures for which they are trained.

The ideal approach for the treatment of patients with peripheral vascular disease is multidisciplinary, requiring the coordinated efforts of cardiologists, vascular surgeons, and radiologists. Turf wars preclude fertilization and exchange of knowledge among the specialties, and patient care suffers from the underutilization of combined efforts. Vascular conferences are encouraged as an important learning tool for exchange of knowledge.

BIBLIOGRAPHY

1. Hannan EL, Racz M, Ryan TJ, et al: Coronary angioplasty volume-outcome relationships for hospitals and cardiologists. JAMA 277:892–898, 1997.
2. Hirshfeld JW, et al: American College of Cardiology training statement on recommendations for the structure of an optimal adult interventional cardiology training program; a report of the American College of Cardiology Task Force on Clinical Expert Consensus documents.
3. Jollis JG, Peterson ED, Nelson CL et al: Relationship between physician and hospital coronary angioplasty volume and outcome in elderly patients. Circulation 95:2485–2491, 1997.
4. Rosenfield K, Isner J: Diseases of peripheral vessels. In Topol EJ (ed): Texbook of Interventional Cardiology. Philadelphia, Lippincott-Raven Publishers, 1998.
5. Spittell J. et al: ACC Policy Statement: recommendations for peripheral transluminal angioplasty: training and facilities. JACC 21:546–548, 1993.

59. THE FUTURE OF CARDIAC SURGERY

Hassan Tehrani, M.B., Ch.B., Kushagra Katariya, M.D., and Tomas Salerno, M.D.

TRAINING

1. What is the current structure of cardiac surgery training, and how is it going to change?

Cardiothoracic surgeons currently complete a 5-year general surgery residency before training for 2 or 3 years in cardiothoracic surgery. At present, they must be certified in general surgery before taking the thoracic board examinations Starting in July 2003, the general surgery certification will no longer be a requirement as a prerequisite for the thoracic boards. The American Board of Thoracic Surgery is looking at a shorter alternative for cardiothoracic training. A 3/3 track has been proposed, in which medical students may directly match into cardiothoracic surgery. The proposed program will consist of 3 years of general surgery training followed by 3 years of cardiothoracic training leading to board certification in thoracic surgery.

CORONARY ARTERY BYPASS GRAFTING

2. What has been the most significant change in coronary artery bypass graft (CABG) surgery in the past decade?

The most significant advance has been the advent of off-pump CABG (Fig. 1). Kolessov first described coronary revascularization on the beating heart in 1966. However, it was not until the late 1990s that it became popularized.

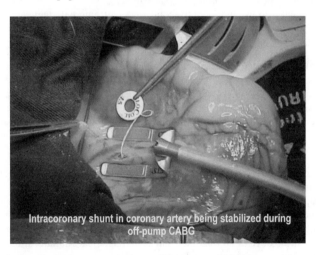

FIGURE 1. Off-pump CABG. Heart and coronary being stabilized by a coronary stabilizer. Intracoronary shunt in coronary artery.

3. Which patients are candidates for off-pump CABG, and what are the keys to success?

In our experience, all patients, including patients undergoing emergency surgery and those with left main disease. The only indication for cardiopulmonary bypass is refractory hemodynamic instability.

The keys to success are twofold. First, the surgeon must have patience and the right mindset. There is typically some blood pressure variation when the heart is initially manipulated into position for performing an anastomosis, but this nearly always stabilizes after a few seconds. Second is having a good anesthesiologist at the head of the bed to monitor the patient at all times during the procedure.

4. Can complete revascularization be performed using off-pump CABG techniques?

Yes. The left anterior descending (LAD) coronary artery and diagonal vessels are revascularized with the heart left in the pericardial cavity. The circumflex and posterior descending vessels are revascularized by lifting the heart out of the pericardial cavity by means of a sling created by placing a stitch attached to strip of packing in the posterior pericardium.

5. Which robots are available for use cardiac surgery?

The Aesop system (Computermotion, Inc., Goleta, CA) is a voice-activated video camera controlled by the surgeon. Aesop has been used in conjunction with regular thoracoscopic instruments and techniques to facilitate mammary artery takedown.

The Zeus system (Computermotion, Inc.) is Aesop combined with surgeon-controlled robotic arms that are able to suture and cut through thoracoscopic sized incisions. The da Vinci system (Intuitive Surgical, Sunnyvale, CA) is similar to the Zeus. For both of these systems, the surgeon may be remotely located, with the assistant remaining at the patient's side to change instruments as necessary.

6. What is the current status of robotic surgery in performing CABG?

Robot-assisted complete coronary revascularization has been described in a few cases. These patients have been placed on percutaneous cardiopulmonary bypass, with the surgery being performed through minimal incisions with the aid of a robot. The downside of this approach is that the patient has had to be placed on cardiopulmonary bypass.

A recent approach is to use the robot to mobilize the left internal mammary artery through the left chest and then use a mini-thoracotomy incision to create anastomoses to the LAD and diagonal branches on a beating heart.

7. What is the hybrid approach to coronary revascularization, and what role will robotic surgery have?

The hybrid approach is using a combination of percutaneous angioplasty and surgery to achieve complete coronary revascularization. The ultimate minimally invasive approach could involve the interventional cardiologist performing angioplasty on the favorable lesions. The surgeon using an off-pump minimally invasive approach with robotic assistance would bypass the complex lesions and occlusions.

8. What is the current status of anastomotic stapling devices in cardiac surgery, and what is their advantage?

Proximal stapling devices are already in clinical use. Currently available devices allow the proximal anastomoses of saphenous vein aorto-coronary grafts to be created without cross-clamping the aorta. Stapling devices for creating distal anastomoses are in the preclinical stages of testing. The advantages of these devices are that they can save time; create a uniform optimally shaped anastomosis; and in the case of the proximal stapler, avoid cross-clamping the aorta, thereby minimizing atheroembolization.

VALVE SURGERY

9. What are the current limitations of available replacement valves, and will they be improved upon?

Replacement mechanical valves have been shown to be extremely durable for more than 25 years, but have drawbacks because of the need for anticoagulation with warfarin. Replacement bioprosthetic valves do not need anticoagulation with warfarin but have a shorter lifespan (10–12 years on average). The ideal valve of the future will be bioprosthetic and have a long lifespan, with minimal degeneration.

10. Does robotic assistance have a place in valve repair?

Yes. Mitral valve repair has been performed using robotic assistance via the right chest, with the patient being placed on cardiopulmonary bypass through the femoral vessels.

11. Will we be ever able to perform valve repair or replacement percutaneously?

Percutaneous mitral valve repair has already been performed in humans. A flexible hemi-ring is delivered through the coronary sinus into the circumflex coronary vein via a femoral venous approach. When the ring is in the correct position, it is then constrained to reduce the anteroposterior diameter and circumference of the mitral ring to reduce or eliminate regurgitation.

Percutaneous aortic valve delivery has been described in animal studies. A freshly harvested valve has been mounted in a vascular stent, which has been delivered into the thoracic aorta. A hurdle to overcome is how to safely remove the native valve through an endovascular approach.

THORACIC AORTIC DISEASE

12. What are the limitations of using stent grafts to treat thoracic aortic aneurysms, and how can they be overcome?

The placement of a stent graft necessitates the presence of satisfactory proximal and distal nonaneurysmal landing zones. In the thoracic aorta, these should ideally be 2 cm in length at either end. Stent grafts can clearly not be placed across major branch vessels (for aneurysms that begin close to the left subclavian takeoff or end close to the celiac axis). In a few cases, stent grafts with side branches have been specially made and deployed successfully to overcome this problem. Future generations of thoracic stent grafts will not only be able to have side branches added if necessary but will also have bonding agents (either biological or chemical) at their proximal and distal ends that will help prevent dislodgement and endoleak.

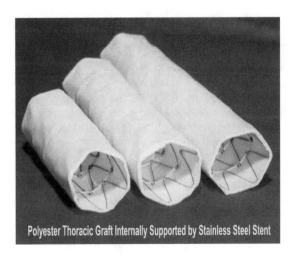

Polyester Thoracic Graft Internally Supported by Stainless Steel Stent

FIGURE 2. Examples of thoracic stent grafts.

13. Will aortic dissections be treated differently in the future?

Certain institutions are already successfully treating type B dissections with a stent graft at the proximal entry point. This reestablishes blood flow in the true lumen, minimizing the potential for distal ischemia and long-term aneurysmal dilatation.

ATRIAL SEPTAL DEFECT AND VENTRICULAR SEPTAL DEFECT

14. Will surgery be the primary treatment for closure of atrial septal defects or ventricular septal defects in the future?

No. Percutaneously placed closure devices are being increasingly used in both pediatric and adult patients with atrial septal defects. These same devices are also being used to close congenital ventricular septal defects and adults with postinfarction or posttraumatic septal defects.

HEART FAILURE

15. How big a problem is heart failure in the United States today?

More than 700,000 people die in the United States each year from heart failure making it the leading cause of death. Currently, there are 6000 to 8000 Americans on the waiting list for heart transplants. But because of a lack of donor organs, only 2000 heart transplants are performed each year in the United States.

16. What will the role be in the future for left ventricular assist devices (LVADs)?

LVADs are currently being used as a bridge to heart transplant in the sickest of patients on recipient waiting lists. Trials are underway to see if they are beneficial for use as destination therapy in view of the discrepancy between donor and recipient numbers.

17. Are total artificial hearts (TAHs) the solution to the problem?

Probably not. Approximately 90% of patients with heart failure only have a failing left ventricle and therefore only need left-sided support. LVADs are smaller, cheaper, and less technically complex than TAHs, making them preferable for these patients.

CARDIAC GENE THERAPY

18. What place will gene therapy have in treating patients with coronary disease (CAD) in the future?

Gene therapy has already been used in clinical trials to treat patients with advanced CAD refractory to medical management who are not candidates for surgery. Genes that encode for proteins such as vascular endothelial growth factor (VEGF) or fibroblast growth factor (FGF) are currently under investigation. These are either directly or percutaneously injected into ischemic myocardium to stimulate angiogenesis. Future trials may involve combined CABG and gene therapy delivery in which the angiogenic genes are injected into areas of ischemic myocardium that do not have good bypass-able targets.

19. Will gene therapy have a place in treating patients with heart failure?

Yes. Experimental findings and early clinical work have demonstrated the feasibility of skeletal myocyte transfer. The hope being that in the future, *ex vivo* gene manipulation of stem cells will allow creation of functional cardiac myocytes that can be transplanted into failing hearts, avoiding cardiac transplantation.

ARRHYTHMIA SURGERY

20. What role can surgery play in treating patients with chronic atrial fibrillation?

Patients with chronic atrial fibrillation and concomitant CAD or valvular disease who need to undergo surgery are particularly good candidates. The traditional maze procedure necessitated the surgeon's making multiple carefully placed incisions in the walls of the left atrium that then needed to be repaired. The recent introduction of radiofrequency and cryoablation probes has simplified the procedure. After the heart is arrested and the left atrium is opened, the probes are run around the orifices of the pulmonary veins and the mitral annulus, preventing initiation or propogation of the arrhythmia. Successful conversion to sinus rhythm has been seen in up to 76% of patients by 6 months after the procedure.

BIBLIOGRAPHY

1. Bauriedel G, Redel DA, Schmitz C, et al: Transcatheter closure of a posttraumatic ventricular septal defect with an Amplatzer occluder device. Catheter Cardiovasc Interv 53:508–512, 2001.
2. Bergsland J: Off-pump beating heart coronary bypass surgery. In: Soltoski PR, Karamanoukian HL, Salerno T (eds): Cardiac Surgery Secrets. Philadelphia, Hanley & Belfus Inc, 2000.
3. Boyd WD, Kodera K, Stahl KD, Rayman R: Current status and future directions in computer-enhanced video- and robotic-assisted coronary bypass surgery. Semin Thorac Cardiovasc Surg 14:101–109, 2002.
4. Inoue K, Hosokawa H, Iwase T, et al: Aortic arch reconstruction by transluminally placed endovascular branched stent graft. Circulation 100(Suppl)316–321, 1999.
5. Kalra GS, Verma PK, Dhall A, et al: Transcatheter device closure of ventricular septal defects: immediate results and intermediate-term follow-up. Am Heart J 138:339–344, 1999.
6. Losordo DW, Vale PR, Symes JF, et al. Gene therapy for myocardial angiogenesis: initial clinical results with direct myocardial injection of phVEGF165 as sole therapy for myocardial ischemia. Circulation 98:2800–2804, 1998.
7. Lutter G, Kuklinski D, Berg G, et al: Percutaneous aortic valve replacement: an experimental study. I. Studies on implantation. J Thorac Cardiovasc Surg 123:768–776, 2002.
8. Menasche P: Cell transplantation for the treatment of heart failure. Semin Thorac Cardiovasc Surg 14: 157–166, 2002.
9. Palma JH, de Souza JA, Rodrigues Alves CM, et al: Self-expandable aortic stent-grafts for treatment of descending aortic dissections. Ann Thorac Surg 73:1138–1141, 2002.
10. Williams MR, Stewart JR, Bolling SF, et al: Surgical treatment of atrial fibrillation using radiofrequency energy. Ann Thorac Surg 71:1939–1943, 2001.

60. GENE THERAPY AND TRANSMYOCARDIAL LASER REVASCULARIZATION

Neerav Shah, M.D., and Alexandre C. Ferreira, M.D.

1. What is gene therapy?

Gene therapy is the introduction of genetic material into a cell in order to alter the pattern of gene expression for that cell for the purposes of a therapeutic response

2. Why are cardiac and vascular tissue considered good targets for gene therapy?

There are many reasons that cardiac and vascular tissue are considered good targets for gene therapy. For the most part, the disease processes, such as ischemia, are very localized processes. Blood vessels allow for easy accessibility. A limited duration of gene expression may only be required to achieve the therapeutic response. Additionally, endothelial injury may allow for increased gene transfection

3. Where do we stand in the clinical usage of gene therapy?

Most gene therapy is still in the early developmental phase. Some applications such as the use of angiogenic growth factors (e.g., vascular endothelial growth factor (VEGF) and fibroblast growth fctor (FGF)) for peripheral vascular disease (PVD) and coronary artery disease (CAD) are undergoing phase II and III clinical trials.

4. What are proposed clinical applications of gene therapy?

- PVD (see Table 1)
- CAD
- Restenosis
- Saphenous vein graft failure
- Congestive heart failure
- Dyslipidemia
- QT prolongation

Table 1. Results of Isner Phase I intramuscular VEGF for PVD Study

Nine patients, 10 limbs with rest pain +/− nonhealing ulcer and ABI < 0.6
ABI 0.33 → 0.48 (surgical revascularization usually improves by 0.1)
Four of seven ulcers improved, allowing for limb salvage
Three of seven below knee amputation

5. What issues still need to be addressed regarding gene therapy?

- Which factors or genes to use
- How to best deliver genes to their targets
- How to best allow genetic material to enter cells (vectors)
- Improving the efficiency of gene transfection
- Safety issues
- Ethical issues

6. What factors or targets are currently being studies for gene therapy applications?

Table 2. Factors Being Studied in Gene Therapy Trials

Angiogenesis	Arterial cytoprotection
FGF	VEGF
VEGF	Nitric oxide synthase
Hepatocyte growth factor	Cyclooxygenase
Angiopoetin	
PDGF (platelet-derived growth factor)	

(continued)

Table 2. Factors Being Studied in Gene Therapy Trials (Continued)

Restenosis
VEGF
TIMP (tissue inhibitor of metalloprotease)
Rb (retinoblastoma gene)
PCNA antisense (prolifferating cell nuclear antigen)
Thymidine kinase
GAX gene (growth arrest homeobox)
E2F decoy
P16, p21, p27

7. What is a vector, and what are the differences between currently used vectors?

Genetic material alone is easily degraded. The vector is the portal that allows the genetic material to resist degradation and enter the cell.

VECTOR	MECHANISM OF ENTRY	PROS AND CONS
a. Plasmid	Short sequence of DNA that is modified to resist degradation; enters the nucleus, resulting in transient gene expression	(+) Safe and easy to produce (−) Low efficiency
b. Retrovirus	Altered nonreplicating virus enters cell via receptor, where its RNA is transcribed into DNA encorporated into the host cell genome	(+) Long-term response possible (−) Cells must be proliferating (−) Low efficiency (?) Gene mutation may lead to replication
c. Adenovirus	Altered virus that enters cell via a receptor where it is broken down by lysosomes, which release the transgene, allowing it to enter the nucleus, where it remains extrachromosomal but results in transient gene expression	(+) Easy to produce (+) Affects nonproliferating cells (+) Transient gene expression (−) Inflammatory reaction (−) Low efficiency

8. What are the proposed mechanisms of gene delivery?

a. Intramyocardial or intramuscular injection
b. Catheter- or balloon-mediated therapy
c. Intracoronary injection
d. Intrapericardial injection
e. Epicardial injection
f. Biodegradable microspheres or ultrasound-guided therapy

9. What is angiogenesis, and what are its limitations?

Angiogenesis is the formation of new vessels that lack a tunica media such as capillaries. It is different from arteriogenesis (i.e., the formation of new arterioles), which is the more desired goal (collateral vessels). Limiting our study of angiogenesis is the fact imaging technology is not sophisticated enough to yet image these small new vessels.

10. How do you bypass the problem of low efficiency gene transfection?

Transfer of genes that encode naturally secreting proteins (e.g., VEGF) can achieve a desired biological effect with minimal gene transfection as long as the transfected cells secrete substantial amounts of gene product. This gene product, in turn, can have a paracrine effect and modulate the bioactivity of a large number of adjacent cells.

11. What limitations exist in the study of gene therapy to fight restenosis?

Restenosis is a complicated process (see Chapter 44) that is not yet fully understood. As a result, we do not know which factors in the restenosis process to target. In order to truly make progress, we need an animal model that replicates the restenosis process in humans. Current animal models may not be adequate because restenosis varies between species. Lastly, most studies are done on normal vessels that are injured with a balloon model; it is unknown whether atherosclerotic arteries will behave in the same manner.

12. Describe the possible risks of gene therapy and the reported incidence during clinical trials.

Mortality—none of the patients in the CAD or PVD studies died as a direct result of gene transfer
- 2-Year mortalities for CAD—high-risk subsets with multiple comorbidities whose mortality may be $> 20\%$
- 2-Year mortalities for PVD—9%

Accelerated atherosclerosis—none seen

Vascular malformations—hemangiomas 0%; one report of transient telangectasias

Neoplasm—small numbers have been reported, but the exact relationship to gene transfer is unclear

Retinopathy—not seen

Peripheral edema—seen in patients with peripheral ischemia (rest pain) ~50%

13. What is transmyocardial laser revascularization (TMR)?

TMR is the use of a high-energy laser either through a left lateral thoracotomy or percutaneously to create channels from the epicardial surface to the left ventricle. It is based on the concept of the reptilian heart, which contains sinusoids that carry oxygenated blood to the myocardium

14. Who are candidates for TMR therapy?

Candidates include patients with refractory angina (CCS III or IV) with objective evidence of ischemia and ejection fraction (EF) of greater than 35% who are not candidates for standard revascularization techniques. Furthermore, TMR may be used as an adjunct to conventional coronary artery bypass grafting (CABG) to cover areas of nonrevascularizable muscle.

Patients Who May be Considered Nonrevascularizable by Standard Techniques

CABG	PERCUTANEOUS CORONARY INTERVENTION
Diffuse disease	Recurrent restenosis
Lack of targets	Ostial lesions
Lack of conduits	Distal branch lesions
Comorbidities	Long stenotic lesions
Multiple thoracotomies	Degenerated SVGs
Degenerated SVGs with patent LIMA	Diffuse disease

15. How does TMR work?

The exact mechanism of action for TMR is unknown. Proposed mechanisms include:

Blood flow via channels→ Autopsy data as early as day 3 after TMR show that most channels are closed

Angiogenesis → Myocardial injury results in the release of angiogenic growth factors

Sympathetetic denervation → Cutting nerve fibers may diminish pain without objective improvement in ischemia

Placebo effect

Clinical Trials Involving TMR and PTMR

	DECREASE IN ANGINA BY 2 CC LEVELS (AT 1 YEAR)		
STUDY	TMR, %	MEDICAL TREATMENT, %	OBJECTIVE DATA
Frazier et al. (1999)	72	43	Small improvement in perfusion defects
Allen et al. (1999)	76	31	No improvement in EF, perfusion defects, mortality
Schoefield et al. (1999)	31	4	No improvement in EF, exercise time, perfusion defects
Osterele (2000) PTMR	34	14	No improvement in EF, perfusion defects; improved exercise time
Whitlow (2001) PTMR	32	10	improved quality of life, exercise time; no mortality benefit

17. What was the significance of the DIRECT (DMR in Regeneration of Endomyocardial Channel) trial?

The blinded trial compared placebo PTMR with low-dose PTMR (10–15 channels) to high-dose PTMR (20–25 channels). All patients showed similar improvement in anginal class, quality of life scores, and exercise time. This study seriously damaged any notion that there was greater benefit to laser revascularization than placebo effect alone.

BIBLIOGRAPHY

1. Allen KB, Dowling RD, Fudge TL, et al: Comparison of transmyocardial revascularization with medical therapy in patients with refractory angina. N Engl J Med 341:1029–1036, 1999.
2. Baumgartner I, et al: Constitutive expression of ph VEGF$_{165}$ following intramuscular gene transfer promotes collateral vessel development in patients with critical limb ischemia. Circulation 1114–1123, 1998.
3. Ferreira AC: Therapeutic angiogenesis: the present and future. Arquivos Brasileros de Cardiologica. 78:145–147, 2002.
4. Frazier OH, March RJ, Horvath KA: Transmyocardial laser revascularization with a carbon dioxide laser in patients with end-stage coronary artery disease. N Engl J Med 341:1021–1028, 1999.
5. Isner JM, et al: Assessment of risks associated with cardiovascular gene therapy in human subjects. Circ Res 89:389–400, 2001.
6. Isner JM: Myocardial gene therapy. Nature 415:234–239, 2002.
7. Kim MC, et al: Refractory angina pectoris—mechanisms and therapeutic options. J Am Coll Cardiol 39:923–934, 2002.
8. Nathan M, Aranki S: Transmyocardial laser revascularization. Curr Opin Cardiol 16:310–314, 2001.
9. Perin E: Eclipe PTMR system study—late breaking trials. Presented at ACC, March 20, 2000, Anaheim, CA.
10. Osterle SN, Sanborn TA, et al: Percutaneous transmyocardial laser revascularization for severe angina: the Potential Class Improvement from Intramyocardial Channels (PACIFIC) randomized trial. Lancet 356:1705–1710, 2000.
11. O'Sullivan MO, Bennett MR: Gene therapy for restenosis: is the enthusiasm justified? Heart 86:491–493, 2001.
12. Schofield PM, Sharples LD, Caine N, et al: Transmyocardial laser revascularization in patients with refractory angina: a randomized controlled trial. Lancet 353:519–524, 1999.
13. Yla-Herttuala S, Martin JF: Cardiovascular gene therapy. Lancet 355:213–222, 2000.

61. INTERVENTIONAL ECHOCARDIOGRAPHY

Juan C. Londoño, M.D., and Miguel Zabalgoitia, M.D.

1. Why has echocardiography, a noninvasive technique, become an interventional tool?

With the introduction of color-flow Doppler-aided transesophageal echocardiography (TEE) in 1987, a new horizon in cardiac imaging and interventions began. The development of multiplane probes helped in improving outcomes in cardiac surgery and percutaneous coronary interventions (PCIs). Further advances in device miniaturization led to intravascular ultrasound (IVUS) imaging of the native vessels and coronary artery bypass graft CABG. Recently, the development of intracardiac echocardiography (ICE) has permitted real-time evaluation of intracardiac structures in guiding PCI.

2. What are the most common applications of echocardiography in the catheterization laboratory?

TEE and ICE allow for the identification of anatomic landmarks easily recognized such as the mitral valve apparatus, mitral annulus, left atrial appendage, and interatrial septum. The most common applications are for monitoring interventional procedures such as percutaneous balloon mitral valvuloplasty (PBMV), nonsurgical septal reduction therapy (NSRT) in patients with hypertrophic cardiomyopathy, and during percutaneous closure of atrial septal communications such as patent foramen ovale (PFO) and atrial septal defect (ASD).

3. Are there other current interventional echocardiographic applications?

Other uses include guidance during electrophysiological studies, endomyocardial and cardiac tumor biopsies, pacemaker insertion; and in assessing pericardial effusion complicating catheter-based interventions. Traditionally, transthoracic echo (TTE) and TEE have assisted in these procedures; however, recent reports suggest that ICE via femoral vein access may take their place.

4. How was intracardiac echocardiography developed?

ICE started with the development of high-frequency transducers in the order of 20–40 MHz used for intravascular imaging. However, with these high frequencies, imaging resolution is superb in the very near field, within millimeters. Thus, for structures within a few centimeters, the image resolution declined and penetration was a significant limitation. Improvement in depth was achieved by using modified lower-frequency (5-MHz) TEE probes; however, their large transducer size limited their clinical use. Subsequent efforts using miniaturized (6- to 10-F), medium-range frequency (10 MHz) transducers were a reasonable compromise; they allow for visualization of intracardiac structures within a few centimeters and yet excellent imaging resolution.

5. Describe the characteristics of currently used ICE systems.

Currently there are two systems commercially available: a 9-Fr, 9-MHz rotating ultrasound element catheter (EP Technologies, Boston Scientific Corp; San Jose, CA); and a 10-Fr (3.2-mm diameter), 5.5- to 10-MHz catheter (Acuson Corporation; Mountain View, CA). The latter is a 64-element vector phased-array intracardiac imaging catheter with Doppler capabilities; it measures 90 cm in length and has been used for both diagnosis and intervention guidance. This transducer has a tissue penetration depth of 12 cm and scans only in a longitudinal plane, which may be a limitation. The two-dimensional images are displayed in a 90-degree sector with the help of a multidirectional catheter tip.

6. How has ICE been used in interventional cardiology?

ICE has been used in the catheterization laboratory during catheter-based interventions such PFO, ASD, and patent ductus arteriosus (PDA) closures, as well as during transseptal puncture in

PBMV and pericardiocentesis. ICE provides real-time imaging guiding for these procedures and for detecting potential complications. Cardiac tumor biopsy under ICE guidance has also been described. Case series have reported both TEE- and ICE-guided closure of ASD and PFO without or with minimal fluoroscopy exposure. Recently, and for the first time, a successful ICE-guided percutaneous ASD closure was performed *without* fluoroscopy in a symptomatic 21-year-old woman during the early stages of pregnancy.

7. Explain the reason behind the use of TEE or ICE during transatrial puncture.

The interatrial septum is ideally visualized from the left atrium with TEE and from the right atrium with ICE. The latter technique may provide better image quality compared with TEE (Fig. 1). A safe puncture of the interatrial septum with a Brockenbrough needle demands exact identification of the fossa ovalis; this has traditionally been done with fluoroscopy. Under radiographic visualization, this procedure requires knowledge of the anatomic landmarks and experience to develop "subtle catheter sensation." This can be challenging when there are anatomical variants such atrial enlargement or ascending aortic dilation. Serious complications such as aortic root and atrial perforation have been reported during transseptal attempts.

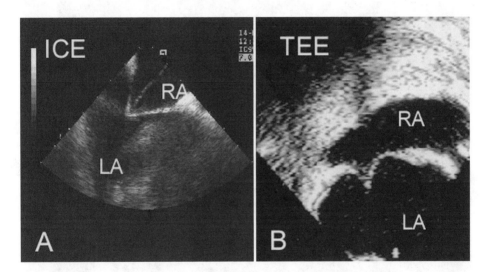

FIGURE 1. AcuNav ICE (*A*) and TEE (*B*) guidance of a transseptal puncture. The TEE probe is positioned at 90° and the tip of puncture needle is well visualized by the tenting of the fossa ovalis. (Part B from Park SH, Kim MA, Hyon MS: The advantages of on-line transesophageal echocardiography guide during percutaneous balloon mitral valvuloplasty. J Am Soc Echocardiogr 13:26–34, 2000; with permission.)

8. What are the advantages of ICE over other imaging modalities?

An important advantage is the immediate identification of procedural complications such as perforation, pericardial effusion, and tamponade. Typically TEE is best performed when the patient is in his or her left lateral decubitus position, which is unsuitable in most cases in the catheterization suite. ICE, on the other hand, is relatively simple and safe; unlike TEE, ICE does not require airway manipulation and anesthesia and is performed while the patient is the supine position. Additionally, ICE may reduce procedural and fluoroscopy time, minimizing both patient and operator exposure.

9. Has ICE ever been compared with TEE during percutaneous interventions?

Yes. Hijazi et al. studied the association between ASD and PFO and cerebrovascular accidents. Eleven patients underwent transcatheter closure, six under TEE and ICE guidance and five under ICE alone. Both TEE and ICE provided similar visualization of the atrial septal communications (Figs. 2 and 3); however, the images obtained with ICE were more found to be more helpful to those obtained by TEE. This advantage is caused by the proximity of the left atrium and left upper pulmonary vein to the esophagus, which limits the near field of the TEE images during different stages of the closure. This study concluded that ICE provides high-quality images similar to those obtained by TEE, suggesting that ICE may replace TEE as the guidance imaging modality of choice.

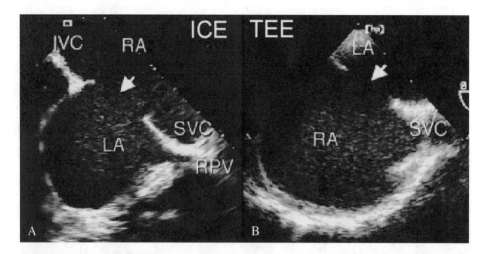

FIGURE 2. ICE (*A*) and TEE (*B*) images of a secundum atrial septal defect. ICE images in a modified long-axis view show a 16.2-mm defect (*arrow*). In the same view, TEE shows the same defect measuring 20 mm (*arrow*). LA-left atrium; RA-right atrium; RPV-right pulmonary vein; SVC-superior vena cava. (From Hijazi ZM, Wang Z, Cao QL: Transcatheter closure of atrial septal defects and patent foramen ovale under intracardiac echocardiographic guidance: feasibility and comparison with transesophageal echocardiography. Cathet Cardiovasc Intervent 52:194–199, 2001; with permission.)

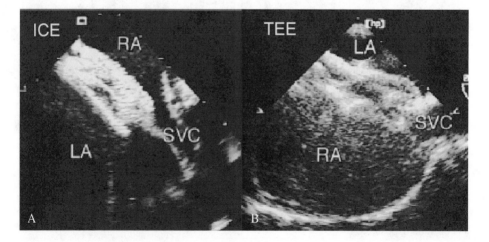

FIGURE 3. ICE (*A*) and TEE (*B*) after successful device deployment (Amplatzer septal). Compared with the TEE images, ICE produces a better image. (From Hijazi ZM, Wang Z, Cao QL: Transcatheter closure of atrial septal defects and patent foramen ovale under intracardiac echocardiographic guidance: feasibility and comparison with transesophageal echocardiography. cathet cardiovasc intervent 52:194–199, 2001; with permission.)

10. In mitral stenosis, which echocardiographic predictors determine probability of success during PBMV?

Leaflet mobility, valvular thickening, subvalvular thickening, and valvular calcification are the predictors used to determine feasibility of percutaneous valvuloplasty. According to the severity, each item is graded from 1 (minimal) to 4 (severe). A score of 8 or less favors PBMV with excellent immediate and long-term results. A greater score usually results in less favorable outcomes, including development of significant mitral regurgitation (MR).

11. How do TEE and ICE assist during PBMV?

Echocardiographic guidance provides a reliable assessment of mitral valve anatomy as well as balloon sizing and positioning (Figs. 4 and 5). It also assists during transseptal puncture and evaluates immediate outcome and complications.

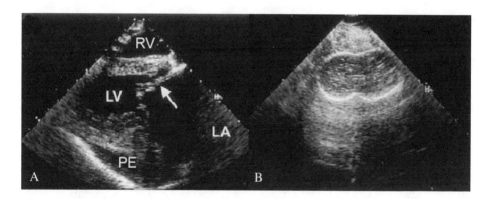

FIGURE 4. ICE images during percutaneous mitral balloon commissurotomy. The ICE catheter is in the same position in the right ventricle (RV) in both images. *A,* The anatomy is well visualized and the *arrow* indicates marked chordal thickening and tethering. *B,* The Inoue balloon catheter (Toray Industries, Inc., Tokyo, Japan) is inflated. PE-pericardial effusion; LV-left ventricle; RV-right ventricle; LA-left atrium. (From Bruce CJ, Nishimura RA, Rihal CS: Intracardiac echocardiography in the interventional catheterization laboratory: preliminary experience with a novel, phased-array transducer. Am J Cardiol 89:635–40, 2002; with permission.)

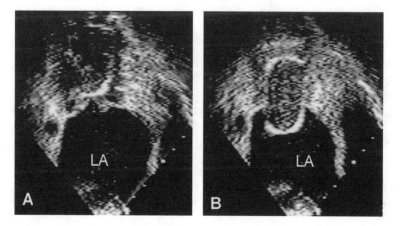

FIGURE 5. TEE monitoring of balloon position before, and during inflation. *A,* The balloon is inflated at the subvalvular position. *B,* The position is corrected with the mitral valve leaflets located at the waist of the balloon. (From Park SH, Kim MA, Hyon MS: The advantages of on-line transesophageal echocardiography guide during percutaneous balloon mitral valvuloplasty. J Am Soc Echocardiogr 13:26–34, 2000; with permission.)

12. Describe the echocardiographic monitoring during PBMV.

These are the mean valve gradient, valve area by planimetry, commissural morphology, and changes in the degree of MR using color-flow Doppler. A significant improvement in LA mean pressure should be seen with a reduction in the transmittal gradient, as cardiac output increases and pulmonary artery pressure decreases. It is important to assess these parameters because of the inaccuracy of Gorlin's formula in the presence of atrial shunts or MR. Furthermore, because the accuracy of Doppler measurements during valvuloplasty is limited, planimetry from two-dimensional echocardiography should be the preferred method.

13. What are the echocardiographic procedural endpoints of PBMV?

a. Mitral valve area (MVA) larger than 1 cm^2/m^2 of body surface area (BSA)
b. Unrestricted opening of at least one leaflet
c. The assessment of MR

14. List the main complications related to PBMV that may be identified echocardiographically.

Until recently, the main indication for TEE imaging in patients undergoing PBMV was to exclude LA thrombi before the procedure. Today, TEE and ICE can help diagnose other complications such as thrombus formation on catheters or at the site of endothelial injury, valve disruption, residual ASD after septal puncture, mitral leaflet tear with estimation of MR, and pericardial effusion.

15. List the limitations of TEE-guided PBMV compared with ICE guidance.

Although the main limitations are related to the need for esophageal intubation, recent studies have shown successful TEE monitoring with mild sedation and intermittent suctioning of secretions. In addition, positioning and handling of the TEE probe can be cumbersome during PBMV, and the use of this technique presents direct radiation exposure to the sonographer during simultaneous fluoroscopy and ultrasound scanning. Currently, ICE allows for similar or better visualization and less fluoroscopy time and obviates the need for anesthesia compared with TEE. On the other hand, the cost and limited number of hospitals with this technology has delayed its widespread use.

16. Is there a role of echocardiography for the assessment of myocardial perfusion with intracoronary contrast injection?

Myocardial contrast echocardiography (MCE) is a research tool that uses microspheres with a mean size of 4 μm (half size of a red blood cell), which can be injected either intravenously or intracoronary. Although most of the work with MCE has been done outside in the echocardiography laboratory, MCE has the potential to be used in cardiac catheterization. Intracoronary injection of

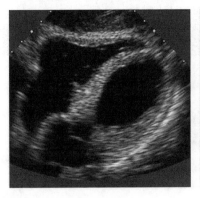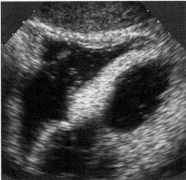

FIGURE 6. Subcostal four-chamber view in a patient with left dominant coronary circulation. *A* represents basal and *B* illustrates imaging during selective injection of diluted Optison into the left main artery. Pronounced microvascular opacification of the septum, lateral wall, apex, and free wall of the right ventricle can be appreciated in this large dominant vessel.

commercially available microspheres (Optison) diluted in normal saline solution may provide an excellent agent for myocardial opacification. Potential clinical applications are to visualize the extent of vascular territory in a left dominant circulation (Fig. 6) and assess perfusion before and after an intervention. Myocardial opacification after an intracoronary injection represents the capillary microcirculation of the territory attributed to the specific coronary artery injected.

17. What is the contribution of echocardiography during septal ablation in patients with hypertrophic cardiomyopathy?

An echocardiography-guided anatomical approach for identifying the target septal branch was introduced in 1996. This has helped to define the vascular territory and identify complications (i.e., acute MR caused by papillary muscle rupture, new wall motion abnormalities). Since its introduction, clinical and hemodynamic results are comparable to surgical myomectomy, and the number of permanent pacemaker implantations caused by trifascicular block has been reduced from 20% to 40% to 5%, which is close to the postsurgical range.

18. Describe the echocardiographic measurements during alcohol septal ablation.

a. The LV outflow tract gradient by Doppler at baseline

b. Myocardial contrast echocardiography, including selective intracoronary injection of diluted sonicated albumin (Optison) into the septal perforator with simultaneous transthoracic imaging

c. The area of myocardial opacification is assessed from the apical and parasternal views in order to verify its spatial relationship and the extension in the anterior-posterior and subaortic-apical directions

d. Mapping of vascular beds of the septal perforators; the septal perforator to inject should spatially match the obstructive jet and include the coaptation region between the septum and the systolic anterior motion (SAM)

e. Careful exclusion of echo-enhanced areas distant from the septal target area to minimize the infarct area

f. Ethanol injection in the selected septal perforators

g. Evaluation of wall motion abnormalities, severity of MR, and changes in the degree of SAM of the anterior mitral leaflet

h. The LVOT gradient by Doppler at the end of the procedure

19. What is the background of echo-guided pericardiocentesis?

It is important to highlight that "echo-guided" pericardiocentesis is when the transducer is used to determine the *exact location* on the chest wall where the pericardial effusion is the largest and the *correct orientation*. After the location and orientation have been defined, the transducer is removed, the area is prepared, and the needle is advanced (see below for more technical details). The most impressive reported series is from the Mayo Clinic experience during 1979 to 1998. More than 28,000 cardiothoracic surgeries were performed, of which 245 (0.8%) required pericardiocentesis for significant pericardial effusion. Therapeutic success was reported in 97% of cases, with 92% occurring during the first attempt. The ideal site of entry was reported as on the chest wall (86%) followed by the subcostal approach (12%). Adverse events included two patients who had chamber laceration requiring surgery and five patients with pneumothorax. Of the few unsuccessful pericardiocenteses, five circumferential effusions were described, three of which were loculated. There were no deaths in either group.

20. How do we treat pericardial effusion complicating a catheter-based procedure?

Based on the Mayo Clinic experience from 1979 to 2000, 116 of 1127 pericardial effusions were related to cardiac perforation from invasive procedures (nine between 1979 to 1986, 36 between 1986 and 1993, and 71 between 1993 and 2000). The incidence of cardiac perforation was greatest with valvuloplasty (3%) and least with diagnostic catheterization (0.01%). With a greater than 97% success rate, echo-guided pericardiocentesis is the procedure of choice for elective and emergency therapy of pericardial effusions.

21. Describe the technique to perform an echo-guided pericadiocentesis.

a. Use two-dimensional echocardiography to assess size, location, and hemodynamic significance.

b. Use a 16 to 18-gauge polytef-sheathed venous intracath, sheath and dilator set (6 to 8 Fr) with floppy-tipped guidewire and a pigtail angiographic catheter.

c. The chosen site of entry is the *closest* point between the transducer and the largest fluid accumulation. This should be the *farthest* point from the internal mammary artery (3 to 5 cm from the parasternal border) and the vascular bundle of the inferior margin of the rib.

d. The needle will follow the trajectory defined by the *angulation* of the transducer.

e. After the polytef-sheathed needle enters the pericardial space, the steel needle core is withdrawn and the sheath is advanced.

f. Agitated saline solution or commercially available microspheres (Optison, Definity) can be used to confirm the catheter position.

g. Measure intrapericardial pressures and send specimens for analysis.

h. If extended drainage is needed, the dilator and introducer sheath are advanced over a guidewire. The guidewire is then removed and the pigtail inserted over the sheath.

i. It is extremely important to be sure that MOST of the fluid is drained. The dryer the pericardium, the higher the success rate in avoiding recurrence. An important "clue" to remember is to roll the patient over his or her left lateral decubitus position and continue to aspirate, repeating the same over the right lateral decubitus position.

j. Daily two-dimensional echocardiography follow-up is performed until a satisfactory outcome is achieved (< 25 cc in 24 hours).

22. What is the role of echocardiography during endomyocardial biopsy?

Miller et al. studied 58 patients with orthotopic cardiac transplantation. A total of 910 TTE-guided biopsies were obtained with a mean number of 14 biopsies per patient (~ 4700 samples). Adequate visualization was possible in all patients, and the bioptome was inserted via a right internal jugular sheath. Only two complications were reported: an apparent RV perforation without significant effusion and one probable tricuspid chordae injury. This study concluded that TTE is a useful alternative to fluoroscopy for guiding endomyocardial biopsy.

23. Has echocardiography ever been compared with fluoroscopy during endomyocardial biopsy?

Yes. Bell et al. compared biplane fluoroscopy-guided endomyocardial biopsies with two-dimensional TTE. Using a femoral approach, only six of 21 (39%) fluoroscopy-guided biopsies were obtained from the septum despite adequate bioptome positioning as described by Grossman, et al. The remaining 15 (71%) were echocardiography-guided with samples obtained from the lateral wall and apex. This study concluded that bioptome location can be more accurately positioned with TTE than fluoroscopy, especially in patients with transplants and in those with cardiomyopathy.

24. Can ICE assist during an endomyocardial biopsy?

Yes. Current reports demonstrate that ICE plays an important role in patients with distorted anatomy in which TTE may be suboptimal (i.e., transplanted patients, post-open heart surgery or breast implants). Because the ICE probe is introduced via the femoral vein and the bioptome goes via the internal jugular or subclavian vein, the maneuverability of each device is unobstructed. The resultant ICE high-resolution images with excellent depth penetration may decrease complications.

25. What are the most common indications for endomyocardial biopsy?

The most common indication is to assess allograft rejection after heart transplantation, and cardiac tumor biopsy. Other less common indications are undiagnosed cardiomyopathies. The indications abandoned by many include anthracycline cardiotoxicity, carcinoid and amyloid heart disease, endocardial fibroelastosis, hemochromatosis, and HIV cardiomyopathy and other infiltrative diseases.

26. How does echocardiography-guided endomyocardial biopsy compare with fluoroscopy?

Echocardiography offers no radiation, provides maximal portability and, greater sampling area, and is less expensive. In contrast, ICE use for this indication has been limited because of increased cost and lack of training.

27. What are the current uses of ICE during electrophysiologic studies and procedures?

Currently, ICE is used in radiofrequency ablation of different arrhythmias. ICE allows precise anatomic location, including normal variants, positioning of the catheter, adequate electrode–tissue contact, detection of electrode migration during ablation, and direct visualization of microbubble or clot formation during the procedure (Fig. 7). ICE also allows visualization for transseptal puncture in the treatment of left-sided arrhythmias (Fig. 1).

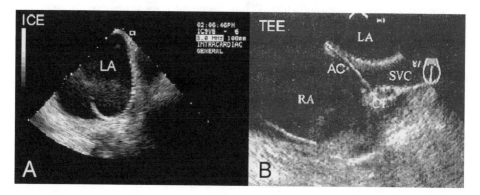

FIGURE 7. ICE and TEE during EP interventions. *A,* AcuNav ICE reveals an ablation catheter in contact with the left atrial (LA) wall. *B,* TEE is performed during modification of the sinoatrial node, and a longitudinal sector from the left atrium (LA) is seen. The ablation catheter (AC) is positioned in contact with the crista terminalis (CT). RA - right atrium; SVC - superior vena cava. (Part B from Haines DE: Catheter ablation therapy for arrhythmias. In Topol EJ (ed): Textbook of Cardiovascular Medicine. Philadelphia, Lippincott Williams & Wilkins, 2002. Electronic version, with permission.)

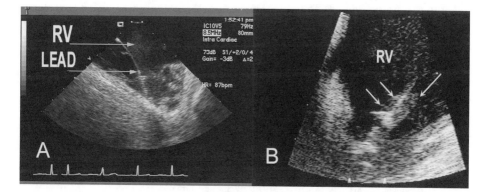

FIGURE 8. ICE images demonstrating right ventricular leads in the apical position. *A,* AcuNav ICE imaging a right ventricular pacemaker lead. *B,* ICE echocardiographic images of a patient with persistent bacteremia and a negative TTE and TEE are demonstrated. A soft tissue echo-density encircling pacemaker lead is noted representing a vegetation (*arrows*). RV - right ventricle. (Part B from Dalal A, Asirvatham SJ, Chandrasekaran K: Intracardiac echocardiography in the detection of pacer lead endocarditis. J Am Soc Echocardiogr 15:1027–1028, 2002; with permission.)

28. Can echocardiography assist during pacemaker implantation?

TEE has been used during permanent dual chamber pacemaker implantation when radiation is believed dangerous, such as in pregnancy. TTE has also been used to confirm placement of electrode catheters within the right ventricle in emergency transvenous pacing. There is not sufficient data to recommend the routine use echocardiography over fluoroscopy during lead implantation; however, with the advent of ICE, improved imaging during pacemaker implantation and diagnosis of pace lead endocarditis may be another clinical application (Fig. 8).

29. Describe the use of echocardiography in direct LV apical puncture and its indications.

TTE helps to identify the location for the thoracic puncture with the apical two-, three-, and four-chamber views. The unique indication for apical puncture is to measure LV pressure and to perform ventriculography in patients with mechanical prosthesis in both the mitral and aortic positions, in whom retrograde arterial and transseptal catheterization is not possible. However, it is recommended to obtain adequate TTE, TEE, and cine-magnetic resonance imaging studies before performing this task because of potential complications.

BIBLIOGRAPHY

1. Bell CA, Kern MJ, Aguirre FV: Superior accuracy of anatomic positioning with echocardiographic-over fluoroscopic-guided endomyocardial biopsy. Cathet Cardiovasc Diagn 28:291–294, 1993.
2. Braunwald E: Valvular heart disease. In Braunwald E, Zipes DP, Libby P (eds): Braunwald Heart Disease: A Textbook of Cardiovascular Medicine, 6th ed. Philadelphia, W. B. Saunders Company, 2001, pp 1394,1651.
3. Bruce CJ, Nishimura RA, Rihal CS: Intracardiac echocardiography in the interventional catheterization laboratory: preliminary experience with a novel, phased-array transducer. Am J Cardiol 89:635–640, 2002.
4. Bruce CJ, Packer DL, Belohlavek M, Seward JB: Intracardiac echocardiography: newest technology. J Am Soc Echocardiogr 13:788–795, 2000.
5. Cafri C, de la Guardia B, Barasch E, et al: Transseptal puncture guided by intracardiac echocardiography during percutaneous transvenous mitral commissurotomy in patients with distorted anatomy of the fossa ovalis. Cathet Cardiovasc Interv 50:463–467, 2000.
6. Cooper JM, Epstein LM: Use of intracardiac ehocardiography guide ablation of atrial fibrillation. Circulation 104:3010, 2001.
7. Dairywala IT, Li P, Liu Z, et al: Catheter-based interventions guided solely by a new phased-array intracardiac imaging catheter: In vivo experimental studies. J Am Soc Echocardiogr 15:150–158, 2002.
8. Faber L, Ziemssen P, Seggewiss H: Targeting percutaneous transluminal septal ablation for hypertrophic obstructive cardiomyopathy by intraprocedural echocardiographic monitoring. J Am Soc Echocardiogr 13:1074–1079, 2000.
9. Hijazi ZM, Wang Z, Cao QL, et al: Transcatheter closure of atrial septal defects and patent foramen ovale under intracardiac echocardiographic guidance: feasibility and comparison with transesophageal echocardiography. Cathet cardiovasc intervent 52:194–199, 2001.
10. Li P, Dairywala IT, Liu Z, et al: Anatomic and hemodynamic imaging using a new vector phased-array intracardiac catheter J Am Soc Echocardiogr 15:349–355, 2002.
11. Miller LW, Labowitz AJ, McBride LA: Echocardiography-guided endomyocardial biopsy. Circulation 78(suppl III):99–102, 1988.
12. Nagueh SF: Role of myocardial contrast echocardiography during nonsurgical septal reduction therapy for hypertrophic obstructive cardiomyopathy. J Am Coll Cardiol 32:225–229, 1998.
13. Park SH, Kim MA, Hyon MS: The advantages of on-line transesophageal echocardiography guide during percutaneous balloon mitral valvuloplasty. J Am Soc Echocardiogr 13:26–34, 2000.
14. Tsang TS, Barnes ME, Hayes SN: Clinical and echocardiographic characteristics of significant pericardial effusions following cardiothoracic surgery and outcomes of echo-guided pericardiocentesis for management. Mayo Clinic experience, 1979–1998. Chest 116:322–331, 1999.
15. Tsang TS, Enriquez-Sarano M, Freeman WK: Consecutive 1127 therapeutic echocardiographically guided pericardiocenteses: clinical profile, practice patterns, and outcomes spanning 21 years. Mayo Clin Proc 77:429–436, 2002.

INDEX

Entries in **boldface type** indicate complete chapters.